THE HISTORY OF MEDICINE SERIES

ISSUED UNDER THE AUSPICES

OF THE LIBRARY OF THE

NEW YORK ACADEMY OF MEDICINE

————————

No. 42

GREAT MEN OF GUY'S

Edited, with an Introduction by

WILLIAM B. OBER

With a Foreword by

LORD BROCK

Published under the auspices of the Library
of The New York Academy of Medicine

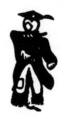

Scarecrow Reprint Corporation
Metuchen, N.J.   1973

Library of Congress Cataloging in Publication Data

Ober, William B   comp.
  Great men of Guy's.

  (The History of medicine series, no. 42)
  "Published under the auspices of the Library of
the New York Academy of Medicine."
  CONTENTS: Addison, T. Observations on the
diagnosis of penumonia. On the constitutional and
local effects of disease of the supra-renal capules.
Anemia, disease of the supra-renal capsules.--
Bright, R. From Reports on medical cases, v. 1, including 24 cases illustrative of some of the appearances
observable on the examination of diseases terminating
in dropsical effusion. ₍etc.₎
  1. Medicine--Addresses, essays, lectures.
2. Guy's Hospital, London. I. Title.
II. Series: ₍DNLM: 1. Medicine--Collected works.
WB5 G786 1973₎
R111.02   616'.008   73-14793
ISBN 0-8108-0676-2

TABLE OF CONTENTS

FOREWORD

IT IS with great pleasure that I write this introduction to Dr. Ober's interesting and valuable anthology of the contributions to medicine and surgery of Great Men of Guy's. His text is admirable in the way it combines brevity with scholarly completeness and accuracy. I find it especially commendable that he has had the vision to select and to present this account of the performance of the Guy's School in the 19th century. It is a truly remarkable story and this anthology serves the very useful purpose of bringing knowledge of it to a wider audience. The explanatory preface that covers each article selected is just what is needed to present this fascinating and informative volume. As I read through it I feared that it contained no reference to that great Guy's surgeon of the early years of the 19th century, Sir Astley Cooper. I need not have feared because he appears in the place of honour at the end; a fitting finale even though his contributory years preceded those of the Great Guy's physicians whose writings form the main substance of this anthology.

His industry, his success and his example must have played their part in setting a standard for these later men who were to be associated with the young, new medical school of Guy's Hospital, the founding of which was occasioned, directed and inspired by Astley Cooper when Guy's separated from St. Thomas's Hospital and the United Borough Hospitals ceased to be anything but a memory.

Even this account of the Great Men of Guy's is incomplete, for several names deserve to be added to this galaxy of talent.

Sir William Gull, to whom we owe the first description of *anorexia nervosa* and of myxoedema, was particularly associated with Bright's great contribution; he carried it one stage further and differentiated the condition now known as essential hypertension. In the Gordon Museum of Guy's Hospital is a specimen jar containing a large heart and a small contracted kidney used by Gull in a lecture given at Guy's and reported in the *British Medical Journal* in 1872. Gull states that the specimen is one of especial historical interest as it was mounted under Richard Bright's own direction. He then states, "I cannot but look upon this work with veneration, but not with conviction. I think with all deference to so great an authority, that the systemic capillaries and, had it been possible, the entire man should have been included in this vase, together with the heart and kidneys; then we should have had, I believe, a truer view of the causation of cardiac hypertrophy and of the diseased kidney."

The clinical recognition of essential hypertension depended upon the discoveries of Dr. Mahomed, another Guy's physician, who succeeded in measuring the blood pressure. In 1881 he wrote an article in the *Guy's Hospital Reports* on "Chronic Bright's disease without albuminuria," in which he completed the story by recognising that high blood pressure might precede anatomical changes in the vessels.

Dr. John Ryle, another distinguished Guy's physician, writing in the Bright Centenary number (1927), states: "We may justly claim that the whole story of high blood pressure, including the little we know of its consequences, were written at Guy's between the years 1827 and 1881."

Sir Samuel Wilks was the first to describe bacterial endocarditis which he does in the *Guy's Hospital Reports* for 1870 under the name of "Capillary embolism or arterial pyaemia."

He claimed to be the first to describe alcoholic peripheral neuritis. He considered his article "On the syphilitic affection of internal organs," written in 1863, gave him one of his highest honours — election as a Fellow of the Royal Society. In this article he corrected the impression hitherto held that syphilis was only a superficial disease. As a result of post-mortem study he revealed that the internal organs were also affected; notably the liver, gummatous disease of which he was the first to describe. He described syphilitic arteritis and how it differed from atherosclerosis.

Constrictive pericarditis is commonly known as Pick's disease but few know of the prior claim of both Wilks, who wrote of it in 1871, and of another even earlier Guy's man, Norman Chevers, whose own contributions deserve far wider recognition than they have had. He gave a clear clinical account of constrictive pericarditis in 1842. Chevers was the first to describe aortic subvalvar stenosis.

We should also recall the names of two other great men who worked at Guy's, E. H. Starling and F. Gowland Hopkins. Starling was a demonstrator of physiology and in 1890 he wrote a short article on "The urine in a case of phosphorous poisoning" with Hopkins, who was then a medical student. In the following year, amongst their other papers was one on "The volumetric determination of uric acid in the urine." Starling left Guy's for the Chair at University College where he continued his important research, and Gowland Hopkins proceeded to Cambridge where he made his epoch-making discoveries of the accessory food factors. He subsequently became President of the Royal Society.

One other Guy's surgeon who deserves mention for his earlier basic work is Arbuthnot Lane. His entirely original observations on skeletal modifications due to occupation were published in 1886 and preceded his great surgical contributions to the treatment of fractures by securing full anatomical correction and his many other contributions.

Although the anthology is concerned with Great Guy's men of the 19th century I feel that acknowledgment should be made of Arthur F. Hurst, that great physician of the earlier decades of the 20th century who made such great contributions to the diagnosis, radiology and understanding of many intestinal disorders and diseases.

I wish this anthology well.

BROCK.

Royal College of Surgeons of England
London
January, 1973.

INTRODUCTION

Two brief quotations from H. C. Cameron's admirable history, *Mr. Guy's Hospital, 1726-1948* (London, 1954), can set the perspective:

> Unlike that of St. Bartholomew's or St. Thomas's, the history of Guy's Hospital does not stretch far back into a shadowy origin in the Middle Ages. Guy's is one of a group of hospitals which were founded almost at the same time, in the second quarter of the eighteenth century. Westminster made a start in 1719, Guy's in 1721, St. George's in 1733, the London in 1740, and Middlesex in 1745. It was the beginning of the voluntary system.

Thomas Guy (1645-1724), its founder, began his commercial career as a bookseller and printer. His chief stock in trade was the Bible printed by the Oxford University Press. Profits from this virtuous trade were invested in government securities and South Sea stock. After counting the profit and the loss for a decade or two, Guy became a philanthropist. Through Sir Richard Mead he became interested in hospitals and was chosen a governor of St. Thomas's in 1704. In 1721 he began to construct the hospital which bears his name on land leased from St. Thomas's but he died before it was completed. He bequeathed £20,000 to carry out the plan, and the first patients were admitted in 1726. Cameron takes pride in pointing out that

> From 1768 to 1815 Guy's *alone* of all the schools in London conducted organized teaching of Medicine and of the sciences on which it rests, and it was at Guy's that the scientific interests of the time were congregated.

Guy's fame and fuller development came from the then novel idea that patient care and teaching were inseparable.

Actually, for pedagogic purposes Guy's and St. Thomas's

joined forces to form the United Hospitals in 1768. Anatomy and surgery were taught at St. Thomas's; medicine, chemistry, materia medica, and physiology at Guy's. When the joint arrangement was dissolved in 1825, it left Guy's with a strong staff of physicians, actively interested in just those fields in which progress would be most rapid during the next few decades. The presiding genius was not a physician but the hospital's Treasurer and chief administrative officer, Benjamin Harrison, whose tenure from 1797 to 1848 spanned the transition from Georgian stability to Victorian progress. A notable contribution to the eminence of Guy's was the establishment, in 1836, of *Guy's Hospital Reports.* A few sporadic attempts to publish a medical journal had been made at other hospitals, but they had not succeeded, and Guy's alone of all hospitals can show an unbroken series of volumes from that date until today.

The present anthology, *Great Men of Guy's,* is designed to supply the late twentieth-century reader with facsimile reprints of some of the more important original communications by such famous physicians as Thomas Addison, Richard Bright, Thomas Hodgkin, and their colleagues. Only by examining the original documents can one comprehend the nature of problems as they presented themselves to mid-nineteenth century physicians, follow the details of their reasoning, and estimate the quality of their analyses. A few biographical and bibliographical notes are in order.

Thomas Addison (1793-1860) was born near Newcastle and came from yeoman stock. He received his M.D. degree from Edinburgh in 1815 and came to London where he was appointed house surgeon to the Lock Hospital and, although already possessing a degree, he entered as a student at Guy's. Addison had neither influence nor connections, but Benjamin Harrison recognized his talents as a clinical observer and teacher and appointed him assistant physician in 1824. His lectures on materia medica attracted many students, and in 1837 he was appointed full physician and joint-lecturer on medicine with Richard Bright. Addison's reputation was established by his study of pneumonia in which he expanded the diagnostic methods of Laennec and demonstrated that the exudate took place not into the interstitial tissue of the lung, as then believed, but into the alveoli themselves. Reprinted here is his "Observations on the Diagnosis of Pneumonia" (*Guy's Hospital Reports,* 1st Series 2: 57-67, 1837,) a landmark in the study of chest diseases during the period between Laennec's discovery of auscultation and the later development of bacteriology and roentgenography. Like Addison's later work, it depends upon careful clinical observation correlated with the findings at post-mortem dissection.

Addison's fame, of course, rests upon the discovery of the disease which bears his name, hypoadrenocorticism. Trying to find the cause of an insidious malady characterized by pallor and asthenia, often associated with a peculiar 'bronzing' of the skin, he found that in a group of these patients the adrenal glands, then called supra-renal capsules, had been destroyed by either tuberculosis or damaged by primary atrophy. He published his account in a monograph titled *On the Constitutional and Local Effects of Disease of the Supra-renal Capsules* (London, Samuel Highley, 1855). This handsomely printed volume is now a collector's item. Since its large quarto size is inconvenient for facsimile reproduction, the text reproduced here has been taken from the collection of Addison's writings published in 1868 by the New Sydenham Society, supplemented by selected reproductions of the original illustrations.

Addison's anemia is a term applied by some to the pernicious anemia, but it is not clear whether the patients Addison studied did or did not have this disease. In retrospect, the clinical features of pernicious anemia had been described by Combe and by Gabriel Andral in 1823, and again in 1837 by Marshall Hall. Anton Biermer, apparently without knowledge of Addison's account, wrote a more comprehensive description in 1872. Shortly thereafter, William Pepper and Julius Cohnheim independently described the changes in the bone marrow, and the characteristic macrocytosis in the peripheral blood was described by Paul Ehrlich. The changes in the spinal cord were described by Lichtheim in 1887. Addison's short paper, "Anemia — Disease of the Supra-renal Capsules"

(*London Medical Gazette 43:* 517-518, 1847) was read at a meeting of the South London Medical Society. Addison probably discussed anemia secondary to failure of the adrenal cortex rather than a primary hematological entity. The term *Morbus Addisonii* was applied by Samuel Wilks (*Guy's Hospital Reports,* 3d Series 5: 89-118, 1859) and apparently restricted to adrenal disease. Armand Trousseau is credited with having popularized the eponym on the Continent.

In contrast to the self-confident, extroverted Richard Bright, Addison was a sensitive, unhappy man, an insomniac and mild depressive. Yet on the lecture platform Addison could communicate enthusiasm to his students while Bright's performance was sound but pedestrian. Cameron describes Addison's manner with patients as "so distant and cold that he has been described as like 'one trying to discover the derangement in a piece of machinery, rather than one who regards his patient as a suffering, sensitive human being . . .'" As a consequence, his practice was not large, but his income from Guy's was sufficient for his simple needs, and he could devote almost his whole time to research and teaching. It seems likely that Addison was a man driven by self-doubt and self-criticism, anxious to maintain the high standard he had set, and that his cold and distant manner was a mask of objectivity he had donned to protect himself from letting his real kindness appear. In 1860, feeling that his health would no longer permit him to carry out his work, he resigned from Guy's, retired to Brighton, and died a few months later.

Richard Bright (1789-1858), the son of a wealthy Bristol banker, began his medical studies at Edinburgh, but interrupted them to join Sir George Mackenzie and Mr. (later Sir) Henry Holland on a journey to Iceland, contributing chapters on botany and zoology to the former's *Travels in Iceland* (London, 1811). He continued his medical studies at Guy's in 1811-1812 but returned to Edinburgh to take his M.D. degree in the latter year. He then entered Peterhouse College, Cambridge, but left after two terms, finding university residence incompatible with his other interests. A trip to Central Europe led to his engaging book, *Travels from Vienna through*

Lower Hungary (London, 1815). In 1816 he received the license of the Royal College of Physicians and was appointed assistant physician to the London Fever Hospital. In 1820 he was appointed assistant physician to Guy's and began "that course of arduous clinical study and indefatigable industry as a teacher which made his own reputation and contributed much to that of the school." He was made full physician in 1824, and occupied that post until 1843, when he was made consulting physician.

Bright's first major contribution was his *Reports on Medical Cases,* the first volume appearing in 1827, the second in 1831, both illustrated by handsome colored plates. The nature of the work is revealed in its subtitle, *Selected with a view of illustrating the symptoms and cure of disease by a reference of morbid anatomy.* As in Addison's work, it was based on the careful correlation of clinical entities with post-mortem observations. The first twenty-four cases are classified as "illustrative of the appearances observable on the examination of diseases terminating in dropsical effusion." It was the observation of edema in the living patient, a damaged kidney found at post-mortem examination, and albumin in the urine when examined in the laboratory that led to what is known as Bright's disease. This material is reprinted here. Regrettably, the limitations of black-and-white reproduction are such that Bright's illustrations can not be included here.

Prior to Bright's publication it was known that the urine of many patients with edema contained albumin, and Morgagni had described cases with small contracted kidneys, but at post-mortem examinations which were not routine at that time, the kidneys were usually laid aside, and the association between albuminuria and renal disease was not appreciated until Bright published his *Reports,* nor had anyone considered kidney disease common or important. Cameron comments that "Bright's predecessors only occasionally asked leave to make a post-mortem examination. As a rule the attitude was that the cause of death was too obvious to need confirmation. Bright and Addison at the time they were doing their great work were much hampered by the difficulty in obtaining post-mortem examinations. It was only later in Wilks's time that arrangements were made for routine examinations."

Tests for proteinuria using heat and acetic acid had been described as early as the end of the seventeenth century by the Dutch physician, Frederik Dekkers, but the significance of the method had not been appreciated because it lacked practical application. In 1757 William C. Wells of Charleston, South Carolina had noted that the urine of patients with dropsy coagulated on heating, but he failed to relate this observation to kidney disease. John Blackall of Exeter had noted in 1813 that dropsy and proteinuria were associated, but he too failed to make a general connection between this observation and a renal lesion. Bright himself had no particular knowledge of chemistry and left the urinalyses to John Bostock, lecturer in chemistry at Guy's. Bostock's contribution to Bright's *Reports* of 1827 showed that the specific gravity of the urine in Bright's cases was lower than average, that the proportion of urea and salts was reduced, and that albumin might be present in large quantities. Bright was able to build upon his predecessors' observations and to utilize his chemist's data to synthesize a new constellation of renal disease marked by proteinuria and edema. His work is a classical example of how a perceptive internist utilizes data from both pathologic anatomy and clinical pathology to delineate a new disease entity.

Bright's interest in kidney diseases did not cease after his first brilliant *Reports*. Almost a decade later he published his observations on the next hundred cases in a major accumulation of clinico-pathologic data titled "Cases and Observations, Illustrative of Renal Disease accompanied with the Secretions of Albuminous Urine" *(Guy's Hospital Reports 1:* 338-379, 1836), followed directly by his systematic recording of the essential data as "Tabular View of the Morbid Appearances in 100 Cases Connected with Albuminous Urine" *(Guy's Hospital Reports 1:* 380-402, 1836). Though Bright's method of tabulating data was not original, his use of it firmly established the method as an indispensable tool for a clinical investigator trying to develop generalizations from empirical data. Bright's work was so sound and meritorious, so widely accepted without demur, that in 1842 he was able to persuade

Mr. Harrison, the Treasurer, to set aside two clinical wards, forty-two beds in all, for a period of six months, for an intensive study of renal disease. This was the beginning of today's "special metabolic ward" and similar hospital units.

Bright's further observations were recorded in two lengthy communications. The first appeared under his own name, and was titled "Cases and Observations, &c.—Memoir the Second" (*Guy's Hospital Reports 5:* 101-161, 1840); the second, by his junior colleagues, George Hilaro Barlow and George Owen Rees, was titled "Account of Observations made under the Superintendence of Dr. Bright on Patients whose Urine was Albuminous" (*Guy's Hospital Reports,* 2nd Series *1:* 189-316, 1843). It is greatly to Bright's credit that he was able to inspire two younger investigators to pursue researches in a subject of his own interest. This may well be the earliest example of a "team" investigating a single problem. Publications by Barlow and Rees reporting research done in their own right (*q.v.*) are also included in this book, partly for the merit inherent in their work, partly as an example of how research projects derive from antecedent observations. It is also to Bright's credit that he gave his juniors latitude to pursue their own investigative lines.

The *Reports of Medical Cases* was reprinted in 1872. Some of the material from *Guy's Hospital Reports* was reprinted by Arnold Osman in his useful book, *Original Papers of Richard Bright on Renal Disease* (London, Oxford University Press, 1937), long out of print. Osman (*Guy's Hospital Reports 83:* 185-193, 1933) and later J. B. Cavanagh (*Ibid. 107:* 390-398, 158) reviewed the histopathology of three of Bright's original cases preserved in the Gordon Museum at Guy's, but the most recent view through the retrospectoscope is by R. O. Weller and B. Nester (*Brit. Med. J. 2:* 761-763, 1972). Contemporary terminology assigns two cases to mesangiocapillary (membranoproliferative) glomerulonephritis and one to renal amyloidosis.

Bright was a cheerful, genial, outgoing man whose easy manner inspired confidence. Well cultivated by both travel and society, he combined an active career as a teacher and assiduous clinical investigator with a large, successful consulting practice. He died at his home in Savile Row after a brief illness, while still active in practice.

Thomas Hodgkin (1798-1866) was born in Middlesex into a well educated Quaker family. He began his medical studies at Guy's, continued them in Paris, but finally took his M.D. degree at Edinburgh in 1823. He returned to London, began practice, and worked at Guy's where he was appointed Curator of the Museum and Demonstrator of Morbid Anatomy in 1825. He made many improvements in the museum, arranging it according to a systematic plan designed to show diseases as they occurred in different organs and tissues. His catalogue of specimens and preparations was published in 1832, the year he published his most important paper, "On some Morbid Appearances of the Absorbent Glands and Spleen" (Medico-Chirurgical Transactions, London 17:68-114, 1832), now recognized as the first description of what is now called Hodgkin's disease. In 1837, when James Cholomely died and Addison was promoted to full physician, Hodgkin was a candidate for the post of assistant physician but was not elected.

Hodgkin did not confine his interests to medicine. He was active in the affairs of the University of London and was a member of its Senate from 1837 until his death. One reason for his interest may have been that the University was founded to provide education and grant degrees to candidates who were debarred from degrees at Oxford or Cambridge because they were not members of the Church of England, a qualification which in effect excluded Quakers, Protestant nonconformists, Roman Catholics, and Jews. Hodgkin was interested in the developing discipline of ethnography and wrote a number of papers on topics then of interest in that field. True to his Quaker background, he allied himself with several organizations devoted to social welfare, notably ones working in behalf of oppressed savages and aborigines, persecuted Jews, and the ill-housed poor. Diversity of interests and "radical" ideas rarely recommend their holder to those whose hands are on the levers of power and hold the key to preferment. There may have been substance to the charge made by Hodgkin's friends that Mr. Harrison, the Treasurer, blocked Hodgkin's appointment to the staff. After this disappointment, Hodgkin's interest in medicine waned. His practice had never been large nor was he ever interested in his fees; his idealistic nature placed higher value on other satisfactions. Most of the last twenty years of his life were devoted to ethnographic studies and philanthropic causes. He died of a sudden attack of enteric fever at Jaffa while visiting the Holy Land with Sir Moses Montefiore.

Hodgkin's discovery of a distinctive form of malignant lymphoma went unnoticed until 1856 when Samuel Wilks (1824-1911), then an assistant physician at Guy's assigned to the museum and morgue, independently rediscovered the same entity. Wilks's paper, "Cases of Lardaceous Disease and some Allied Affections" *(Guy's Hospital Reports, 3d Series 2: 103-132, 1856)*, which added fifteen cases to Hodgkin's seven, was ready for press when he came upon Hodgkin's article, written only twenty-four years previously. Medical libraries and methods of retrieval were not then so efficient as they later became. In a generous footnote Wilks mentioned Hodgkin's work, regretting that the latter had not been able to affix a distinctive name to the entity so that he might have recognized the contribution earlier. In the subsequent paper titled "Enlargement of the Spleen and Lymphatic Glands" *(Trans. Path. Soc., London 10: 259-263, 1859)* Wilks applied Hodgkin's name to the entity, honoring his predecessor in the then embryonic department of morbid anatomy at Guy's.

In 1926, Herbert Fox re-examined tissue from four of Hodgkin's original cases, reporting in "Remarks on the Presentation of Microscopical Preparations from some of the Original Tissue described by Thomas Hodgkin, 1832" *(Ann. Med. Hist. 8: 370-374, 1926)*. He confirmed the diagnosis by finding Reed-Sternberg cells in three cases (Cases II, IV, and VII), but in one case (Case VI) the sections showed either leukemic infiltration or lymphosarcoma. Reviewing Hodgkin's case histories, Fox concluded that Case I was tuberculosis, Case III syphilis, and Case V systemic lymphomatosis. Hodgkin, of course, had no microscopical preparations to study, and the assortment of diagnoses underscores the difficulty in assigning

Hodgkin's disease to the category of malignant lymphoma *vs.* progressive, systemic granulomatous disease.

Also reprinted in the present book is an early article by Hodgkin "On the Object of Post Mortem Examination" (*London Medical Gazette 2:* 423-431, 1828) which demonstrates not only the value placed on autopsies by the school of clinicians then developing at Guy's, but also shows what pathologists during the years between Morgagni and Virchow regarded as diagnostic clues and how they explained the mechanisms of disease.

George Hilaro Barlow (1806-1866), the son of an Exeter clergyman, came to Guy's in 1830, fresh from Trinity College, Cambridge, where he had been graduated B.A. the year before. He worked diligently in the clinic and laboratory and became interested in Bright's recent advances in the study of kidney disease. In 1836, along with James Babington, he was appointed editor of *Guy's Hospital Reports* and continued to edit and supervise production of that valuable journal for many years. On receiving his M.D. degree from Guy's in 1840 he was appointed assistant physician and assisted Bright in managing the patients on the specially allocated kidney ward. In 1843 with Rees, he published an account of these cases observed "under the superintendence of Dr. Bright" (*Guy's Hospital Reports*, 2nd Series 1: 189-316, 1843) and was appointed full physician. Earlier he had published the paper reprinted here, "Cases of Albuminous Urine Illustrative of the Efficacy of Tartar Emetic, in Combination with other Antiphlogistic Remedies, &c." (*Guy's Hospital Reports 5:* 167-184, 1840), an example of the type of laboratory study which derived from the clinical experience of that day and also an early effort to select a suitable form of therapy.

Cameron describes Barlow as "shy and retiring . . . clasping and unclasping his hands as he slowly gave vent to his opinion." Wilks, who knew him personally, found him a penetrating thinker, noting that "The superior men . . . always sought out Barlow, as in him they found a congenial mind with whom they could converse over some of the more abstruse subjects in medicine." He died of pneumonia in 1866 while still actively engaged in teaching.

George Owen Rees (1813-1889) was born at Smyrna, the son of a Welsh merchant in the Levant who served as British consul. He began his medical studies at Guy's in 1829 but took his M.D. degree at Glasgow in 1836. Returning to London, he became medical officer at Pentonville prison and was appointed assistant physician at Guy's in 1843. During that period he attracted Bright's attention and was given laboratory space as well as clinical duties. His first major contribution was a method for detecting sugar in the blood of diabetics, "On Diabetic Blood" (*Guy's Hospital Reports* 3: 398-400, 1838), reprinted here. Also included in the present collection are two later papers stemming directly from his laboratory studies of Bright's patients: "On the Proportion of Urea in Certain Diseased Fluids" (*Guy's Hospital Reports 5:* 162-166, 1840), the forerunner of the blood urea nitrogen determination of today, and "Observations on the Blood, with Reference to its Peculiar Condition in Morbus Brightii" (*Guy's Hospital Reports,* 2nd Series *1:* 317-330, 1843). He was not appointed full physician until 1856, and he retired in 1873. Rees had a diversity of skills; in addition to his work at Guy's, he was consulting physician to the Queen Charlotte Lying-in Hospital, and he worked closely with Alfred S. Taylor (*q.v.*) on many criminal investigations, notably the case of William Palmer, the Rugeley poisoner. He was disabled by a stroke in 1886 and died in 1889.

Cameron describes him: "Rees, who was always faultlessly dressed, was often to be found at the Athenaeum and was a welcome guest in the houses of many great men. His green brougham and red-faced coachman were long remembered at Guy's."

Golding Bird (1814-1854) was born at Downham, Norfolk and was educated privately. He showed precocious brilliance as a youthful chemist and came to London in 1829 as an apprentice to an apothecary. He entered Guy's as a student in 1832 but took his M.D. degree at St. Andrews in 1838. He returned to London where he combined clinical practice with chemical research at Guy's. Bird was in the forefront of chemical methods of his day. He used nitric acid to test for bile in the urine and an alkaline copper reagent to test for glycosuria. His detailed studies on urinary sediments and renal calculi were more sophisticated than any up to that time, and their value endured for more than half a century. Reprinted here is his "Observations of Urinary Concretions and Deposits" (*Guy's Hospital Reports 7:* 175-233, 1842) which he expanded into a monograph titled *Urinary Deposits, their Diagnosis, Pathology, and Therapeutical Indications* (London, 1844). Also reprinted here is his short paper, "Remarks on Cystine, or Cystic Oxide, and its Existence in Urinary Deposits" (*Guy's Hospital Reports 1:* 486-494, 1836), not so much for its substance as for its implications. William Wollaston had isolated cystine in 1808 but was more interested in its chemical properties. Bird's interest was that of a physician, a biochemist before that field was defined. Studies like Bird's paved the way for Sir Archibald Garrod's prophetic Croonian lecture of 1908, *Inborn Errors of Metabolism,* from which stems present day interest in aminoacidurias, genetic transmission of metabolic disease, and even the "one gene, one enzyme" theory.

Ill health prevented Bird's brilliant promise from reaching full flower. He suffered from both rheumatoid arthritis and rheumatic heart disease. Cameron suggests that "Perhaps it was because his frail body was stiffened and rigid from chronic rheumatism that he was one of the first to introduce a stethoscope with a flexible attachment; or it may have been that he wished himself to listen to the ominous sounds which proceeded from his own heart." It was probably aortic regurgitation that caused his breakdown in health in 1849, but he rallied and was able to work until 1851 when another breakdown took place. He resigned from Guy's in 1853 and died little more than a year later.

Alfred Swaine Taylor (1806-1880) came as a boy from Kent to Guy's and St. Thomas's as a student in 1823. When the two schools separated, he continued his studies under Sir

Astley Cooper. After being licensed by the Society of Apothecaries in 1828, he went abroad for an extended tour of medical schools and hospitals. Taylor was in Paris during the July Revolution of 1830 and had the opportunity, then rare for British students, to see gunshot wounds and their treatment on a large scale. He returned to Guy's and in 1831 was created professor of medical jurisprudence, a new chair, which he occupied until 1877. In 1832 he was appointed joint lecturer in chemistry with Arthur Aikin and held that post alone from 1851 to 1870.

Taylor can be called the father of British forensic medicine. His textbook, *The Principles and Practice of Medical Jurisprudence,* was first published in 1865 and went through many editions. Its influence was still evident a hundred years later, as generation after generation of students, pathologists, and medical examiners learned the elements of their craft from it. For over forty years Taylor published accounts of medico-legal cases in *Guy's Hospital Reports* as well as other medical journals. His forte was poisoning, then a popular method of homicide, but his publications ranged widely over death by foul play from any number of causes. Taylor frequently appeared as a witness for the Crown; his best known testimony was in the case of William Palmer, who used strychnine. By their very nature, Taylor's reports are anecdotal and, taken in bulk, are a set of variations on a now familiar theme. Their impact over the years made the medical public aware of medico-legal problems and raised the standards of forensic medicine. Reprinted here is Taylor's account of a "Trial for Murder by Poisoning by Arsenic" *(Guy's Hospital Reports,* 2nd Series 3: 187-196, 1854), selected as typical of this genre. It contains some perceptive comments on the nature of medical testimony, and aficionados of crime and its detection may be startled by the reason Taylor advances for not using the Marsh test in the case. This classical test had been developed in 1836 by James Marsh (1789-1846), a chemist, and Taylor was among the first to use it and popularize it. However, like any other laboratory test, it can be applied indiscriminately, and Taylor makes the point adroitly.

Taylor became a Fellow of the Royal Society in 1845 and was awarded an M.D. degree honoris causa by St. Andrews in 1852. He retired from active work in 1877 and died in his home overlooking Regent's Park in 1880. It is plain that Taylor's work, like that of Barlow, Rees, and Bird, was based on chemistry, in contrast to that of Addison, Bright, and Hodgkin whose intellectual roots lay in clinico-pathological correlation.

Not all the brilliant men who were trained at Guy's could be accommodated with appointments to the staff. Among these was Thomas Williams (1819-1865), who came to London from South Wales and entered Guy's in 1837. He was a talented student and took his degree, the newly created M.D. at the University of London in 1840, the first Guy's man to do so. He was also one of the first at Guy's who could be said to understand the importance of microscopical observations. Early in his career he grasped the new cell theory of Schwann, and reprinted here is his paper, "On the Pathology of Cells" (*Guy's Hospital Reports*, 2nd Series *1*: 423-461, 1843), which foreshadows the later and more extensive studies by Virchow along comparable lines. Wilks and Bettany, in their *Biographical History of Guy's Hospital* (London, 1892), describe him as " . . . striking in appearance and manner; indeed, he came under the domination of genius. It was grand to see him at the Physical Society standing up with long, flowing, black hair, making a speech on some abstruse question, having an air of inspiration as the eloquent phrases flowed from him. But it was not all talk; he was eminently scientific . . . "

Williams held the post of tutor at Guy's, but seeing no prospect of advancement, joined the staff of Grainger's School in Webb Street as demonstrator of anatomy circa 1843. When that institution closed a few years later, he returned to South Wales and began practice at Swansea. His practice flourished and he developed a considerable reputation, but he found time to continue his studies of natural history. Unfortunately, his days were numbered. He had had "renal dropsy" as a child and apparently recovered, but he died at the age of forty-six. He may well have been a victim of Bright's disease.

No anthology of Guy's would be complete without a memento of the bravura surgery of Sir Astley Cooper (1768-1841). A generation older than Addison, Bright, and Hodgkin, he was established as the leading surgeon in England before any of them began to study medicine. The events of his life are so numerous, his honors so plentiful, and his career so familiar that they require no repetition. One need only recall that in 1784 he was apprenticed to his uncle, William Cooper, surgeon to Guy's, but soon transferred to Henry Cline, surgeon to St. Thomas's. A year at Edinburgh under Gregory, Cullen, Black, and Fyfe, followed by anatomical studies with John Hunter, completed his basic training. The rest he learned by diligent dissection, his daily practice. It would be easy to attribute Cooper's success to a combination of charm and flair, and these he had in abundance. But in an age when a surgeon's skill depended on manual dexterity and speed, Cooper's pre-eminence was the result of continuous industry. One has but to examine his handsome books on hernias (*The Anatomy and Surgical Treatment of Inguinal and Congenital Hernia,* 1804 and *The Anatomy and Surgical Treatment of Crural and Umbilical Hernia,* 1807), to recognize the nature of his skill as a dissector and his ability to teach from direct experience. Parenthetically, these two volumes were published by Longmans, Rees, Orme, Brown & Green, the same house which brought out Bright's *Reports on Medical Cases;* so lavish was their production department that Cooper was £1,000 out of pocket after the press run sold out.

Cooper played a decisive role in the separation of Guy's from St. Thomas's in 1825, when he found that his nephew Bransby Cooper would not be chosen to succeed him as surgeon to St. Thomas's. Sir Astley helped persuade Benjamin Harrison to set up Guy's as an independent school and became its consulting surgeon. By that time he was on the verge of retirement, but he never quite managed to discontinue practice. It was quite natural, when *Guy's Hospital Reports* began publication 1836, to include some mention of his earlier triumphs. Reprinted here are two short articles to document his legendary skill: "Case of Femoral Aneurysm" (*Guy's Hospital Reports 1*: 43-50, 1836) and the justly famous "Account of the First Successful Operation, Performed on the Carotid Artery for Aneurysm in the year 1808" with the "Post-Mortem Examination in 1821" *(Ibid. 1:* 53-57, 1836). They were prepared for publication by (Charles) Aston Key, who married Astley Cooper's niece (Bransby Cooper's sister) and who also became a leading surgeon at Guy's. In the twentieth century, especially during the past two decades, surgery for aneurysms and upon major vessels has become commonplace, but it was Cooper who in 1816 — sans anesthesia, sans blood transfusion, sans aseptic technique, sans antibiotics — first attempted to ligate the abdominal aorta for aneurysm. When we criticize surgeons for "grandstand heroics," let us not forget that today's fantasy is tomorrow's fulfilled wish. One of the oldest lessons of medical history is that barriers to progress are forever being breached, and new frontiers do not remain intact for long. The point becomes self-evident when we look backward at the nature of medical practice, clinical investigation, and laboratory research at Guy's Hospital during the first part of the nineteenth century.

PRODUCTION NOTE

Bright's *Reports of Medical Cases* is illustrated by a set of splendid color lithographs, five of which depict the gross appearance of the kidney in his cases of dropsy and albuminuria. Regrettably, black and white reproduction fails to do them justice, and rather than present them badly we have decided not reproduce them at all. Likewise, Addison's monograph contains eleven plates. Six of them are designed to show the characteristic yellowish pigmentation of the skin associated with adrenocortical failure, and the delicate color values are lost in black and white reproduction. However, Plates IV, VII, and VIII demonstrate visceral lesions, and Plates X and XI demonstrate hyperpigmentation and depigmentation respectively. Because they retain their didactic value, we have chosen to reproduce them.

WILLIAM B. OBER, M.D.

OBSERVATIONS

ON THE

DIAGNOSIS

OF

PNEUMONIA.

BY DR. ADDISON.

Any attempt at a further elucidation of pneumonia, after the splendid performances of Laennec, may probably appear presumptuous; and especially so, when made by one who acknowledges himself indebted for almost all that he knows of thoracic diseases to that truly great man, at once the most distinguished and most successful cultivator of medical science that ever adorned the profession. When, however, it is recollected how vast and barren was the field of his inquiries when he commenced his brilliant career—and when our former ignorance is compared with the knowledge that resulted from his unprecedented discoveries—our astonishment is, not that he should have left something undone, but that he should have done so much. It is with the most profound deference and respect for his memory, therefore, that I venture to add this tributary mite to the riches of one of his favourite essays. I cannot but feel, also, that some apology is due to the profession, for presuming to direct attention to a subject with which the works of Laennec must already have made them familiar; and particularly to those who have so far resisted the influence of prejudice as to have made themselves conversant with the use of the stethoscope. My apology is, that the very familiarity of the subject appears to have lulled medical men in general, and even the stethoscopist, into a too passive confidence in what is already known: and has probably proved a check to that correction and improvement which Laennec himself was at all times so eager to accomplish.

The main object of this brief communication is, to make

some addition; however trifling, to the ordinary means of diagnosis ; since experience has forced upon me the conviction, that there are few acute diseases more frequently mistaken or overlooked than pneumonia, to the detriment of the patient, and the no small embarrassment of the practitioner.

In order to make myself understood, I may perhaps be permitted to take a very slight survey of the pathology, signs, and symptoms of the disease ; merely observing, at the outset, that, in doing so, I shall adhere as closely as possible to the purely practical tenor of our Reports ; indulging in theory no more than is unavoidable, in arranging and reasoning upon facts derived from the sick chamber and the dissecting-room. To the facts, or supposed facts, alone, do I attach any importance. The use of these facts must be left to the judgment and discernment of the reader.

In pneumonia, the inflammation is manifestly seated in or around the air-cells, or in both situations. It is perhaps of little importance, whether we conclude it to be seated primarily and essentially in the one or in the other of these structures : although, for my own part, I entertain no doubt whatever of its being primarily and essentially seated in the interior of the cells themselves—a belief drawn from the successive local changes observed to take place as the disease advances. In the first stage of the disorder, we find the cells red, and filled with a serous-looking and sometimes bloody fluid, rendering the lungs more heavy, dense, and œdematous, whilst they still retain their tenacity. At a more-advanced period, or second stage, the cells are found filled up with red solid matter, which appears to consist of the thickened parietes of the cells themselves : for if the lung be torn, and the torn surface examined with a magnifying-glass, it seems to be made up of innumerable minute red grains, just such as one might conceive to result from a filling-up of the cells in the manner supposed. At this period, the serous-looking fluid has disappeared, the lung is comparatively dry, and the tenacity of the solidified part is so far diminished, that it may be readily broken down by forcing the finger into it : this is what has been called red hepatization. At a later period, and sometimes apparently without having been preceded by the red granules, the solidified lung presents a grey appearance, an albuminous matter seems to occupy the place of the granules, or rather their centres, constituting the grey hepatization. This albuminous matter is sometimes firm and fixed, at other times it is less plastic, and occasionally, especially in bad constitutions, takes on a more decidedly purulent aspect, and may be squeezed out by pressure ; or, as the cohesion of the pulmonary tissue is often, under such circumstances, very much diminished, the slightest pressure of the finger causes it to break down into a semi-fluid mass, resembling an abscess.

It is not necessary to be more minute in describing the pathological changes which take place in the progress of pneumonia: it is sufficient to remember, that, in the first stage, the cells contain air and a serous-looking and sometimes bloody fluid, as shewn by the peculiar crackling sound, and escape of the fluid on squeezing a cut surface ;—that, in the second stage, the cells are solidified, comparatively dry, and, sooner or later, have poured into them an albuminous matter, either solid and fixed, or, more rarely, a matter approaching the character of pus. The stethoscopic signs indicative of these respective changes are such as might be expected, and are easily understood. Whilst the cells contain air and serous fluid, there is little or no dulness of sound on percussion, but during respiration, we hear the crepitating rattle—a rattle which undoubtedly depends upon the presence of air and fluid in the cells, for it is observed in cases of œdema of the lungs, and in some instances of pituitous catarrh, as well as in the first stage of pneumonia. When the cells are solidified, and admit no air, we have dulness of sound on percussion, bronchophony, and bronchial respiration, at least when the consolidation is considerable, and seated near the surface. Such are the stethoscopic signs of simple pneumonia : they are quite characteristic, and are pretty uniformly present, except under very peculiar circumstances.

If an opportunity present itself of examining the body, when a lung consolidated by pneumonia is retrograding towards a recovery of its normal state, we commonly find the cut surface of the portion previously hepatized of a pale or pinkish hue ; or we find it presenting a mixture of pale, pink, and grey : it is still more friable or lacerable than natural ; and the cells are again more or less loaded with serous-looking fluid, rendered frothy by squeezing the lung, in consequence of the presence of a considerable number of air-bubbles. It would also appear, that the further changes consist in the absorption of the effused fluids, a gradual increase of the tenacity of the pulmonary tissue, and a more or less complete restoration of the normal state. In some instances, however, when the albuminous matter thrown out is of the more plastic or organizable kind, it fails to be entirely absorbed, and part of it permanently remains. Under these circumstances, we find it, at an after-period, either in small, detached, and more or less rounded masses, or more extensively and more irregularly diffused through the pulmonary tissue. When distributed in small insulated portions, I believe it to constitute one of the forms of albuminous deposit, indiscriminately called tubercles ; whereas, when more extensively and irregularly diffused, it has, in like manner, been regarded as a form of tubercular infiltration. The history, however, of the patient's case, in many instances, as well as the local appearances themselves, lead me to the conclusion, that they are merely the result of a previous attack of pneumonia. We often learn, on inquiry, that, at some former period, perhaps years before, the patient had had an attack of inflammation within the chest ; whilst, if he die of some other disease, we almost uniformly discover, on dissection, unequivocal evidence of antecedent inflammation. The evidence consists in thickening and adhesions of the pluræ, especially in the neighbourhood of the appearances in question, together with induration and puckering of the pulmonary tissue immediately surrounding each albuminous deposit : or, when the deposit is irregular and extensive, we often have an actual deformity and puckering of the pleura above the infiltrated parts. This view of the origin of these albuminous deposits will probably serve, in some measure, to explain why they are much less uniformly found in the apices of the lungs than ordinary tubercles.

It has been observed, that these deposits may remain

passive for an unlimited period, and without undergoing any very appreciable change, except perhaps a conversion of some of them into calcareous or chalky masses, especially when deposited in the upper lobe of the lung : it would nevertheless appear, that the vital influence by which they are maintained in their integrity is so extremely slender, that if inflammation happen to be set up around them by any accidental cause, and especially if the vital powers of the patient have been greatly impaired, that influence is so far exhausted, that they lose their cohesion, and soften ;—the softening commonly first taking place in those portions most remote from the more highly organized living structures : they soften in the centre; the softening proceeds outwards, and, in the end, causes the formation of a vomica, and so produces one of the modifications of phthisis pulmonalis. Such, at least, are the conclusions to which repeated observation of the living, and dissection of the dead, have led me, in regard to this part of the subject.

Having premised these very superficial remarks, I shall now proceed to the reputed functional signs or symptoms of pneumonia; for it is to the unsteadiness and fallaciousness of these, that errors in diagnosis are chiefly attributable; and, consequently, it is to them more particularly that I am desirous of directing attention.

The characteristic symptoms of pneumonia enumerated by Laennec, are, an *obtuse and deep-seated pain in the chest, dyspnœa, hurried respiration, cough,* and *peculiar expectoration :* but, in reference to these, he tells us, that each of them individually may occasionally be absent, and, indeed, that they may all be absent in the same case. Now, were it quite correct to assume that the character of pneumonia is that which is expressed by the above symptoms, that the reputed deviations and exceptions alluded to by Laennec are only of very rare occurrence, and that obscurity happened only in the pneumonia of old people, and in cases complicated with other diseases, there might probably be some excuse for resting satisfied with the present position of the subject: but if it be as true, as I am convinced it is, that these reputed deviations and exceptions, regarded as obscure, are of extremely frequent occurrence, that they

are met with at every period of life, and in every variety of
constitution; and that they are very far indeed from being
limited to old persons, and to what have been called complicated cases; I hope to be pardoned if I make an attempt,
in some degree to unravel the difficulty, and place the subject, if not in a more correct, at least in a more safe and
practical point of view.

I have been led to the conclusion, that cases of pneumonia
characterized by obtuse and deep-seated pain, dyspnœa,
hurried respiration, cough, and peculiar expectoration, are,
in truth, themselves the exceptions, in a pathological sense;
and that, although most frequently met with in practice,
they are, in fact, cases of complication.   It may be said, if
such cases of complication be those most commonly en-
countered in practice, why interpose a mere pathological
subtlety, to disturb the practical rule?   To this I oppose my
belief, that it is an adherence to such a general character of
pneumonia that has led, and is constantly leading, to an over-
sight—to a neglect of the disease, when it occurs in what I
am disposed to regard as its more *simple form:* and as cases
partaking more or less of this simple form of pneumonia are
of frequent occurrence, I am willing to persuade myself that
what follows may have the effect of diminishing the liability
to the errors alluded to.

In *simple pneumonia,* after chilliness, shivering, feebleness,
and depression, the patient experiences, for the most part,
strongly-marked symptoms of febrile re-action, giddiness,
confusion, and sometimes intense pain in the head; occasionally delirium, especially towards night; *the skin acquires
a pungent heat,* generally accompanied by dryness, more
rarely by moisture; the pulse is full and strong, perhaps
labouring and sluggish; the face is usually more or less
suffused with a livid flush, accompanied by an expression of
distress; the tongue is foul; its substance is more injected
than in ordinary phlegmasiæ, and in a short time it manifests a tendency to become dry and brownish; the respiration is somewhat hurried, but *there is seldom any very obvious
cough or expectoration, and sometimes none at all;* in short,
the whole assemblage of symptoms bears a most striking
resemblance to those of a severe attack of common continued

fever of the typhoid type, for which it is so repeatedly mistaken. If this form of the disease occur in moderately good constitutions, and is overlooked, especially if stimulants be administered on the supposition of its being a severe case of typhoid fever, it very commonly happens that the general prostration increases, the delirium or oppression of the brain is aggravated, the tongue gets dry and black, and the teeth covered with sordes; the breathing becomes more hurried, occasionally with a frequent slight hacking cough, and now and then a little bloody expectoration; the pulse gets flaccid, frequent, and feeble; and at length the patient dies.

Notwithstanding its close resemblance to a severe attack of continued fever—a resemblance so great, that even the stethoscopist is occasionally thrown off his guard—attentive observation will, in most cases, enable us to recognise the difference. The attack, in general, is more abrupt, and often follows some manifest exposure to cold or wet. The countenance, though congested and somewhat distressed, has not the dejection and stupidity so remarkable in fever: it displays more intelligence; and, although confused and perhaps slightly delirious, the patient, on being roused, commonly evinces a clearness and vigour of intellect not found in fever. The condition of the tongue also furnishes a valuable diagnostic sign. We know that, at the onset of fever, the contrast between the vividly-injected tongue and its white or grey fur is very striking: it is, in general, much less so in pneumonia. In the latter, if I may be allowed the expression, it is more the tongue of a phlegmasia: the hurry of respiration in pneumonia is often not more than we commonly perceive amid the general distress of fever; and I repeat, that neither cough nor expectoration is necessarily present in a very appreciable degree. But of all the symptoms of pneumonia, the most constant and conclusive, in a diagnostic point of view, is *a pungent heat of the surface.* By this symptom alone, the first stage of pneumonia may, in most instances, be readily recognised: by this symptom alone, I have repeatedly pronounced the existence of pneumonia, before asking a single question, or making the slightest stethoscopic examination of the chest. The presence of this symptom has scarcely ever yet deceived me, even in the most complicated forms of inflammation within the chest.   I by no means contend that it is necessarily present at some period of every case, although I do not know to the contrary ; but I feel justified in affirming, that when inflammation is confined to the chest, however varied may be the tissues involved in the inflammatory process, provided this symptom be present, pneumonia may be confidently pronounced to form a part, in nineteen cases out of twenty, and I believe in a much larger proportion.

A similar pungent heat of the surface is now and then observed in certain forms of renal dropsy; more frequently in continued fever, especially in children ; and still more commonly in the eruptive fevers of the exanthemata and erysipelas : and, as such cases may supervene upon already existing disease within the chest, the fact ought to be carefully remembered, lest a most valuable diagnostic sign should rather mislead than assist us.   It is in original inflammation within the chest that it proves so constant and conclusive a sign of pneumonia, but on every occasion, when present, it ought to lead to a most careful scrutiny, by means of the stethoscope.

I am unwilling to swell this communication by a detailed recital of individual cases : but were it otherwise, it would be easy to introduce a very great variety of instances, in which simple pneumonia has been mistaken for common fever of a typhoid type.   I have repeatedly witnessed it in children ; the first suspicion of it having generally been suggested to me by recognising, on applying the hand to the surface, the peculiar pungent heat already noticed.   I not long ago had an example in a young woman who was supposed to be labouring under a severe attack of bilious fever ; so called, because pneumonia of the right lung was accompanied, as is not unfrequently the case, by a sallowness, or almost jaundiced aspect of the patient's countenance.   I have a very similar case in Miriam's Ward at this time, also occurring in a young female.   In elderly persons it is so common, that when a case of typhus is represented to have occurred in any individual above fifty years of age, without evidence of the existence of the disease in other branches of the family, I confess that I consider it at all times an equal chance that it is, in reality, a case of pneumonia. An instance of this kind I saw very recently: the person was upwards of 60, but of a hale constitution, and presented most of the ordinary signs of continued fever, whilst the pulmonic symptoms were so slight as never to have attracted the least attention. This brief representation may probably suffice to fix attention upon the likelihood of the presence of pneumonia in cases of supposed continued fever.

The more simple form of pneumonia not unfrequently assumes another appearance, which has occasionally led to a belief that the brain was the seat of the disorder; the original affection of the lungs being so obscure as to be entirely overlooked. I have, within a short period, seen two cases of acute pneumonia in vigorous adults, in which, at the commencement, and for some days, the disturbance of the brain was such, that remedies were applied exclusively for the relief of that organ. In both instances, the inflammation was very intense, and was, at a latter period, attended with cough, expectoration, and other signs commonly regarded as characteristic of pneumonia.

Some time ago, I was requested to see an elderly man, who appeared to be labouring under obscure symptoms of mental aberration, and was supposed to have become insane. He looked pale, his countenance was somewhat anxious, his tongue was loaded, slightly brown, and disposed to become dry, he was occasionally incoherent, and wandered about the ward in a wild and unaccountable manner, but had neither cough nor expectoration sufficient to attract any particular attention. On examination, I found him labouring under pneumonia already advanced to hepatization. He recovered. A similar case is now under treatment in the hospital.

In infants and very young children, such cases are by no means rare, and simulate hydrocephalus. In one instance, where hepatization had taken place, the most prominent symptom was convulsions, for which various applications had been made to the head.

Such are some of the affections of the brain, to which pneumonia not unfrequently gives rise—secondary affections, calculated to mislead the most wary; and such as must inevitably distract the attention, and perplex the judgment of those who do not habitually have recourse to the stethoscope.

If the representations I have made be correct, they certainly lead to an inference, that even acute disease does not, when confined to the air-cells, necessarily give rise either to cough or expectoration—symptoms, perhaps, too much relied upon, in recognising, or even suspecting, affections of the lungs.

Without arguing the question, whether it be possible to expectorate a thin watery fluid, which must necessarily gravitate in the cells of the lungs, I may venture to state, that I entertain very strong suspicion that the cough and expectoration so commonly observed in pneumonia depend altogether upon the accidental implication of the bronchial tubes, and that, without a doubt, the degree of these symptoms depends upon the degree of that implication. Certain it is, that the most intense pneumonia may exist, even in hale constitutions, with cough and expectoration so slight as to pass unnoticed; and it is not difficult to suppose, that, when so slight, they may depend rather upon mere sympathetic irritation of the minute bronchial tubes in the immediate neighbourhood of the inflamed tissue, than upon any considerable degree of actual inflammation set up in them. It is true, that, on dissection, we very commonly find the mucous membrane of the smaller tubes reddened; but whether from inflammation, or not, is by no means so easily determined. I am disposed to think, that, in simple pneumonia, the small tubes are either not at all inflamed, or only inflamed in a very slight degree, and that, when more decidedly involved, their inflamed state gives rise to the cough and peculiar viscid expectoration described as characteristic of pneumonia in general. This complication is indisputably more frequently present than absent; a circumstance little calculated to excite surprise, and one probably sufficient to account for the symptoms which attend the complication, having usually been described as those essential to, and characteristic of, pneumonia.

When cough and expectoration are as well marked as

ON THE

CONSTITUTIONAL AND LOCAL EFFECTS

OF

DISEASE

OF THE

SUPRA-RENAL CAPSULES.

BY

THOMAS ADDISON, M.D.,

SENIOR PHYSICIAN TO GUY'S HOSPITAL.

LONDON:

SAMUEL HIGHLEY, 32 FLEET STREET.

1855.

TO

THE RIGHT HONOURABLE LORD HAWKE,

AS A TRIBUTE OF RESPECT,

AND IN GRATEFUL ACKNOWLEDGEMENT OF A LONG, CORDIAL,

AND MOST DISINTERESTED FRIENDSHIP,

THIS LITTLE WORK

IS DEDICATED

BY HIS LORDSHIP'S OBLIGED FRIEND AND HUMBLE SERVANT,

THOMAS ADDISON.

-12-

PREFACE.

IF Pathology be to disease what Physiology is to health, it appears reasonable to conclude, that in any given structure or organ, the laws of the former will be as fixed and significant as those of the latter; and that the peculiar characters of any structure or organ may be as certainly recognized in the phenomena of disease as in the phenomena of health. When investigating the pathology of the lungs, I was led, by the results of inflammation affecting the lung-tissue, to infer, contrary to general belief, that the lining of the air-cells was not identical and continuous with that of the bronchi; and microscopic investigation has since demonstrated in a very striking manner the correctness of that inference,—an inference, be it observed, drawn entirely from the indications furnished by pathology. Although Pathology therefore, as a branch of medical science, is necessarily founded on Physiology, questions may nevertheless arise regarding the true character of a structure or organ, to which occasionally the pathologist may be able

-13-

to return a more satisfactory and decisive reply than the physiologist,—these two branches of medical knowledge being thus found mutually to advance and illustrate each other. Indeed, as regards the functions of individual organs, the mutual aids of these two branches of knowledge are probably much more nearly balanced than many may be disposed to admit; for in estimating them, we are very apt to forget how large an amount of our present physiological knowledge, respecting the functions of these organs, has been the immediate result of casual observations made on the effects of disease. Most of the important organs of the body, however, are so amenable to direct observation and experiment, that in respect to them the modern physiologist may fairly lay claim to a large preponderance of importance, not only in establishing the solid foundation, but in raising and greatly strengthening the superstructure of a rational pathology. There are still, however, certain organs of the body, the actual functions and influence of which have hitherto entirely eluded the researches and bid defiance to the united efforts of both physiologist and pathologist. Of these not the least remarkable are the "Supra-Renal Capsules,"—the *Atrabiliary* Capsules of Caspar Bartholinus; and it is as a first and feeble step towards an inquiry into the functions and influence of these organs, suggested by Pathology, that I now put forth the following pages.

T. A.

24 New Street, Spring Gardens,
    May 21, 1855.

CONSTITUTIONAL AND LOCAL EFFECTS

OF

DISEASE OF THE SUPRA-RENAL CAPSULES.

IT will hardly be disputed that at the present moment, the functions of the supra-renal capsules, and the influence they exercise in the general economy, are almost or altogether unknown. The large supply of blood which they receive from three separate sources; their numerous nerves, derived immediately from the semilunar ganglia and solar plexus ; their early development in the fœtus; their unimpaired integrity to the latest period of life ; and their peculiar gland-like structure; all point to the per-formance of some important office : nevertheless, beyond an ill-defined impression, founded on a consideration of their ultimate organization, that, in common with the spleen, thymus and thyroid body, they in some way or other minister to the elaboration of the blood, I am not aware that any modern authority has ventured to assign to them any special function or influence whatever.

To the physiologist and to the scientific anatomist, therefore, they con-tinue to be objects of deep interest, and doubtless both the physiologist and anatomist will be inclined to welcome, and regard with indulgence, the smallest contribution calculated to open out any new source of inquiry respecting them. But if the obscurity, which at present so entirely conceals from us the uses of these organs, justify the feeblest attempt to add to our scanty stock of knowledge, it is not less true, on the other hand, that any one presuming to make such an attempt, ought to take care that he do not, by hasty pretensions, or by partial and prejudiced observation, or by an over-statement of facts, incur the just rebuke of those possessing a sounder and more dispassionate judgement than himself. Under the influence of these considerations I have for a considerable period withheld, and now venture to publish, the few facts bearing upon the subject that have fallen within my own knowledge; believing as I now do, that these concurring facts, in relation to each other, are not merely casual coincidences, but are such as admit of a fair and logical inference—an inference, that where these concurrent facts are observed, we may pronounce with considerable confidence, the existence of diseased supra-renal capsules.

As a preface to my subject, it may not be altogether without interest or unprofitable, to give a brief narrative of the circumstances and observations by which I have been led to my present convictions.

For a long period I had from time to time met with a very remarkable form of general anæmia, occurring without any discoverable cause whatever; cases in which there had been no previous loss of blood, no exhausting diarrhœa, no chlorosis, no purpura, no renal, splenic, miasmatic, glandular, strumous, or malignant disease. Accordingly, in speaking of this form of anæmia in clinical lecture, I, perhaps with little propriety, applied to it the term "idiopathic," to distinguish it from cases in which there existed more or less evidence of some of the usual causes or concomitants of the anæmic state.

The disease presented in every instance the same general character, pursued a similar course, and, with scarcely a single exception, was followed, after a variable period, by the same fatal result. It occurs in both sexes, generally, but not exclusively, beyond the middle period of life, and so far as I at present know, chiefly in persons of a somewhat large and bulky frame, and with a strongly-marked tendency to the formation of fat. It makes its approach in so slow and insidious a manner, that the patient can hardly fix a date to his earliest feeling of that languor, which is shortly to become so extreme. The countenance gets pale, the whites of the eyes become pearly, the general frame flabby rather than wasted; the pulse perhaps large, but remarkably soft and compressible, and occasionally with a slight jerk, especially under the slightest excitement; there is an increasing indisposition to exertion, with an uncomfortable feeling of faintness or breathlessness on attempting it; the heart is readily made to palpitate; the whole surface of the body presents a blanched, smooth and waxy appearance; the lips, gums and tongue seem bloodless; the flabbiness of the solids increases; the appetite fails; extreme languor and faintness supervene, breathlessness and palpitations being produced by the most trifling exertion or emotion; some slight œdema is probably perceived about the ankles; the debility becomes extreme, the patient can no longer rise from his bed, the mind occasionally wanders, he falls into a prostrate and half-torpid state, and at length expires: nevertheless to the very last, and after a sickness of perhaps several months' duration, the bulkiness of the general frame and the amount of obesity often present a most striking contrast to the failure and exhaustion observable in every other respect.

With, perhaps, a single exception, the disease, in my own experience, resisted all remedial efforts, and sooner or later terminated fatally. On examining the bodies of such patients after death, I have failed to discover any organic lesion that could properly or reasonably be assigned as an adequate cause of such serious consequences; nevertheless, from the disease having uniformly occurred in fat people, I was naturally led to entertain a suspicion that some form of fatty degeneration might have a share at least in its production; and I may observe, that in the case last examined, the heart had undergone such a change, and that a portion of the semilunar ganglion and solar plexus, on being subjected to microscopic examination, was pronounced by Mr. Quekett to have passed into a corresponding condition. Whether any, or all, of these morbid changes are essentially concerned, as I believe they are, in giving rise to this very remarkable disease, future observation will probably decide.

The cases having occurred prior to the publication of Dr. Bennett's interesting essay on "Leucocythæmia," it was not determined by microscopic examination whether there did, or did not, exist an excess of white corpuscles in the blood of such patients.

It was whilst seeking in vain to throw some additional light upon this form of anæmia, that I stumbled upon the curious facts, which it is my more immediate object now to make known to the Profession; and however unimportant or unsatisfactory they may at first sight appear, I cannot but indulge the hope, that by attracting the attention and enlisting the cooperation of the Profession at large, they may lead to the subject being properly examined and sifted, and the inquiry so extended, as to suggest, at least, some interesting physiological speculations, if not still more important practical indications.

The leading and characteristic features of the morbid state to which I would direct attention, are, anæmia, general languor and debility, remarkable feebleness of the heart's action, irritability of the stomach, and a peculiar change of colour in the skin, occurring in connexion with a diseased condition of the " supra-renal capsules."

As has been observed in other forms of anæmic disease, this singular disorder usually commences in such a manner, that the individual has considerable difficulty in assigning the number of weeks or even months that have elapsed since he first experienced indications of failing health and strength; the rapidity, however, with which the morbid change takes place, varies in different instances. In some cases that rapidity is very great, a few weeks proving sufficient to break up the powers of the constitution, or even to destroy life; the result, I believe, being determined by the extent, and by the more or less speedy development, of the organic lesion. The patient, in most of the cases I have seen, has been observed gradually to fall off in general health; he becomes languid and weak, indisposed to either bodily or mental exertion; the appetite is impaired or entirely lost; the whites of the eyes become pearly; the pulse small and feeble, or perhaps somewhat large, but excessively soft and compressible; the body wastes, without, however, presenting the dry and shrivelled skin, and extreme emaciation, usually attendant on protracted malignant disease; slight pain or uneasiness is from time to time referred to the region of the stomach, and there is occasionally actual vomiting, which in one instance was both urgent and distressing; and it is by no means uncommon for the patient to manifest indications of disturbed cerebral circulation. Notwithstanding these unequivocal signs of feeble circulation, anæmia, and general prostration, neither the most diligent inquiry, nor the most careful physical examination, tends to throw the slightest gleam of light upon the precise nature of the patient's malady: nor do we succeed in fixing upon any special lesion as the cause of this gradual and extraordinary constitutional change. We may indeed suspect some malignant or strumous disease; we may be led to inquire into the condition of the so-called blood-making organs; but we discover no proof of organic change anywhere,—no enlargement of spleen, thyroid, thymus or lymphatic glands,—no evidence of renal disease, of purpura, of previous exhausting diarrhœa, or ague, or any long-continued exposure to miasmatic influences: but with a more or less manifestation of the symptoms already enumerated, we discover a most remarkable, and, so far as I know, characteristic discoloration taking place in the skin,—sufficiently marked indeed as generally to have attracted the attention of the patient himself, or of the patient's friends. This discoloration pervades the whole surface of the body, but is commonly most strongly manifested on the face, neck, superior extremities, penis and scrotum, and in the flexures of the axillæ and around the navel. It may be said to present a dingy or smoky appearance, or various tints or shades of deep amber or chestnut-brown; and in one instance the skin was so universally and so deeply darkened, that, but for the features, the patient might have been mistaken for a mulatto.

In some cases this discoloration occurs in patches, or perhaps rather certain parts are so much darker than others, as to impart to the surface a mottled or somewhat checkered appearance; and in one instance there were, in the midst of this dark mottling, certain insular portions of the integument presenting a blanched or morbidly white appearance, either in consequence of these portions having remained altogether unaffected by the disease, and thereby contrasting strongly with the surrounding skin, or, as I believe, from an actual defect of colouring matter in these parts. Indeed, as will appear in the subsequent cases, this irregular distribution of pigment-cells is by no means limited to the integument, but is occasionally also made manifest on some of the internal structures. We have seen it in the form of small black spots, beneath the peritoneum of the mesentery and omentum—a form which in one instance presented itself on the skin of the abdomen.

This singular discoloration usually increases with the advance of the disease; the anæmia, languor, failure of appetite, and feebleness of the heart, become aggravated; a darkish streak usually appears upon the commissure of the lips; the body wastes, but without the extreme emaciation and dry harsh condition of the surface so commonly observed in ordinary malignant diseases; the pulse becomes smaller and weaker, and without any special complaint of pain or uneasiness, the patient at length gradually sinks and expires. In one case, which may be said to have been acute in its development as well as rapid in its course, and in which both capsules were found universally diseased after death, the mottled or checkered discoloration was very manifest, the anæmic condition strongly marked, and the sickness and vomiting urgent; but the pulse, instead of being small and feeble as usual, was large, soft, extremely compressible, and jerking on the slightest exertion or emotion, and the patient speedily died.

My experience, though necessarily limited, leads to a belief that the disease is by no means of very rare occurrence, and that were we better acquainted with its symptoms and progress, we should probably succeed in detecting many cases, which, in the present state of our knowledge, may be entirely overlooked or misunderstood ; and, I think, I may with some confidence affirm, that although partial disease of the capsules may give rise to symptoms, and to a condition of the general system, extremely equivocal and inconclusive, yet that a more extensive lesion will be found to produce a state, which may not only create a suspicion, but be pronounced with some confidence to arise from the lesion in question.   When the lesion is acute and rapid, I believe the anæmia, prostration, and peculiar condition of the skin will present a corresponding character, and that whether acute or chronic, provided the lesion involve the entire structure of both organs, death will inevitably be the consequence.

If this statement be correct, and I quite believe it to be so, the chief difficulty that remains to be surmounted by further experience in this, I fear, irremediable disease, is a correct and certain diagnosis ;—how we may at the earliest possible period detect the existence of this form of anæmia, and how it is to be distinguished from other forms of anæmic disorder. As I have already observed, the great distinctive mark of this form of anæmia is the singular dingy or dark discoloration of the skin ; nevertheless at a very early period of the disorder, and when the capsules are less extensively diseased, the discoloration may, doubtless, be so slight and equivocal as to render the source of the anæmic condition uncertain.   Our doubts, in such cases, will have reference chiefly to the sallow anæmic conditions resulting from miasmatic poisoning or malignant visceral disease ; but a searching inquiry into the history of the case, and a careful examination of the several parts or organs usually involved in anæmic disease, will furnish a considerable amount of at least negative evidence ; and when we fail to discover any of the other well-known sources of that condition, when the attendant symptoms resemble those enumerated as accompanying disease of the capsules, and when to all this is superadded a dark, dingy or smoky-looking discoloration of the integument, we shall be justified at least in entertaining a strong suspicion in some instances,—a suspicion almost amounting to certainty in others.   It must, however, be observed, that every tinge of yellow, or mere sallowness, throws a still greater doubt over the true nature of the case, and that the more decidedly the discoloration partakes of the character described, the stronger ought to be our impression as to the capsular origin of the disorder.

The morbid appearances discovered after death will be described with the cases in which they occurred; but I may remark that a recent dissection (March 1855) has shown that even malignant disease may exist in both capsules, without giving rise to any marked discoloration of the skin; but, in the case alluded to, the deposit in each capsule was exceedingly minute, and could not have seriously interfered with the functions of the organs: extensive and fatal malignant disease had, however, affected other parts. It may be observed in conclusion, that on subjecting the blood of a patient, who recently died from a well-marked attack of this singular disease, to microscopic examination, a considerable excess of white corpuscles was found to be present.

CASE I.*—Reported by Mr. THOMAS FULLER.

James Wootten, æt. 32, admitted into Guy's Hospital, under Dr. Golding Bird, Feb. 6, 1850, has been residing at Long Alley, Moorfields, and is by occupation a baker. States that he was attacked with a cough three years since, which he was unable to get rid of by ordinary remedies, and was finally cured at St. Bartholomew's, after taking pills for one week. From this time, his skin, previously white, began to assume a darker hue, which has been gradually increasing. Twelve months after leaving the above hospital he was laid up from excessive weakness, the result of his cough, which had again appeared, and incapacitated him for his work. He now became an out-patient of St. Thomas's, under Dr. Goolden, who cured his cough, and thinking that the colour of his skin depended on jaundice, treated him for that disease, but to no purpose. He left the hospital in tolerable health, but subsequently lost flesh, and became so excessively weak, the colour of his skin at the same time getting rapidly darker, that he applied for admission here, which was granted him.

Present Appearances.—The whole of the skin on the body is now of a dark hue, and he has just the appearance of having descended from coloured parents, which he assures me is not the case, nor have any of his family for generations, that he can answer for, manifested this peculiarity. The colour of the skin does not at all resemble that produced by the absorption of the nitrate of silver, but has more the appearance of the pigment of the choroid of the eye; it seems to have affected some parts of his body more than others, the scrotum and penis being the darkest, the soles of the feet and palms of the hands the lightest; the cheeks are a little sunken, the nose is pointed, the conjunctivæ are of a pearly white-

* The cases generally are given in the language and style of their respective reporters.

ness ; the voice is puny and puerile, the patient speaking with a kind of indescribable whine, and his whole demeanour is childish. He complains of a sense of soreness in the chest about the scrobiculus cordis. The chest is well-formed and perfectly resonant ; the sounds of the heart are also healthy ; there is some slight fullness in the region of the stomach. The urine is of a proper colour, and he has passed in twelve hours one and a half pint, which has a specific gravity 1008, an acid reaction, and contains neither albumen nor sugar ; there is also some pain on pressure in the left lumbar region.

Feb. 8.—Dr. Bird wished a likeness to be taken, so as to be able to watch any alterations in his colour ; and considering the case one of anæmia, ordered Syr. Ferri Iodidi 3j ter die ; and middle diet. These he took the whole of the time that he was in the hospital, and was discharged in April, rather stronger, but the colour remaining precisely the same.

Shortly after his discharge from the hospital, he was seized with acute pericarditis and pulmonic inflammation, under which he speedily sank and died.

The following is a report of the post-mortem examination :—

Lungs universally adherent, the adhesions being very old. The upper lobe of the right lung contained some small defined patches of recent pneumonia, about the size of a crown-piece, surrounded by tolerably healthy structure. The lower lobe was extremely fleshy and without air. The left lung was bound down by old pleuritic adhesions, which were very tough and difficult to be torn through. The substance of this lung was fleshy, and contained but little air. There was no tubercle or cavity. The mucous membrane of the bronchial tubes was considerably injected, and, I believe, rather thickened. The pericardium was distended with fluid of a deep brown colour, amounting to about half-a-pint ; recent lymph was effused over the whole serous surface. The liver and spleen were both of weak texture, and easily broken down ; the structure of the liver rather coarse. The gall-ducts pervious. The gall-bladder contained the usual quantity of bile, which was thin, watery and clear. The thoracic duct was pervious throughout; and there was no obstruction to any of the veins or arteries that I could discover. The colour of the blood in the arteries had an unusually dark appearance. The kidneys were quite healthy and of full size. The supra-renal capsules were diseased on both sides, the left about the size of a hen's egg, with the head of the pancreas firmly tied down to it by adhesions. Both capsules were as hard as stones. Intestines pale. Lumbar glands natural. No tubercular deposit was discovered in any organ. The head was not examined. (Vide Pl. I.)

In some of the cases about to be given, the capsules merely participated in disease affecting other organs, either of a strumous or malignant character, and it might consequently be doubtful whether the peculiar symptoms depended upon such complications, or upon the special disease of the capsules.

In the above instance, however, no such doubt could reasonably be entertained, inasmuch as there was found no abnormal condition whatever of any other organ, to which these peculiar symptoms could by any means be attributed. The slow and gradual inroads of the disease, and the remarkable excess of pigment, were sufficiently accounted for by the universality of the change that had taken place in the structure of both capsules ; at least such would be the legitimate conclusion to be drawn from a comparison of the present with other cases about to be related.

CASE II.

James Jackson, æt. 35. The subject of this case was admitted into the Clinical ward, under my own care, November 11, 1851, and died December 7, 1851. For the particulars of its history and result, I am indebted to my former pupil and present distinguished colleague, Dr. Gull, who was the first to suspect the true nature of the malady during the life of the patient.

A married man, residing at Gravesend, and occupied as a tide-waiter in the Customs. Of a bilious temperament, dark hair and sallow complexion, which since his illness has much deepened, so that now it is of a dark olive-brown. His wife says, " This obvious change in his complexion has been from the beginning of his illness, and gradually came on at that time."

There can be no doubt as to this change in the complexion depending upon increase of pigment, for if the lips be turned down, the mucous membrane is seen to be mottled by a deposit of pigment, and a closer examination shows that the dark colour of the lips, which at first had the appearance of sordes, is dependent upon the presence of a black pigment, which is not moveable by moistening or washing the lips. There is an expression of anxiety in the face, and the brow is contracted. He gives the following history of himself :—

His occupation subjects him to much anxiety; he is exposed to all the vicissitudes of the weather, both night and day, and sometimes his food for weeks together consists of salt provisions. Eight years ago he had rheumatism, accompanied with great nervous depression ; since that time he has enjoyed general good health, with the exception of some attacks of bilious vomiting. His present illness came on six months ago with headache, vomiting and constipation. About the sixth day of his illness he became delirious, and was insensible for twenty-four hours. On recovering his consciousness, he was unable to move the fingers of either hand, nor could he move the legs below the knees; the same parts were numb, as was also the tip of the tongue. He continued weak during the whole summer.

Two months ago he resumed his occupation, and remained at it until ten days back, when the old symptoms of headache, vomiting and constipation returned. Dr. McWilliam saw him at this time, and found his symptoms to have an intermittent character, and regarded the case as one of miasmatic poisoning, not only from his general symptoms, but also from the dark poisoned look of his face, not altogether unlike that presented on the approach of the asphyxic stage of cholera.

On his admission into the hospital, the pulse was extremely small and feeble, the expression of the face pinched, the brows knitted. He vomited mucus containing altered blood of a dark brown colour; tongue clean; epigastric region full, especially towards the left side, where he has had some twitching pain and slight tenderness on pressure. Urine natural in colour and quantity, of a light brown colour, not coagulable by heat. He went on, day by day, with but slight symptoms of change. Skin cool; pulse moderate in frequency, but extremely feeble, so as scarcely to be felt at the wrist. On several occasions the depression was so great as to require the exhibition of decided stimulants. There was a continued tendency to sickness. The abdomen soft, with marked aortic pulsation. Bowels constipated; chest everywhere resonant; heart's sounds normal; extent of dullness on percussion not increased. Slight traces of intermittence in the symptoms; the surface in the evening being cool, or even cold, and the following morning warm, as if from reaction.

Probable diagnosis.— The epigastric tenderness and pulsation, with frequent vomiting, and the ejected mucus and altered blood, point to an inflammatory condition of the gastric mucous membrane. But what

-27-

condition of system is it which favours the production of black pigment ? Is it some affection of the liver; or is it, as Dr. Addison supposes, disease of the supra-renal capsules ?

Sectio Cadaveris.

The lining membrane of the stomach was finely injected into minute puncta and stellæ of a bright red colour, with two or three spots of ecchymosis. The structure of the membrane was thickened and pulpy, and the surface covered with tenacious mucus. In some parts there were irregular superficial abrasions ; these appearances of the mucous membrane becoming very distinct by examining it under water by aid of sunlight, and seeming, moreover, unequivocally to demonstrate the existence of a gastritis. The brain, lungs, heart, spleen, liver and kidneys were normal.

The supra-renal capsules contained both of them compact fibrinous concretions, seated in the structure of the organ ; superficially examined they were not unlike some forms of strumous tubercle.   (Vide Pl. II. and Pl. VIII. figs. 4, 5.)

The slow and insidious approach and progress of the constitutional loss of strength, the extreme feebleness of the pulse, the absence of all evidence of any lesion sufficient to account for the patient's declining condition, the loss of appetite, the uneasiness and irritability of the stomach, and the indications of disturbed cerebral circulation, were all so strongly marked, and so exactly corresponded in kind with what have been observed to accompany the most extensive disease of the capsules, that, coupled with the excess of dark pigment in the integument, we did not hesitate to anticipate with much confidence an extensively diseased condition of these organs.

CASE III.—Reported by Mr. WILLIAMS.

Henry Patten, æt. 26, a carpenter and window-blind maker, residing at 13 Brandon Street, Walworth, was admitted Nov. 9, 1854, having been for some time an out-patient under Dr. Rees.

His habits have been somewhat intemperate; his drink chiefly malt liquor and spirits. With the exception of a sister, who died of phthisis, all his relations are healthy. He has been married four years. The patient states that up to six months ago, he enjoyed very good health, but then began to be troubled with what he calls "rheumatic" pains in the right leg, which, without laying him up, gradually extended to his hips and side, and thence to the bottom of the spine. His back latterly has been very tender, a jerk or jarring movement giving him great pain at that part. He has noticed his lips to have become dark-coloured for the last three months, and more lately his face to be similarly discoloured in patches. For the last month he has discontinued work on account of attacks of giddiness and dimness of sight, accompanied by a peculiar pain at the back of the head and partial loss of consciousness. These attacks would occur several times in the course of the day, upon any unusual exertion, always whilst in the standing posture, and were instantly relieved by sitting or lying down. Since he has discontinued his employment, they have only occurred on getting out of bed in the morning.

It is for the pains and tenderness at the back, and occasional attacks, as above described, with general debility, that he has been attending this hospital as an out-patient.

Present condition.—The patient presents a highly strumous appearance, being thin, pale, and the hair dark and dry. Over the face and forehead, which are of a general yellowish hue, are several patches of darkened skin, and similar black patches on the lips. There is angular curvature at the second, and great tenderness on pressure over the upper three lumbar vertebræ ; he complains also of pain at this part upon moving in bed. There is no paralysis, but considerable general debility. His bowels are regular, and the tongue clean, but the appetite is impaired ; the urine is clear, moderate in quantity, and not albuminous. Heart-sounds normal, but the impulse feeble. Pulse 80, small and weak.

Nov. 10th.   ℞   Quinæ Disulph. gr. iss.

> Aquæ distill. ʒj.
>
> Syr. Rhœados ʒss.
>
> Acid. Sulph. dil. m. v.
>
> Ft. Haustus ter die s.-Vin. Alb. ʒiv.

With these medicines and middle diet he continued with no appreciable change until the 24th, when he had a kind of fainting fit upon rising to have his bed made, contrary to an order that he should keep in the recumbent posture. This day his diet was changed to milk, at his own request. He has been once or twice sick after taking his food.

28th.—The sickness has continued, and he today has a troublesome hiccough, for which he was ordered

> Jul. Ammon. p. r. n.

29th.—He has had little sleep, the hiccough, unrelieved by the Julep. Ammon., annoying him much. Dr. Barlow, who now took the ward, ordered him   Æther. Chlor. m. v.

> Vini Opii m. v.
>
> ex Mist. Camph. t. d. s.

30th.—He is today about the same. Has been sick this morning, the vomited matter consisting of food and drink. The hiccough occasionally ceasing.

Dec. 1st.—Hiccough still very harassing.

> ℞   Vini Opii m. x.
>
> Tinct. Castorei m. x.
>
> ex Julep. Pimentæ p. r. n.

This was found to relieve the hiccough somewhat.

2nd.—He seems considerably weaker, and upon approaching him, his eyelids, half-closed, allowed the lower sclerotic of the raised eyeballs to be seen. The tongue was moist and clean, and pulse 80, very weak. On speaking to him he roused up and appeared quite as usual, but soon relapsed into the torpid state again. His blood under the $\frac{1}{4}$-inch object-glass presented from forty to sixty white corpuscles in each field, mostly scattered about, but some in patches of two or three and six or eight together.

3rd.—Slept better, although the hiccough did not cease. He complains of a constricting pain about the waist; he is tender on pressure over the spleen, where no tumour is to be felt. The tongue today is dry, and beginning to be sordid, teeth dirty, pulse weak. He presents the same typhoid appearances.

4th.—Pulse weaker, dicrotic, 96; roused from the torpid state with more difficulty than yesterday. He talks very sensibly, but his wife, who watches by his bedside, states that he wanders in the night.

Jul. Ammon. c. Tinct. Castorei m. v. p. r. n.

The blood presented the same appearances under the microscope as before.

5th.—Hiccough continues, is more feeble, pulse scarcely perceptible, lies in a torpid and typhoid state. When roused, said he was sore all over the body. Tongue and teeth sordid.

6th.—Died quietly at 5 A.M.

SECTIO CADAVERIS.

Nine and a half hours after death in cold wet weather. Rigor mortis, but no decomposition. There was not much emaciation, and the axillæ were slightly discoloured. The countenance was paler than in life, but presented the same olive hue, with the dark patches on the face, forehead and lips. There was a psoas abscess on the right side, extending from Poupart's ligament to the diseased vertebræ, and holding about a pint of flaky pus.

The disease was between the first and second vertebræ, commencing in the cartilage, and nearly destroying the neighbouring vertebræ at their centres. The bone surrounding the cavity was red, soft, and infiltrated with strumous matter.

Pleura and bronchi healthy.

Both lungs contained hard masses of grey strumous pneumonic deposit, mostly in the apices, but also in the lower lobes; these masses presented the appearance of a conglomeration of tubercles, held together by inflammatory matter. Heart and pericardium healthy. Heart's weight 7½ oz. The blood on microscopic examination contained the same excess of white corpuscles observed in life. Stomach healthy, slightly adherent to the left supra-renal capsule; its structure was not affected. Spleen large, firm, 7½ oz. in weight. Corpuscles visible. The pancreas and all other abdominal organs were healthy. The head was not examined.

Each supra-renal capsule was completely destroyed and converted into a mass of strumous disease, the latter of all degrees of consistency. The left supra-renal capsule had formed at the upper part a close connexion with the outer coat of the stomach. The upper part of this capsule seemed fluid, and of the colour of pus; the lower firmer, and of the consistency of putty. The right capsule had all degrees of consistency from the bottom to the top; the lower part almost fluid and resembling pus, the centre putty-like, and above this the matter could be detached in flakes; and at the top it was quite earthy, separate angular pieces being easily detached. Vide Plates III. and IV.

Although this patient was known to be labouring under a serious affection of the spine, the ordinary indications of disease of the supra-renal capsules were sufficiently prominent to justify the prediction, which was so satisfactorily confirmed by the post-mortem examination. It is also worthy of remark, that although the patient, as usual, suffered considerably from irritability of stomach, there was but little change observable in that organ after death.

CASE IV.—Reported by the WARD CLERK.

John Iveson, æt. 22, admitted into Guy's Hospital, March 20, 1854, and died the following day. A stonemason, residing at Lambeth. Last winter he had pain in the stomach and vomiting. He slightly improved, but the day after Christmas was confined to his bed with great pain and vomiting; the vomited matter consisting of a watery fluid. At that time he had " tic douloureux." On admission his extremities were cold, he was almost pulseless, his hands were blue; he had not had any diarrhœa; he had slight pain, or rather soreness in the hypogastric region; he was quite sensible; the pupils were much dilated. He rallied a little after his admission; had no purging, but vomited bilious matter; had no diabetes or albumenuria. He appeared to die from syncope.

SECTIO CADAVERIS.

Seventeen hours after death, weather cold, limbs rigid, body tolerably nourished, face of a dingy colour, also the axillæ and hands. Abdomen not distended.

Head.—The dura mater and sinuses were found to be healthy, the membranes injected and the veins full. There was slight subarachnoid effusion. The grey matter of the cerebrum was rather deep in colour. The brain was in other respects normal.

Chest.—Trachea granular and congested. The right pleura adherent at the posterior and lower parts; on the left side there were firm adhesions at the apex. The bronchi granular; the left apex was a little puckered, and presented several lobules, with iron-grey consolidation and calcareous deposit. The right lung was healthy, with the exception of a single iron-grey consolidation at the apex. The bronchial and mediastinal glands were healthy.

Heart.—Pericardium healthy. There was a white patch on the right ventricle. The right side of the heart was moderately distended with clot, the left entirely and firmly contracted. The valves were healthy, and the muscular fibre, though flaccid, appeared healthy. No fat was found about the heart. Weight 7 oz.

Abdomen.—Peritoneum healthy, viscera moderately contracted. Stomach not distended; at the cardiac extremity there was post-mortem solution of the mucous membrane: towards the lesser curvature it was granular, in some parts destroyed, ulcerated; quite superficially there was arborescent injection. On microscopical examination, mucous and granule-cells were observed. Brunner's glands were very prominent. Ileum with much mucous congestion. Peyer's and solitary glands very distinct, but only hypertrophied. The mesenteric glands were enlarged, firm and white, full of nuclei, hypertrophied.

Large intestines were healthy.

Liver was of normal form and condition; there was a small amount of fat in the cells; weight 2 lbs. 14 oz., containing no arsenic. Gall-bladder healthy; ducts free, but not enlarged. Spleen enlarged, weight 6 oz. Pancreas was healthy.

The two supra-renal capsules together weighed 49 grains; they appeared exceedingly small and atrophied; the right one was natural, firm; the left deformed by contraction; each adherent to surrounding parts by dense areolar tissue. The section gave a pale and homogeneous aspect; it presented a fibrous tissue, fat and cells about the size of white blood-corpuscles. The lumbar glands were enlarged. The kidneys coarse, weighing 10 oz. The bladder and prostate were healthy. Vide Plate V.

The history of this man's case renders it probable that his disease commenced several months prior to his admission into the hospital, and it is not a little remarkable that his earliest complaint was of sickness, vomiting and pain in the region of the stomach; symptoms which have constituted a more or less prominent feature in every case that has fallen under my notice, and which in the present instance were so urgent as to suggest a suspicion of some acrid poison having been received into the stomach.

How far these gastric symptoms when present are referrible to sympathy existing between the diseased capsules and the stomach—how far they depend upon disturbed circulation within the head—how far they are attributable to accidental or essential gastric inflammation—and how far the inflammatory aspect of the gastric mucous membrane is the mere result of severe and repeated vomiting, a more extended observation will probably determine hereafter. It was from the presence of these gastric symptoms, the extreme and peculiar prostration of the patient's strength, the great feebleness and smallness of the pulse, the anæmiated eye, the absence of any discoverable lesion to account for the patient's condition, and more especially the dingy discoloration of the face, that led before death to a belief that we should on post-mortem examination find disease of the supra-renal capsules.

It is, moreover, of some significance and importance to observe, that in the present instance, the diseased condition of the supra-renal capsules did not result as usual from a deposit either of a strumous or malignant character, but appears rather to have been occasioned by an actual inflammation,—that inflammation having destroyed the integrity of the organs, and finally led to their contraction and atrophy.

CASE V.

The following, taken from Dr. Bright's Reports of medical cases, presents, according to my belief, a very good illustration of the disease under consideration, and is headed :

"Serous effusion under the arachnoid and into the ventricles in a case of emaciation, with bilious vomiting and diseased renal capsules."

"*Ann Roots* was admitted in July 1829, under one of the surgeons, into Guy's Hospital, on account of a tumour in the left breast and a swelling of the right parotid ; but as it was perceived that she was greatly emaciated and apparently sinking, and therefore quite unfit to undergo any operation, she was transferred to the care of the physician.

" *Her complexion was very dark,* her whole person emaciated ; she had no cough, and neither tension nor tenderness of abdomen ; she had great difficulty in opening her jaw, owing to the glandular swelling, and could not protrude her tongue. There was no indication but to support the strength. Her stomach soon became irritable ; she had bilious vomiting, which reduced her strength, and for a day or two before her death, which took place on the 18th of August, she became drowsy, yet capable of being roused ; complaining of some pain over the forehead, and occasionally wandering a little in her intellects.

" In the absence of all positive symptoms, I concluded that it was possible some glandular disease, similar to that which had shown itself below the mammæ and under the jaw, might exist internally, giving rise to emaciation and vomiting ; and it appeared probable that serous effusion had been going on in the head for the last few days.

- 36 -

" Sectio Cadaveris.

" Considerable emaciation; and on removing the integuments the scalpel opened into an abscess, containing an ounce or two of pus, situated beneath the mamma of the left side. The dura mater was firmly attached to the skull at the vertex, where the bone was remarkably thin, and indented by the glandulæ Pacchioni, and the ordinary opake deposit which surrounds them; on raising the dura mater several small opacities were observable on the arachnoid, and a very considerable quantity of serous fluid was effused under the arachnoid, raising it into bladders, as well as filling up the hollow between the convolutions.

" The whole brain was soft and watery, and many vessels showed themselves where horizontal sections were made. In the ventricles about half an ounce of fluid was collected. The choroid plexus was quite exsanguine.

" Slight adhesions of the pleura pulmonalis and pleura costalis were found, but not sufficient to prevent the lungs from collapsing pretty completely when the air was admitted into the chest. The upper lobe of each lung was in an unhealthy state, looking puckered and containing one or two masses of earthy matter, besides several small incipient tubercles; the greater part of the lungs, however, was in a very healthy condition. Heart small, but healthy. In the abdomen slight old adhesions had taken place in various parts, but they were composed of the finest transparent cellular tissue; even the omentum, which was glued by them to various parts both of the intestines and the parietes, had lost none of its natural delicacy and transparency. The intestines were healthy, but stained with bile; the mucous membrane healthy; the liver healthy, and the gall-bladder full of bile; the pancreas healthy, and the spleen also, but just between the pancreas and the spleen a few absorbent glands were enlarged The glands of the mesentery were also slightly enlarged. The only marked disease was in the renal capsules, both of which were enlarged, lobulated, and the seat of morbid deposits apparently of a scrofulous character; they were at least four times their natural thickness,

-37-

feeling solid and hard ; on the left side one part had gone into suppuration, containing two drachms of yellow pus. The kidneys themselves healthy. The uterus held down by adhesions in the pelvis."

It does not appear that Dr. Bright either entertained a suspicion of the disease of the capsules before death, or was led at any period to associate the colour of the skin with the diseased condition of these organs, although his well-known sagacity induced him to suggest the probable existence of some internal malignant disease. In this, as in most other cases, we have the same remarkable prostration ; the usual gastric symptoms ; the same absence of any very obvious and adequate cause of the patient's actual condition, together with a discoloration of the skin, sufficiently striking to have arrested Dr. Bright's attention even during the life of the patient.

CASE VI.

R. H., Esq., was a member of the bar, somewhere about middle age. I had the satisfaction of attending him in consultation with Dr. Watson and Mr. Barker, when I was informed that he had been getting thin and emaciated during a period of about twelve months. His appearance and symptoms were very remarkable. He was certainly thin, but not strikingly emaciated, and the surface was soft, loose and supple. He was greatly anæmiated ; his eyes were pearly ; he complained of extreme languor and faintness ; his pulse, contrary to what is usual in capsular disease, was of good size, but exquisitely soft and compressible ; the impulse of the heart was feeble, and palpitation or throbbing with scrobicular pulsation was immediately produced by the slightest exertion ; without pain, the stomach was exceedingly irritable, and vomiting was both urgent and distressing.

With these symptoms, the surface generally presented a dark dingy aspect, and there were observed, chiefly on the face, neck and arms, patches of a rather deep chestnut-brown colour ; these chestnut-brown patches were of various sizes and shapes, and were associated here and there with others presenting a singularly white or blanched appearance, arising either in consequence of the latter portions of the integument having remained unaffected, and so contrasting with the surrounding discoloration, or, what is more probable, from their having received a less supply of pigment than natural. A patient inquiry and most careful examination failed to elicit any information, or to detect any lesion, sufficient to afford even a plausible explanation of the patient's singular condition. The violent vomiting pointed to organic, perhaps carcinomatous disease of the stomach : nevertheless the general condition and

- 39 -

symptoms did not in other respects seem to warrant such a conclusion; and coupling the existing condition and symptoms with the irregular deposition of dark pigment in the skin, a suspicion was entertained that the whole might arise from disease of the supra-renal capsules. To the last, however, considerable doubt prevailed amongst us as to the true nature of the case,—chiefly in consequence of the severity and persistence of the vomiting, and from the vomited mucous matters having been occasionally tinged with blood. The patient speedily sank, and the following report of the morbid appearances discovered after death was furnished, I believe, by my distinguished friend Dr. Hodgkin,

"The morbid specimens consisted of part of the stomach and duodenum,—the termination of the small, and the commencement of the large intestines, with the appendix vermiformis, and the renal capsules with a small portion of the kidney. They were taken from a man rather beyond middle life, who for a considerable time had suffered from obstinate derangement of the stomach.

"The coats of the stomach taken unitedly did not produce any preternatural thickness, but rather the reverse; yet there might be a little thickening or increased development of the mucous membrane. The peculiarity of its appearance consisted in a spotted character not very easily described. Near the pylorus it seemed to consist of a very slight degree of that irregularity which Louis has described as the *état mamelonné*, and which appears to be nothing more than the increased development of a natural structure; but in this instance the elevations were smaller in size, and consequently more numerous, though less prominent than those generally seen towards the middle of the stomach, where this appearance is most frequently noticed.

"Further from the pylorus, in the direction of the smaller curvature, smaller spots were seen more scattered and distant from each other, and apparently consisting of opake lighter-coloured matter, within the semitransparent substance of the mucous membrane itself, which was generally of a faint dusky reddish colour. It could not be decided whether these spots depended on any glandular apparatus, yet the idea suggested itself that they might be connected with the follicles of Lieberkühn. Immersion under water, with the intention of facilitating the examination with the microscope, rendered these spots less conspicuous. The largest might equal a small pin's head ; the smaller ones scarcely a quarter so large. The duodenum appeared healthy. The portion of small and large intestine, of which the next specimen consisted, offered nothing remarkable in texture. The mucous membrane was tinged with the dingy olive-green of the fæcal contents, and the ileo-colic valve was rather more prominent than usual in the cæcum. The appendix vermiformis was about three inches in length, but much distended, being about an inch in diameter at its commencement, and becoming gradually less towards the free extremity, where it but little exceeded the normal size. Its peritoneal coat was quite healthy ; its general thickness was very little increased ; its mucous membrane apparently healthy, of greyish colour, from a little black pigment towards the upper part. Its follicular apparatus was nearly or quite imperceptible. It was completely cut off from the interior of the intestine, the mucous membrane forming a cul-de-sac at both extremities, although there was no apparent want of continuity on the exterior ; the septum between the two cavities being merely composed of the two mucous membranes united by cellular tissue. No appearance of cicatrix was discovered, indicating that the separation was of long standing, if not congenital. The contents of the appendix consisted principally of a transparent colloid or thick mucoid secretion, partly of a light straw colour, partly tinged with blood. Interspersed through it, but especially towards the upper part, was an opake white substance of the same consistence, resembling coagulated milk or ground white lead. A few points were blackened by pigments. Examined with the microscope, the transparent portion exhibited no determinate structure, but a slight tendency to filamentous arrangement. The whole portion was made up of a congeries of oil-globules, varying in size, but all very minute. The black pigment appeared to pervade some of the oil-globules, rather than itself to compose distinct corpuscles. The basis of this collection was undoubtedly the mucus of the appendix itself, retained by the want of any excretory passage.

" The small fragment of kidney appeared to be of healthy structure, but both the renal capsules were enlarged, (the united weight of the two being one and a half ounce,) of rather irregular surface and considerably indurated. When cut into, instead of exhibiting the ordinary appearance of combination of dark and yellow substances, they seemed to consist of a firm, slightly transparent reddish basis, interspersed with irregular spots of opake yellow matter, the whole bearing a strong resemblance to an enlarged mesenteric gland, mottled with tubercular deposit. Such was probably the nature of the change which the organ had undergone. The naked eye could discover no trace of cystiform arrangement, and the opake matter when examined with the microscope exhibited a copious amount of fatty matter, but no nucleated cells."

It was to me a matter of much regret that I had not an opportunity of employing an artist to make an exact representation of the singular discoloration observed upon the skin, and the more so, because, although agreeing in general character with those observed in other cases, there was a manifest peculiarity, as well in the intensity, as in the mode of distribution of these discolorations. With universal dinginess of the surface, there were, especially about the neck, hands and arms, several well-defined patches of a deeper, or somewhat chestnut-brown hue, inter-spersed here and there with blanched or almost dead-white portions of integument, contrasting in a very remarkable manner with both the general dinginess and deeper brown patches ; and what is very remark-able, wherever the integument presented the blanched or dead-white appearance, the hairs upon its surface were observed to have turned completely white.

The superiority of a coloured drawing over the most elaborate verbal description, in conveying a correct idea of any morbid appearance, is so universally felt and acknowledged, that I have great satisfaction in being now able to furnish one, which may most fairly and faithfully be applied to the above case.

Very recently March 1855—I was requested to visit a patient (Mr. S.) about 60 years of age, who presented, in a strongly marked degree, the indications of diseased renal capsules. The history, mode of attack, the progress, the anæmia, the extreme feebleness of the heart's action, the uneasiness and irritability of the stomach, and the discoloration of the skin, were all such as characterize the disease generally, and bore the closest resemblance to the above case in particular. My belief was that the capsules were affected with malignant disease, and that probably some other structures about the posterior mediastinum might have been in a similar condition, as the patient had slight œdema of both the upper extremities, whilst the lower limbs remained free. Anxious as I was to procure a post-mortem examination, it was most firmly and peremptorily refused, and it was only through the kind and persevering efforts of my friend, Mr. Parrott of Clapham, that I succeeded in gaining permission to have a sketch taken of the discoloured integument. Of course this representation does not carry along with it such authority and conviction as one taken from a subject actually proved to have had diseased capsules. Nevertheless I entertain no doubt whatever that the capsules were diseased; and even if they were not, I hold myself answerable for the most perfect resemblance between the two cases, so far as the affection of the integument was concerned. Vide Pl. XI.

CASE VII.

The following case, having been under the care of one of the surgeons for " carcinoma" of the mamma, I have not been able to furnish any record of the symptoms during life. The corpse, however, presented appearances sufficiently striking to arrest the attention, and call forth the correct prediction of Dr. Lloyd the inspector, who kindly furnished me with the following report.

" SECTIO CADAVERIS.

" *M. T.*, æt. 60. Cancerous disease of the mamma, with cancerous degeneration of the supra-renal capsules.

" Sixteen hours after death. Body extremely emaciated ; the left mamma presented a very extensive ulcerated phagedænic malignant tumour, occupying the whole of the upper part of the left side of the chest, infiltrating the cellular tissue, the skin and intercostal muscles with carcinomatous material. *The colour of the skin covering the face, arms and chest was of a peculiar light brown swarthy hue.*

" *Chest.*—On raising the sternum and cartilages, it was found that the malignant growth had passed through the pleura and invaded the lung on the left side, for a space of the size of the palm of the hand, by direct continuity of structure. The pleural cavity of the side contained about 16 oz. of dark-coloured fluid. The lower lobe of the left lung was compressed, and sank in water. The upper lobe was healthy. The right lung was healthy.

" *Heart*—was small and flabby.

" *Abdomen.*—The liver was contracted, irregular on its surface, of yellow

-44-

colour, containing abundance of fat, burning brilliantly in the spirit-lamp; upon its surface were several nodules of cancerous development. The gall-bladder was occupied in its entire extent by a calculus, and did not contain any bile.

" Both supra-renal capsules contained a considerable amount of cancerous deposit, invading their entire structure, and almost obliterating their cavities.

" The kidneys were contracted and granular. The uterus healthy, but atrophied."

I have already expressed my belief that the urgency of the symptoms, and the quick or slow progress of the disease, are determined by the activity or rapidity of the morbid change going on in the capsules, and by the actual amount or degree of that change; and that universal disease of both capsules will in all probability be found to prove uniformly fatal. These views appear to be countenanced by the character, progress and termination of the cases already given, and receive additional confirmation from the history of the following, in which the morbid change was limited to a single capsule, and in which the constitutional and local consequences indicated a corresponding result.

CASE VIII.—Reported by the WARD CLERK.

Elizabeth Hannah Lawrence, æt. 53, admitted into Guy's Hospital under
Dr. Babington, March 30, 1853.

Appearance.—A short woman ; emaciated and feeble; skin harsh and
dry, and of a darkish hue. The folds of the axillæ were remarkably dark :
coloured patches, the size of the palm of the hand, were observed, raised
in wrinkles, and resembling a slight Ichthyosis. Also a very dark brown
areola around the umbilicus. Hair grey; much long hair on lips and
chin.

Previous History.—Is a single woman, has always been a servant, and
has been living of late in Trinity Street, Borough. Was always thin,
but yet always enjoyed good health.

Present History.—Four months ago an eruption appeared on her body,
for the cure of which she went to the Cutaneous Infirmary at Blackfriars.
In a short time she was cured, and just as the eruption disappeared, the
present stomach symptoms began. For three months she has had
vomiting, with pain in the abdomen and back, particularly in the latter.
She has thrown up no blood. She was sent to the hospital as a case of
malignant disease of the stomach. The stomach can be felt as a hard
tumour in the abdomen : no remains of eruption on the skin. The
vomiting continued after admission, and in three days she died from
exhaustion.

SECTIO CADAVERIS.

External Appearance.—The body that of a small emaciated woman, with
a fair skin and dark hair, presenting certain peculiar discolorations. On

either side of the neck there was a tawny appearance, which would not have been remarked, had it not been for three still more marked tawny patches, one on the centre of the sternum, the other two under either axilla. The skin also, besides presenting this yellowish-brown appearance, was somewhat raised and wrinkled or corrugated. These marks led me to prognosticate disease of the supra-renal capsules before opening the body, believing them to be the marks pointed out by Dr. Addison.

Thorax.—The lungs were congested, exuding a frothy serum, and easily lacerable.

Heart.—Small and lacerable. The mediastinal glands in one or two instances carcinomatous.

Abdomen—was shrunk and contracted.

Stomach.—The walls of the stomach from the pylorus through the lesser curvature were thickened, presenting on the surface externally a peculiar network appearance, containing a transparent stroma; beneath this, another layer, with its fibres longitudinally arranged, of strong cellular material; within this, the mucous membrane whole and intact; the entire thickness being about three-quarters of an inch at the pylorus, gradually decreasing to a quarter at the commencement of the cardia. The mucous membrane lower down was here and there destroyed by ulceration, and this ulceration in one instance of an eighth of an inch in size. The stomach was contracted and empty; externally to the stomach several of the glands were affected, even to the head of the pancreas, but the pancreas itself was not affected. Several of the lumbar glands were enlarged.

The left supra-renal capsule was infiltrated with malignant material, and closely adherent to the vessels of the kidney. The kidney itself was healthy. The uterus contained three fibrous tumours, the size of walnuts. Vide Pl VIII. fig. 1, and Pls. IX. and X.

Although this woman only survived four days after her admission into

- 47 -

the hospital, we were led by the partial discoloration of the skin to anticipate disease of the capsules, one only of which, however, was found to
be implicated. It will have been perceived, that in a certain number of the
cases already given, either strumous or malignant disease existed in other
parts or organs, as well as in the capsules; and of course, in the midst
of such complications, there is often more or less difficulty in satisfactorily
unravelling the case in all its details during life; nevertheless as we know,
that without any such complication whatever, mere disease of the capsules
themselves has proved sufficient to produce such alarming symptoms
and such serious consequences, it cannot with any show of reason be
alleged that these peculiar symptoms, when present, arise exclusively from
the accidental complication of other organs.

In the present instance, as in some others, the immediate cause of
death, as well as of many of the most distressing symptoms during life,
was unquestionably carcinomatous disease of the stomach.

CASE IX.

Thomas Clouston, æt. 58, admitted into Guy's Hospital, February 11, 1852, under Dr. Barlow. A muscular and strong-built man, of a sanguine temperament and dark complexion. He has been a married man, but his wife died about twenty years ago. His occupation has been that of a sailor, and according to his own statement, he has led a very sober life. His general health has been very good. About five years since, he had a hernia in the left inguinal region, for which he has since worn a truss. This has never given him any difficulty to return. About two months ago he came from Liverpool, in which place he had settled, not intending to go to sea again ; and was taken on board the Dreadnought for stricture. His general health was quite good at this time, but while in the Dreadnought he began to lose his appetite and to feel generally unwell ; he had likewise some affection of the left eye, in which he is now nearly blind.

On Saturday the 8th he left the ship at his own request, thinking that he might be better on land ; after waiting two or three days, he found that he got no better, and his friends advised him to come to the hospital.

Present Symptoms.—He complains of a sensation of sickness, without actual vomiting ; and tightness over the epigastrium. His countenance is anxious. He has no pain in any part. He has rigors, followed by mild sweats, every five or six hours, the rigors usually lasting about an hour. The abdomen is tense and tympanitic ; not tender to the touch, excepting over the upper part. The liver does not appear enlarged. His chest is broad and well-formed ; the motion of the ribs moderate, resonant on percussion ; and the lungs are apparently sound. The heart's sounds are normal. Pulse rather feeble, 80. Tongue injected at the tip and edges, coated with a light brown fur, very dry. Urine of about average quantity, rather large than otherwise ; of a high colour, acid, and does not coagulate by heat. The bowels have been regular. After . he had been in a few hours, he brought up a large quantity of beer. Ordered

Mist. Efferves. 4tis horis.

Feb. 12.—The sickness has not returned, but he is without any appetite. He slept but little.

Feb. 13.—He is much the same, but has a more sallow and sunken expression of countenance. He complains of nothing but loss of appetite and general debility. His tongue continues dry and coated with a brownish fur. His bowels have been relaxed, and he passed his motions partly involuntarily.

Feb. 14.—No special change.

Feb. 17.—He seems rather better; he had a little breakfast, and enjoyed it.

Feb. 18.—He has relapsed into his former state, having no appetite and complaining of great debility and thirst. He has ʒiv of sherry daily.

Feb. 20.—There is but little change in him, *his countenance appears to grow darker,* and his strength seems gradually failing. His bowels are rather irritable. Ordered

Enema Amyli c. Syr. Papav. ʒss.

Inf. Cuspariæ ʒiss t. d.

Feb. 25.—He has been getting gradually weaker, without showing any special symptoms in addition to those mentioned. He died this morning.

SECTIO CADAVERIS.

None was allowed beyond the brain and abdomen ; of the former there was considerable softening, and a large amount of subarachnoid fluid. The kidneys were slightly enlarged, mottled, and in some parts the cortical substance was entirely degenerated into fat. A few tubercles were observed on the surface. The tunic was very easily taken from the surface. Tubercles were also observed on the spleen, and on the peritoneum covering the termination of the Ileum. Tubercular deposit was likewise found in one of the supra-renal capsules. Vide Pls. VI. VII.

The development of tubercles on various parts, as well as in one of the supra-renal capsules, sufficiently attests the strumous character of the patient's disease ; and it is difficult to divest oneself of the notion that the disease in the supra-renal capsule had some share in producing the peculiar symptoms which immediately preceded the fatal result, whatever importance may be attached to the state of the kidneys and cerebral complication. At all events, the discoloration of the skin indicated before death the existence of capsular disease ; and it is worthy of remark, that in this instance the deposition of pigment-cells was not limited to the integument, but was found scattered in small masses over the omentum, the mesentery, and the cellular tissue on the interior of the abdominal parietes.

CASE X.

Jane Roff, æt. 28. This person was admitted into the Obstetric Ward, labouring under cancer of the uterus, Feb. 4, 1852. She died Feb. 8, and on the 9th the body was placed on the table for inspection. When proceeding to perform this duty, Dr. Lloyd was struck with the peculiar dingy appearance of the skin, and in consequence, prior to commencing, sought me to look at it. The appearance, though not very strongly marked, was certainly such as to create a strong suspicion that something was wrong with the capsules. On exposing the organ on the right side, it presented a perfectly healthy appearance, and we felt disposed to conclude that our anticipation would turn out to be erroneous. On proceeding to examine the left capsule, however, we were much surprised to find a very extraordinary, and, I suspect, an extremely rare condition of parts. A malignant tubercle had been developed at that precise point, where the large vein escapes from the organ; this tubercle projected into the interior of the vein, so as almost or entirely to obstruct it, and had moreover led to rupture and effusion into, or a sort of apoplexy of the capsule itself.

This case would render it probable that the excess of dark pigment, so characteristic of renal capsular disease, depended rather upon an interruption to some special function, than upon the nature of the organic change; for, with the exception of the manifestly recent sanguineous effusion into its tissue, the capsule itself did not appear to have undergone any considerable deterioration. Vide Pl. VIII. figs. 2, 3.

-52-

CASE XI.

I may observe in conclusion, that very recently there was examined at Guy's Hospital the body of a person—*William Godfrey*—who had died of cancer, affecting the thoracic parietes, and extending through to the lungs. Quite unexpectedly there was found extensive disease of one of the supra-renal capsules ; the organ being very much enlarged, and converted into a hard mass of apparently carcinomatous disease. On referring to the notes of the case as taken by the clinical clerk, I found it stated that "*the patient's face presented a dingy hue*," although he was naturally of a fair complexion, with reddish or sandy hair on the pubes; and, moreover, the face of the corpse was ascertained to present a freckled and dingy appearance, with a slight brown discoloration at the root of the nose and at each angle of the lips. Vide Pl. VIII. figs. 6, 7, 8.

EXPLANATION OF THE PLATES.

PLATE IV.

Fig. 1. The Liver of Henry Patten, with the diseased supra-renal capsules *in situ*.

Figs. 2 & 3. Sections of the diseased supra-renal capsules.

PLATE VII.

Separate parts from Thomas Clouston.

Fig. 1. Portion of small intestine and mesentery with deposits of dark pigment.

Fig. 2. Ditto   ditto.

Fig. 3. Portion of omentum with deposits of dark pigment.

Fig. 4. Deposit of dark pigment in the adipose tissue on the inner surface of the internal oblique muscle.

Figs. 5 & 6. Microscopic views of the dark pigment taken from fig. 1, ($\frac{1}{4}$-inch).

Fig. 7. Natural size of the deposit represented in fig. 6.

PLATE VIII.

Fig. 1. The left kidney and diseased supra-renal capsule of Elizabeth Lawrence. CASE VIII.

Fig. 2. The left supra-renal capsule of Jane Roff, exhibiting a fungoid growth obstructing the vein of the capsule at its entrance into the renal vein. CASE X.

Fig. 3. Section of the same, exhibiting sanguineous infiltration of the organ.

Fig. 4. Section of one of the supra-renal capsules of James Jackson, with strumous deposit. CASE II.

Fig. 5. Exterior view of the same.

Fig. 6. Kidney and diseased supra-renal capsule of William Godfrey. CASE XI.

Fig. 7. Microscopic view displaying meshes composed of a delicate stroma of transparent and fibrous tissue, containing cancer-cells, taken from the diseased supra-renal capsule of William Godfrey.

Fig. 8. Cancer-juice, consisting of well-formed cells, with large nuclei and nucleoli, from the same.

PLATE X.

Abdomen of the same, exhibiting general dinginess of the integument, with several small circumscribed deposits of darker pigment.

PLATE XI.

Head, neck and trunk of Mr. S., exhibiting peculiar discolorations and white patches of the integument, similar to those observed in Case VI.

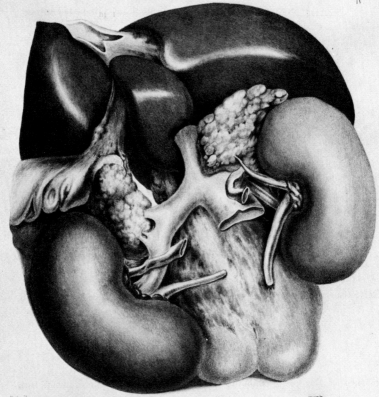

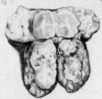

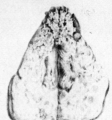

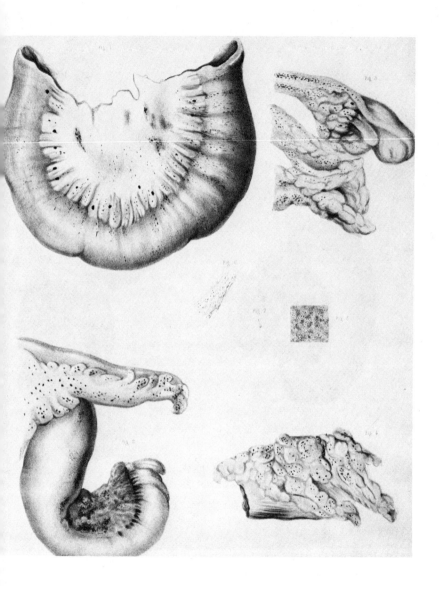

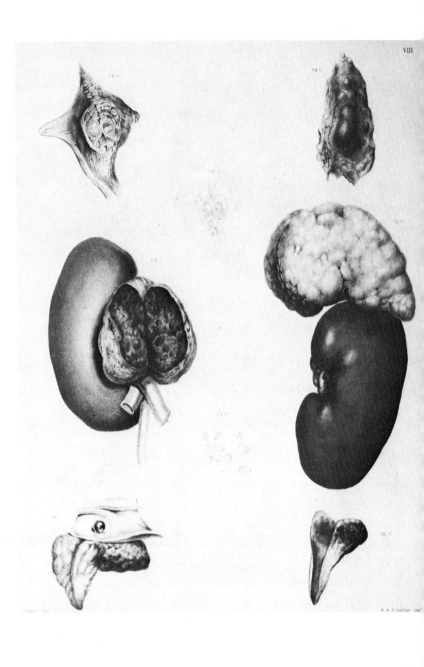

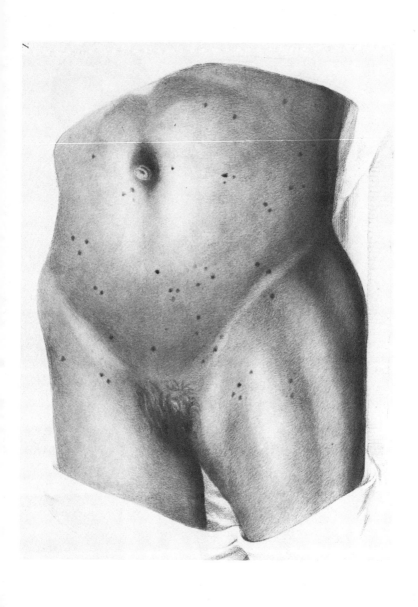

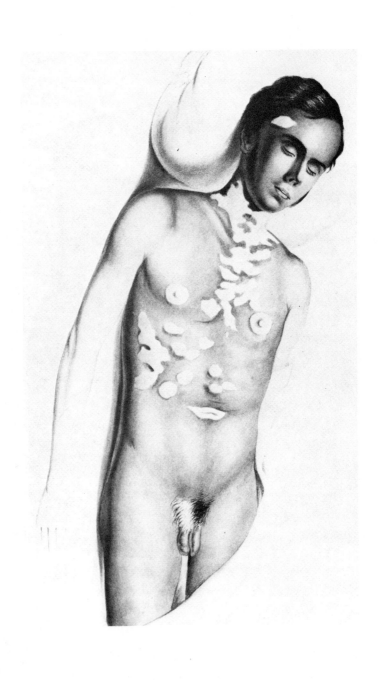

Thursday, March 15th.

Anæmia—Disease of the Supra-renal Capsules.

Dr. ADDISON, at the request of the President, proceeded to describe a remarkable form of anæmia, which, although incidentally noticed by various writers, had not attracted, as he thought, by any means the attention it really deserved. It was a state of general anæmia incident to adult males, and had for several years past been with him a subject of earnest inquiry and of deep interest. It usually occurs between the ages of twenty and sixty; sometimes proceeding to an extreme degree in a few weeks, but more frequently commencing insidiously, and proceeding very slowly, so as to occupy a period of several weeks, or even months, before any very serious alarm is taken either by the patient or by the patient's friends. Its approach is first indicated by a certain amount of languor and restlessness, to which presently succeed a manifest paleness of the countenance, loss of muscular strength, general relaxation or feebleness of the whole frame, and indisposition to, or incapacity for, bodily or mental exertion. These symptoms go on increasing with greater or less rapidity: the face, lips, conjunctivæ, and external surface of the body, become more and more bloodless; the tongue appears pale and flabby; the heart's action gets exceedingly enfeebled, with a weak, soft, unusually large, but always strikingly compressible pulse; the appetite may or may not be lost; the patient experiences a distressing and increasing sense of helplessness and faintness; the heart is excited, or rendered tumultuous in its action, the breathing painfully hurried by the slightest exertion, whilst the whole surface bears some resemblance to a bad wax figure: the patient is no longer able to rise from his bed; slight œdema perhaps shows itself about the ankles; the feeling of faintness and weakness becomes extreme, and he dies either from sheer exhaustion, or death is preceded by signs of passive effusion or cerebral oppression. With all this, the emaciation or wasting of the body, though sometimes considerable, is not unfrequently quite disproportionate to the failure of the powers of the circulation—relaxation and flabbiness, rather than wasting of the flesh, being one of the most remarkable features of the disorder.

Dr. Addison next proceeded to give the details of several cases which had fallen under his own immediate observation. In only two of these did the patients recover: the one, a man below the middle period of life, who was looked upon as past all hope, and suspected to be suffering from some latent malignant disease, slowly but steadily recovered under the free use of brandy, but with the singular result of the hair of one side of his head turning permanently grey, whilst the other retained its original brown colour. The second case of recovery occurred in a gentleman above middle age: it was by no means far advanced, but was sufficiently well marked to excite alarm. He left his business, quitted London, and sought recreation in the country. After a time he returned, and appeared to have shaken off the disorder almost entirely. In three cases only was there an inspection of the body after death, and *in all of them was found a diseased condition of the supra-renal capsules.* In two of the cases no disease whatever could be detected in any other part of the body. Dr. Addison inquired if it were possible for all this to be merely coincidental? It might be so, but he thought not, and making every allowance for the bias and prejudice inseparable from the hope or vanity of an original discovery, he confessed that he felt it very difficult to be persuaded that it was so. On the contrary, he could not help entertaining a very strong impression that these hitherto mysterious bodies—the supra-renal capsules —may be either directly or indirectly concerned in sanguification; and that a diseased condition of them, functional or structural, may interfere with the proper elaboration of the body generally, or of the red particles more especially. At all events, he considered that the time had arrived when he felt himself warranted in directing the attention of the profession to these curious facts. In thanking the Society for the patient hearing with which they had favoured him, he ventured to bespeak their interest not only in regard to the anæmia he had described, but also in cases of purpura, and some of the more anæmiated forms of chlorosis in the female, which he could not but regard as being more or less allied to the morbid state to which he had directed their attention. Indeed, not only had he found the anæmia in question occasionally occurring in connection with purpura, but had observed in cases of the latter disorder certain local symptoms which pointed somewhat significantly to the seat of the supra-renal capsules; whilst the bloodless and waxy appearance of certain chlorotic females bore so close a resemblance to the anæmia described, that it was difficult not to suspect the existence of something common to both.

REPORTS

OF

MEDICAL CASES,

SELECTED

WITH A VIEW OF ILLUSTRATING

THE SYMPTOMS AND CURE OF DISEASES

BY A REFERENCE TO

MORBID ANATOMY.

By RICHARD BRIGHT, M.D. F.R.S. &c.

LECTURER ON THE PRACTICE OF MEDICINE,

AND ONE OF THE PHYSICIANS TO

GUY'S HOSPITAL.

———

LONDON:

PRINTED BY RICHARD TAYLOR, RED LION COURT, FLEET STREET.

PUBLISHED BY LONGMAN, REES, ORME, BROWN, AND GREEN.
———
1827.

TO

BENJAMIN HARRISON, Esq. F.A.S. &c.

TREASURER TO GUY'S HOSPITAL,

UNDER WHOSE SUPERINTENDENCE

THE BENEVOLENT VIEWS OF THE FOUNDER

HAVE BEEN INCALCULABLY EXTENDED,

AND TO

WILLIAM BABINGTON, M.D. F.R.S. &c.

ONE OF THE GOVERNORS OF GUY'S HOSPITAL,

THE EARLY AND ABLE SUPPORTER

OF THE MEDICAL SCHOOL OF THAT ESTABLISHMENT,

THIS VOLUME

IS MOST RESPECTFULLY DEDICATED

BY THEIR OBEDIENT AND FAITHFUL

FRIEND AND SERVANT

THE AUTHOR.

PREFACE.

The volume which I now offer to the Profession may be considered as the commencement of a work to be continued at irregular periods, receiving additions upon the same plan, more or less frequently, according to the various circumstances which must necessarily influence such an undertaking. It is my wish, in thus recording a number of Cases, to render the labours of a large Hospital more permanently useful, by bringing together such facts as seem to throw light upon each other; and it is more particularly my wish to preserve and explain by faithful Engravings the recent appearances of those morbid changes of structure which have been connected with the symptoms or have influenced the treatment of the disease. Fortunately, I have not in the present day to explain the utility of Hospital Reports; nor am I now called upon to speak of the importance of that information which our profession derives from the study of Morbid Anatomy. To connect accurate and faithful observation after death with symptoms displayed during life, must be in some degree to forward the objects of our noble art: and the more extensive the observation, and the more close the connexion which can be traced, the more likely we are to discover the real analogy and dependence which exists, both between functional and organic disease, and between these, and the external symptoms which are alone submitted to our investigation during life.

Amongst the observations contained in this volume, there are some of which I must bear the responsibility alone. Such are the statements and conjectures regarding the dependence of a peculiar class of Dropsies on disease and irritation of the Kidneys; such are some observations on peculiar changes in the structure of the liver; in the investigation of which however, as in many other cases, I have been kindly assisted by my friend DR. BOSTOCK; and such are the hints thrown out on the influence of the peculiar state of the mesenteric absorbents on the symptoms of Phthisis. There are other subjects, on the contrary, where I write with greater confidence, because borne out by the corresponding testimony of my cotemporaries. Such are the observations on different diseased conditions of the Lungs, many of which, if not all, have fallen under the notice of the diligent pathologists of France; and such are more particularly the observations on the diseased condition of the Mucous Membrane of the Intestines during Fever, a fact long known in particular cases, but never suspected to be so general till brought into view by the French physicians, and which has lately been illustrated in this country with great beauty by the pens of my able and assiduous friends DR. CHAMBERS and DR. HEWETT.

It will form no part of my plan in future volumes, any more than it has done in this, to lay before my readers a succession of striking novelties. Utility is my first object; and the work which I now commence will not, in theory at least, be thoroughly completed, until every disease which influences the natural structure, or originates in its derangements, has been connected with the corresponding organic lesion. Extensive as this undertaking may appear, I do not despair of its completion, to the utmost that the present state of our knowledge will admit. The few months which have been seriously engaged in the task, have enabled me not only to bring together the present volume, but to make large preparations for a second; and at all events

I have the satisfaction of feeling, that each volume, whether it finally form a part of an extensive work on Morbid Anatomy or not, will in the mean time be complete within itself, as a volume of Hospital Reports.

The execution of the Plates I can safely leave without one word of praise; and for the accuracy with which they represent the objects they are intended to illustrate, I cheerfully make myself responsible. The drawing and the engraving were executed under my own immediate superintendence; and in every case, except one, from the recent subject. I have carefully avoided having separate organs represented in the same plate, in order that if any one should hereafter wish to arrange them systematically, unconnected with the cases to which they belong, no difficulty might be experienced; and I trust that the fulness of the index will remove in some degree the inconvenience which necessarily arises, in the employment of a volume of Reports as a book of reference.

It is pleasing, and yet no easy task, to acknowledge the kindness of those many friends who in various ways have assisted me in this undertaking. I may truly say that I have met with the most cheerful compliance in all my wishes from every one connected with our establishment; but in a more particular manner I must confess my obligations to my immediate colleagues DR. CHOLMELEY and DR. BACK; not because they have been more willing to assist me than others, but because without their kind and ready permission I must have been deprived of many of the valuable facts and illustrations which have been largely drawn from cases under their care.

14, Bloomsbury Square, August 10th, 1827.

CONTENTS.

SELECT REPORTS

OF

MEDICAL CASES.

CASES

ILLUSTRATIVE OF SOME OF THE APPEARANCES OBSERVABLE ON THE EXAMI-
NATION OF DISEASES TERMINATING IN DROPSICAL EFFUSION.

THE morbid appearances which present themselves on the examination
of those who have died with dropsical effusion, either into the large cavities of the body or into the cellular membrane, are exceedingly various:
and it often becomes a matter of doubt how far these organic changes
are to be regarded as originally causing or subsequently aiding the production of the effusion, and how far they are to be considered merely as
the consequence either of the effusion or of some more general unhealthy
state of the system. If it were possible to arrive at a perfect solution of
these questions, we might hope to obtain the highest reward which can
repay our labours,—an increased knowledge of the nature of the disease,
and improvement in the means of its treatment.

One great cause of dropsical effusion appears to be obstructed circulation; and whatever either generally or locally prevents the return of the
blood through the venous system, gives rise to effusions of serum more or
less extensive. Thus, diseases of the heart which delay the passage of
the blood in the venous system, give rise to general effusion, both into the
cavities and into the cellular tissue. Obstructions to the circulation through
the liver, by causing a delay in the passage of the blood through the veins

connected with the vena portæ, give rise to ascites.   The pressure of tumours within the abdomen preventing the free passage of blood through
the vena cava, gives rise to dropsical effusion into the cellular tissue of the
lower extremities : and not unfrequently, the obliteration of particular
veins from accidental pressure is the source of the most obstinate anasarcous accumulation.

These great and tangible causes of hydropic swellings betray themselves
obviously after death, and are often easily detected during life ;—yet they
include so great a variety of diseases, that they still present a very wide
field for the observation of the Pathologist.   The different diseases of the
heart and of the lungs on which dropsy depends, and the various changes
to which the liver is subject rendering it a cause of impediment to the
circulation, are still open to much investigation.   In fatal cases of dropsy
we likewise find the peritoneum greatly diseased in various ways ; frequently covered with an adventitious membrane more or less opake, and
capable of being stripped from the peritoneum, which is then left with
its natural shining and glossy appearance.   At other times the peritoneum
is itself altered in structure, or is affected with tubercular or other diseases,
presenting an accumulation of morbid growth.

There are other appearances to which I think too little attention has
hitherto been paid.   They are those evidences of organic change which
occasionally present themselves in the structure of the KIDNEY; and
which, whether they are to be considered as the cause of the dropsical
effusion or as the consequence of some other disease, cannot be unimportant.   Where those conditions of the kidney to which I allude have
occurred, I have often found the dropsy connected with the secretion of
albuminous urine, more or less coagulable on the application of heat.   I
have in general found that the liver has not in these cases betrayed any
considerable marks of disease, either during life or on examination after
death, though occasionally incipient disorganization of a peculiar kind has
been traced in that organ.   On the other hand, I have found that where
the dropsy has depended on organic change in the liver, even in the most
aggravated state of such change no diseased structure has generally been
discovered in the kidneys, and the urine has not coagulated by heat.   I
have never yet examined the body of a patient dying with dropsy attended
with coagulable urine, in whom some obvious derangement was not discovered in the kidneys.

Whether the morbid structure by which my attention was first directed to this subject, is to be considered as having in its incipient state given rise to an alteration in the secreting power, or whether the organic change be the consequence of a long continued morbid action, may admit of doubt: the more probable solution appears to be, that the altered action of the kidney is the result of the various hurtful causes influencing it through the medium of the stomach and the skin, thus deranging the healthy balance of the circulation, or producing a decidedly inflammatory state of the kidney itself:—that when this continues long, the structure of the kidney becomes permanently changed, either in accordance with, and in furtherance of, that morbid action; or by a deposit which is the consequence of the morbid action, but has no share in that arrangement of the vessels on which the morbid action depends.

The observations which I have made respecting the condition of the urine in dropsy, are in a great degree in accordance with what has been laid down by Dr. Blackall in his most valuable treatise.

Where anasarca has come on from exposure to cold, or from some accidental excess, I have in general found the urine to be coagulable by heat. The coagulation is in different degrees: it likewise differs somewhat in its character: most commonly when the urine has been exposed to the heat of a candle in a spoon, before it rises quite to the boiling point it becomes clouded, sometimes simply opalescent, at other times almost milky, beginning at the edges of the spoon and quickly meeting in the middle. In a short time the coagulating particles break up into a flocculent or a curdled form, and the quantity of this flocculent matter varies from a quantity scarcely perceptible floating in the fluid, to so much as converts the whole into the appearance of curdled milk. Sometimes it rises to the surface in the form of a fine scum, which still remains after the boiled fluid has completely cooled. There is another form of coagulable urine, which in my experience has been much more rare; when the urine on being exposed to heat assumes a gelatinous appearance, as if a certain quantity of isinglass had been dissolved in water. I have indeed met with this in one or two cases only.

During some part of the progress of these cases of anasarca, I have in almost all instances found a great tendency to throw off the red particles of the blood by the kidneys, betrayed by various degrees of hæmaturia from the simple dingy colour of the urine, which is easily recognized; or the slight brown deposit;—to the completely bloody urine, when the whole appears to be little but blood, and when not unfrequently a thick ropy deposit is found at the bottom of the vessel.

Besides these cases of sudden anasarcous swelling being generally accompanied by coagulable urine, I have found another and apparently a very opposite state of the system prone to a secretion of the same character; namely, in persons who have been long the subjects of anasarca recurring again and again, worn out and cachectic in their whole frame and appearance, and usually persons addicted to an irregular life and to the use of spirituous liquors. In these cases the albuminous matter has coagulated, in the more ordinary way, in flakes and little curdled clots; but instead of rendering the whole milky, the flocculi often incline to a brown colour, looking like the finest particles of bran more or less thickly disseminated throughout the heated urine. Occasionally in these cases the urine has been much loaded with saline ingredients becoming turbid by standing, but rendered quite clear by the application of a much lower degree of heat, than is necessary to coagulate the albumen.

In all the cases in which I have observed the albuminous urine, it has appeared to me that the kidney has itself acted a more important part, and has been more deranged both functionally and organically than has generally been imagined. In the latter class of cases I have always found the kidney decidedly disorganized. In the former, when very recent, I have found the kidney gorged with blood. And in mixed cases, where the attack was recent, although apparently the foundation has been laid for it in a course of intemperance, I have found the kidney likewise disorganized.

It is now nearly twelve years since I first observed the altered structure of the kidney in a patient who had died dropsical; and I have still the slight drawing which I then made. It was not however till within the last two years that I had an opportunity of connecting these appearances with any particular symptoms, and since that time I have added several observations. I shall now detail a few Cases, beginning with the two first, in which I had an opportunity of connecting the fact of the coagulation of the urine with the disorganized state of the kidneys.

CASE I.

JOHN KING, æt. 34, was admitted October 12, 1825, into the Clinical ward of Guy's Hospital, under my care. He had been a sailor till within the last four years, and was accustomed to take considerable quantities of spirits;—but he said he had since avoided taking them, and had been engaged in turning a cutler's wheel. He was pale, and of an unhealthy appearance.

About three weeks before admission he was seized with pain in his loins, knees, and ankles;—his legs soon became much swollen, and his hands and face occasionally œdematous. When admitted, the abdomen was painful on pressure. Pulse 78, rather hard; tongue natural, but pale. Bowels somewhat purged; dejections rather light coloured. Urine scanty, about one pint in twenty-four hours. Appetite good.

R. Hydrarg. Oxydi cinerei gr. j,
    Pilul. Scillæ compos. gr. xij,
    Opii purificat. gr. j;
Contunde et in Pilulas iij divide hora somni quotidie sumendas.

The reports of the five following days represent him as rather improving with regard to the quantity of urine. The œdema little reduced; and he lay easiest when raised in bed to nearly a sitting posture;—lying flat, however, produced neither cough nor irregularity of pulse. The state of his bowels was improved by an occasional dose of castor oil with tincture of opium.

20th. Attacked with severe febrile and inflammatory symptoms, with tenderness of the abdomen, pain in the chest, cough, and difficulty of lying down. Tongue furred. The pulse rose to 112 and even 120, and this accompanied with a red and turgid state of the face as if erysipelas were coming on.

Mittatur sanguis e brachio ad uncias duodecim.
Foveatur Abdomen.
Sumat Mist. effervesc. cum Vini Ipecacuanhæ ℳ xv; sexta quaque hora, et habeat Olei Ricini f. ʒvj cum Tinct. Opii ℳ v vespere.

21st. The bleeding gave him relief; the blood, which was taken in a full stream, was covered with a sizy coat nearly half an inch thick, but was not the least cupped. In the evening the symptoms returned with severity.

Repetatur sanguinis detractio ad f.ʒxij.

24th. The inflammation of the face had put on all the characters of well marked *Herpes labialis* of most unusual severity, covering not only both lips but the alæ and the point of the nose.   Some blood had been passed in his motions; his urine had become more copious, and the sediment which subsided to the bottom had diminished.

> ℞. Pulv. Ipecacuanhæ gr. j,
> Hydrarg. cum Creta gr. iij;
> Fiat Pulvis ter quotidie sumendus.
> Foveatur Abdomen.

25th. Urine much more copious, amounting to three pints : it has assumed the *dingy brown colour which marks an admixture of the red particles of the blood.*

26th. Eruption taking its natural course of scabbing,—has not extended since the first day of its appearance.   He continues improving, but has some *pain and weakness of his loins;* a little pain occasionally in the shoulders and left side;—he lies down easily;—legs continue to swell.   Pulse 78, soft and of good strength.   Tongue moist, but rather furred.   One small dejection with slight trace of blood.   The tenderness of abdomen gone.   Urine in good quantity, tolerably clear, but *coagulates by heat.*

27th. Gums sore from the mercury.

> Continuantur Pulvis Ipecacuanhæ et Mistura.

28th. Complains of sore-throat, but there is scarcely a blush of redness to be perceived.

29th. Throat still sore.

31st. Is decidedly better—the eruption is nearly gone.   Legs continue to swell, though less; lies down without inconvenience, and only complains of *weakness and pain of the small of the back.*   Bowels confined.   Urine pretty copious, slightly turbid.   Pulse 86, of good strength.   Tongue moist, very slightly furred.

He was removed on the 2nd of November to another ward so much improved as to be able to walk about; he was taking a grain of ipecacuanha three times a day with reference to the disordered secretion of his bowels.

On the evening of the 10th, Mr. Stocker, the skilful and experienced apothecary of the hospital, was called, on account of a sudden attack of dyspnœa with symptoms of inflammation in the chest.

> Mittatur sanguis ad f. ℥x.   Applicetur Empl. Cantharidis Sterno.

11th. He had been relieved by the bleeding.   Blood covered with sizy buff, slightly coagulated.   Was quite unable to lie down in bed,—his pulse 120, rather indistinct in the right wrist, but not so in the left.   He complains of no particular pain, but the dyspnœa is very urgent and apparently increasing.—The urine scanty.

> ℞. Hydrarg. Oxydi cinerei gr. j,
> Pilul. Scillæ comp. gr. xij,
> Opii purificat. gr. j;

In Pilulas iij divide hora somni sumendas.

Repetatur sanguinis detractio ad eandem qua heri quantitatem et applicetur Emplastrum Cantharidis Sterno.

The bleeding gave only temporary relief; the blister was repeated on another part of the chest in two or three days. The œdema increased, and his appearance became more depressed.

15th. ℞. Mistur. Camphoræ f. ʒx,
  Liquor. Ammoniæ Acetat. f. ʒiij,
  Spir. Æther. nitr. f. ʒſs;

Misce, fiat Haustus ter quotidie sumendus.
Repetantur Pilulæ.

Nov. 18th. The symptoms had suffered little change: he sat erect in bed, leaning a little forward, during the day, and at night always wished to sit by the fire. His countenance pallid, rather shrunken, a little puffy about the eyes, and expressive of great anxiety. Hands and legs œdematous; urine very scanty. Pulse 120, quite regular. Respiration 36, with great effort. From the anxiety of his countenance coupled with the position of his body I was led to consider the mischief to be in the pericardium.

20th. The symptoms unaltered, but he loses flesh and grows weaker. Urine very scanty. Pulse 104, quite regular, and of considerable strength.

On the 22nd a grain of digitalis was added to each dose of his pills.

24th. Still as before, never lying down; he complains of some tenderness in the situation of the liver. Resp. 32, performed with great effort and a slight groan on exspiration, which however appears voluntary. Pulse 108, full, strong. On percussion the chest appears quite resonant, except about the region of heart and pericardium. Dejections reported healthy.

25th. Was lying nearly flat in the bed, inclined to the left side. Pulse 104. Resp. 40. Rather more urine.

29th. Lies, slightly raised in bed, rather on his left side. There is considerable œdema of the lower extremities. Resp. 32.—Pulse 86, firm, hard, with a bound, perfectly regular. Urine scanty, but clear and of a natural colour. Great tenderness in the upper part of abdomen, which, he says, came on since the morning. And he likewise speaks of a sense of water rolling about in the right side of the chest, as having come on since the morning. On percussion the right side of the chest is more sonorous than the left, which is rather dull. By assistance of the stethoscope I thought the sound of the heart's beat was as if performed through fluid. Head perfectly free from any thing like delirium or wandering.

He died a few hours after the visit.

Sectio Cadaveris.—Nov. 30th.

Countenance purplish, bloated; some œdema of legs. The pericardium contained four ounces and a half of clear serum, which became gelatinous a few minutes after being removed. Both portions of the pericardium had many patches of a villous deposit of fibrin, thrown out recently so as to be easily peeled off in some parts, in others the fibrin was more firmly fixed. This coating of fibrin covered with a thin pellicle some inches of continuous surface on the posterior and lower part of the loose portion of the pericardium: it was also remarkable that it was attached very firmly and thickly on the heart in the course of the coronary vessels; it occurred likewise in patches of half the size of a sixpence on many parts; not forming adhesions, but presenting a rough villous surface. The heart was large and firm; the only valvular disease was in the semilunar valves of the aorta, where, in the angle between two of the valves, a triangular and solid deposit of bone of the size of a pea was found. The left lung adhered very firmly throughout most of its extent, and was in every part converted into a gray hepatized structure, very few portions admitting partially the entrance of air. There was some effusion into such parts of the cavity of the chest on this side as the nature of the adhesions admitted. The right lung was soft, and in structure not unnatural, but œdematous; filled by the effusion of serum, so that the fluid ran out mixed with innumerable fine bubbles of air immediately it was cut into. The whole cavity of the chest on this side was filled with serum, but the lung not compressed by it.

A pint or two of clear and transparent serum was effused into the cavity of the abdomen. The intestines and stomach were greatly distended with flatus, and there was an appearance as if the vessels running along the large curvature of stomach were distended with air; an oblique hernia was found on the right side; a few of the mesenteric glands were enlarged to the size of horse-beans. The peritoneal coat of the liver covered and rendered somewhat opake by a very thin coating of fibrin apparently not very recent, and a number of flocculent deposits of the same kind. In the size and substance of this organ no obvious disease; rather pale coloured, of a purplish drab throughout, and not of a firm consistence. The gallbladder full of healthy bile, and larger than natural. The pancreas healthy.

The spleen dark coloured, with a slight adventitious covering. The KIDNEYS were completely granulated throughout (Plate I.): externally the surface rough and uneven; internally all traces of the natural organization nearly gone, except in the tubular parts, which were of a lighter and more pink colour than usual.

In this case we have a very well marked example of a granulated condition of the kidneys, connected with the secretion of coagulable urine. If we can form any judgement of the priority of disease from the more advanced state of organic change, we shall be inclined to consider that the disease in the kidney was first established, and had probably laid the foundation for that effusion into the cellular membrane which had taken place previously to his admission.

There was no evidence whatever of organic disease in the liver from the beginning, except the account he gave us of his mode of life. Examination after death afforded no ground for the opinion that either the viscera of the chest or the liver were in the first place materially diseased. On the contrary, the organization of the liver and its functions, as far as any means of judging could be afforded by inspection after death or observation during the progress of the disease, remained unimpaired to the very last; and the morbid appearances of the heart, though evidently connected with the fatal result of the case, were of a nature to evince recent inflammatory action on the pericardium, and not that state of disease which has commonly been observed in connexion with general dropsical effusion. The diseased state of the left pleura was evidently a matter of longer standing, and the firmness of the adhesion gave ground for supposing that some pleuritic attack must have existed previously to his admission: it is not however at all improbable, that greater part of the mischief done to the substance of the left lung had taken place between the 20th of October, when he suffered the severe inflammatory attack, and the 29th of November, when he died. The serous effusion which was found more particularly in the right lung, might have been, and most probably was, one of the last circumstances which took place near to the close of life. At the time this case came under my care, my mind was not made up as to the indications which were to be derived from the albuminous quality of the urine; and therefore, though I noticed the fact, I did not afterwards so regularly mark the progressive changes of this secretion as I have since been in the habit of doing. I have however n‹ reason to suppose that it lost its tendency to coagulate. The dingy colou occasionally communicated to the urine in this case by admixture of blood serves further to connect it with the other cases of dropsy with disease‹ kidney which I have seen; and it is worthy of remark, that the patien complained often of pain and weakness in the loins, a symptom which i not unfrequently connected with this peculiar disease of the kidneys.

The tendency to inflammatory affection in this man was a striking feature in his case, and appears to me connected immediately with the condition of the kidneys; for when the secretion of these organs is greatly deranged, the serous membranes seem always ready to become the seat o‹ inflammatory action. The most severe instance of pleuritis I ever witnessed was in a case of diabetes, where the inflammatory disease carried off the patient in two days. In the present case the tendency to inflammation was such as would have authorized larger depletions, but I was deterred from repeating the bleeding by the decided and rapid increase of the effusion.

CASE II.

ELIZABETH BEAVER, æt. 37, was admitted November 23rd, 1825, into the Clinical ward, with swelling of the whole abdomen, attended by evident fluctuation; but depending in part on tympanitic distention. The more marked effusion was into the cellular membrane of the parietes of the abdomen, and into that of the lower extremities, which were greatly swollen; and there was considerable erythematous inflammation above the ankles. Her face and arms had likewise occasionally swollen. Severe cough was excited by deep inspiration; causing some pain in the abdomen, which was slightly tender on pressure, and she complained of pain under the ribs on the left side. Her breathing was short; she was unable to lie in the horizontal posture; she slept little, but was refreshed by it; and she did not start. Pulse 112, regular. Tongue furred at the back part; clean at the edges. Bowels relaxed. The quantity of urine uncertain, and quite clear.

She had been ill altogether about six months, her illness commencing with pain in the chest, and the increase of a cough to which she had been subject for four or five years. She was at that time under medical treatment, which removed the pain of the chest; but the cough was not cured. The catamenia had stopped about four months, and a week after the last time she was regular the left leg first began to swell, afterwards the right leg; and in two months the abdomen likewise. For the last three months the bowels had been much relaxed. The state of great depression in which this woman was, and the constant diarrhœa, induced me to order the following prescription.

℞ Hydrarg. cum Cret. gr. v,
    Confect. Opii gr. x ;
Fiant Pilulæ ter quotidie sumendæ.
Habeat Julepi Ammoniæ Subcarbon. ʒifs cum Confect. Aromat. ʒfs sexta quaque hora.

24th. Bad night; breathing a little more easy; cough not severe; is obliged to be supported by pillows in bed; legs very painful; inflammation above the ankles increased; complains of pain in the abdomen and across the loins; four or five dejections, curdly, fœtid, and rather scanty. Tongue rather furred at centre and base. Not much thirst. Pulse 112, very weak, quite regular; hands cold and purplish.

25th. Tolerable night; cough less; expectoration tough puriform mucus, moderate in quantity. *Urine coagulates by heat*, for the last two days scanty, passes frequently and unconsciously. Two watery dejections, much improved in character. Pulse from 108 to 120, weak. Tongue a little furred, and red at its edges.

The reports for the next three days were very nearly the same; but she gradually became weaker. The respiration increased to 32 in the minute, the pulse to 132. Vesications arose on various parts of her lower extremities, and she died on the evening of the 29th. The only remedy which was given with immediate reference to the dropsical symptoms, was a little squill pill and gray oxide of mercury, with a grain of opium twice a day for the last three days; while at the same time her strength was supported to the utmost by mild diet and by cordials.

SECTIO CADAVERIS.—Nov. 30th.

Whole surface greatly œdematous, and light purple ecchymoses covered with vesications on the upper parts of both thighs, and on the sides of the abdomen. Some effusion had taken place into the cavity of the chest on both sides, but the lungs throughout were in a tolerably healthy condition. Heart unusually small, and feeble in its structure; the cavity of the left ventricle very small, and the parietes of the right very thin, but not distended. In the pericardium about one ounce and a half of serum.

The cavity of the abdomen contained a very considerable quantity of limpid straw-coloured serum. The intestines were somewhat distended with flatus, but presented no unhealthy appearance. The liver externally gave the idea of being granulated with some yellowish granules; but this

appearance was very much confined to the surface; so that on making
a section, although in some parts where this was most marked, there was a
little of the same disorganization seen, for the eighth or tenth of an inch in
depth, yet the rest of the liver was throughout tolerably healthy, but
flaccid; the superficial appearance was partial.   The gall-bladder contained healthy bile of very natural colour.   The pancreas and spleen
healthy, or not manifestly otherwise.

The KIDNEYS were both of unusual size, certainly half as large again
as most commonly seen; the right was the largest: on an external view
they were obviously granulated with a large proportion of yellow granular
matter: on taking off the proper tunic this was more distinctly seen; and
on cutting in, the whole of the cortical structure seemed to be converted
into a yellow substance in appearance like fat in many parts; though in
other parts the change had not gone so far.   In the pelvis, the uterus and
bladder small and contracted; some of the lumbar glands looked dark,
and were of the size of large French beans.

————

In this case we have an example of dropsy with coagulable urine, connected with no other organic derangement except that which had taken
place to so great an extent in the kidneys; unless indeed we take into view
the small size of the heart, which appears to have been an original formation, or the result of a continued state of debility.   The size of the
kidneys considerably larger than usual, certainly suggested the idea that
the fatty and granular substance had been the effect of the deposit of fresh
matter in the interstices of the natural structure.

CASE III.

MARY SALLAWAY, aged about 25, was admitted into Guy's Hospital, November 8th,
labouring under anasarcous swellings.   Jan. 7th, when passing through the ward, I
was requested to see her, on account of a severe diarrhœa under which she was suffering: this was the first time I had observed her.   I found on inquiry that about
two months before her admission into the hospital she had perceived the swelling of
her limbs, which she ascribed entirely to low living and having during a period of
much privation drunk a great quantity of water: however, it appeared that she had
lived a very irregular life, and no doubt had at some period been in the habit of taking
spirits.   She lay at this time on her right side, coughing very frequently, and pant-
ing as if effusion had already taken place into the chest.   Her face was bloated and

swollen, of a livid colour; her legs œdematous;—but I was told that they were much reduced since she had been in the hospital. Both her stools and her urine were passed chiefly in bed, so that I could not then procure a specimen of the urine. The stools were not unhealthy in colour. On the following day I found the urine *to coagulate very considerably by heat.* She was then lying on her left side, and her breathing was exceedingly embarrassed. On the 12th she died.

With regard to treatment, a very fair and careful trial had been made of the squill and mercury for nearly a month; and various combinations of squill and opium, with the occasional use of other diuretics, had been cautiously adapted to the changes in her circumstances.

Sectio Cadaveris.—Jan. 12th.

In the left cavity of the thorax nearly two pints of turbid serum of a brownish colour were effused. The left lung on its upper part was very œdematous, so as to feel hard, it appeared almost fleshy when cut into, and in some parts the earliest stage of tubercular disease was taking place. On opening the right side of the chest some air made its escape. A considerable quantity of serum was found effused, and the lung was very much condensed, so that only a small portion admitted air. A thick adventitious membrane surrounded the greater part; and it was firmly glued to the pleura. The apex of the right lung was completely tuberculated, and two cavities as large as walnuts were there formed by suppuration. Most of the tubercles were in an early stage of their progress. The heart was healthy; the commencement of the aorta slightly diseased, with bony deposit.

In the abdomen about two pints of clear straw-coloured serum were effused. The liver was pale, yellowish, rather firm, and inclined to granulation; but not greatly altered in its structure, size, or consistence. The gall-bladder contained a small quantity of thin saffron-coloured bile. The spleen and stomach healthy; the intestines externally appeared healthy, but the ilium near to the valve was ulcerated, a number of small round ulcers forming amongst the aggregate mucous glands.

The KIDNEYS externally somewhat misshapen from the tubercular character of their structure: the form did not depend upon any disease analogous to true tubercles, but upon a general change in the substance of the kidney, some parts projecting of a white colour upon a pinkish ground, the small starlike vessels running over them. The size was but little altered. The proper tunic adhered very closely. Internally the whole

cortical structure was of a pretty uniform yellowish colour with many sma.
opake and indistinct yellow spots.　On injecting the arteries with fine size
it was found that considerable spaces were left free from injection exter
nally, and on making a section the same partial distribution of the vessel
was also observed (Plate II. Fig. 1, 2, 3.).

———

This case was one where, in addition to the hydropic effusions which ha
so prominently forced themselves on our observation, symptoms of cor
firmed phthisis pulmonalis had supervened.　The urine was decidedl
coagulable, and the kidney in a state of degeneration, which I have i
other instances remarked as connected with a cachectic state of body, bot
attended with anasarca, and unaccompanied by it.　In Plate II. where
have given a representation of this kidney, I have also introduced th
section of a kidney in what I conceive a less confirmed state of the sam
degeneration (Fig. 4.).　The patient (Cadmore) from whom this was taker
and whose case I may hereafter more particularly detail, died after a mos
protracted illness, from a tumour connected with the left ovary, whic
contained the imperfect rudiments of a foetus.

CASE IV.

DANIEL PEACOCK, a bricklayer, was admitted into the Clinical ward, Nov. 22nd, 182(
It appeared both from his own account and that of his relations, that he was by n
means a man of intemperate habits, having very seldom taken spirits : he was i
tolerable health until about two months before his admission ; when being very hc
by carrying a great weight, he drank some cold beer and lay on the damp grass ;—
the following day, or the day after, his legs began to swell.

At the time of his admission he was anasarcous over his whole body, but his leg
were most particularly swollen, and some effusion appeared to have taken place int
the cavity of the abdomen ; his breathing was much oppressed.　He had taken n
medicine except an emetic, which had been administered on account of the sicknes
which attended his first attack.

> ℞ Hydrarg. Oxydi cinerei gr. j,
> 　Pilul. Scillæ compos. gr. xij ;
> Contunde et in Pilulas iij divide hora somni quotidie sumendas.

> ℞ Misturæ Camphoræ ℥j,
> 　Spirit. Æther. nitr. ʒſs ;
> Misce, fiat Haustus ter die sumendus.

23rd. Three copious watery dejections, with griping. Urine very scanty, and high-coloured, *coagulating by heat.* Pulse 120, small. Tongue clean. The quantity of urine in a few days increased considerably; it was of *a brown colour, apparently from admixture of the red particles of blood.*

On the 26th, half a grain of opium was added to his pills; and on the 29th, a dram of the stronger mercurial ointment was ordered to be rubbed daily upon his abdomen. The stools were always copious and watery.

Dec. 1st. The abdomen much less tense, swelling of legs and thighs nearly gone; breathing still continues short. Pulse 120, small. Tongue rather white. Urine very scanty, turbid, and high coloured. Appetite good.

Although for a time there was considerable appearance of improvement, yet the symptoms soon became stationary, and the swellings occasionally returned; and it was found necessary to adopt a variety of treatment;—for a time elaterium combined with opium produced a good effect;—the extract of taraxacum was also tried;—and a combination of calomel with antimony and opium. All, however, failed in changing the character of the urine, which still continued scanty, coagulating very strongly so as to form a complete white curd on the application of heat.

On the 12th of December Erysipelas made its appearance on the right leg and foot; an exhausting diarrhœa came on: and he sunk upon the 16th.

Sectio Cadaveris.—Dec. 18th.

Very little œdema except in the legs. The right cavity of the chest contained about three pints of clear yellowish serum. The lung on that side was slightly puckered and hardened at the apex of the upper lobe: the whole lung was rather condensed owing to the pressure of the fluid, but in no way disorganized, or hardened, or œdematous. The left cavity contained about a pint and a half of serum; the left lung was healthy. The heart small but quite healthy, and its valves perfect. The aorta natural, and its internal lining beautifully white and smooth. In the abdomen no fluid was effused. The intestines to external appearance were natural, but internally showed marks of irritation throughout. The mucous glands in the small intestines enlarged; the colon as if smeared with blood; no ulcerations were discovered. The liver rather misshapen, with one or two scars upon it; and at the upper part of the right lobe a small collection of tubercular bodies, in a circumscribed group; a similar collection near the thin edge of the small lobe. The whole substance of the liver was nearly in a healthy state; a little inclined to be granulated, of a pale colour, the acini differing rather more from the surrounding parts than in perfect health. The gall-bladder not well supplied with bile. The spleen had, imbedded in its substance, a white mass half an inch deep and an inch long, otherwise it was of its ordinary appearance. The KIDNEYS afforded throughout their whole cortical structure a curious specimen of disease, apparently the commencement of granulation; they were rather large and soft; their general colour was pale, and on taking off the tunic, the whole surface was seen speckled with minute yellowish bodies: on making a longitudinal section the same bodies were seen pervading the whole cortical substance, assuming near the surface somewhat of the striated arrangement observed in the structure of the kidney at that part, and irregularly disseminated through the other parts. (Plate III. Fig. 3.)

We carefully examined the state of some of the principal arteries and veins of the body, and found them all free from the slightest marks of disease.

―――――

The appearances thus presented on examination were in the most perfect accordance with what I had anticipated, and even previously committed to writing. I had been able to trace very little evidence of disease either in the heart, the lungs, the liver, or any other organ to the derangement of which we usually ascribe dropsy; but I had observed the well marked symptoms of renal irritation and disorder, from which I have of late been led to look for decided changes in the kidney: the invasion of the disease had been sudden, apparently from repressed perspiration; the urine had been highly coagulable, and had at different times been loaded with the red particles of blood; and the ordinary medicines exhibited with unusual care and skill had failed in making any favourable impression on the disease.

CASE V.

HUGH THOMAS, a stout-looking sailor, about 34 years of age, was admitted Nov. 29th. Not unhealthy in countenance: he denies having been intemperate, but has taken a good deal of spirits-and-water. Three years ago he caught a severe cold, and since that time has never felt well. About five months ago first began to swell. At present there is the most decided œdema of the lower extremities, thighs and legs, which are soft and pitting; occasionally his whole body is said to swell. Urine scanty, very little is passed in the day, more at night; high coloured and clear; *coagulates into a complete gelatinous mass by heat.* He was cupped in the region of the liver, and was ordered to take a combination of the gray oxide of mercury with squills at night, and to make use of a solution of tartrate of potash with a little of the tincture of digitalis. Under this treatment he improved for some days; his urine rather increased, and became less coagulable, so that occasionally the application of heat produced merely an opalescence. It was necessary to give purgatives, and for this purpose powders of jalap and supertartrate of potash were found best. It was remarkable that his skin was almost always perspirable. The urine continued to increase and to become less coagulable, so that occasionally the application of heat produced simply an opacity in the fluid. On the 22nd of December very urgent dysenteric symptoms came on, and from that time the greatest care was necessary to regulate the condition of the bowels.

27th. The dysenteric attack subsiding; the secretion of the kidneys rather more copious. I saw about eight ounces of high coloured urine; by exposure to heat it became covered with a fine pellicle, such as is seen on boiled milk when cooling; œdema of the legs and thighs continues.

31st. Is much better with regard to his bowels, but he passes very little urine; looks pallid and ill, and the œdema remains as it was : it is chiefly confined to the legs and thighs, which are not tense, but very soft and yielding under pressure.

Jan. 4th. Urine exceedingly scanty; on the application of heat a pellicle is formed stronger than before.

12th. Swelling increased. Urine scanty, and becomes throughout milky by heat.

22nd. Anasarcous swellings rather increase about the hands as well as the legs; he always appears low in spirits, and is pallid. Urine scanty, of a very light straw colour; becomes quite milky by heat, and remains like milk-and-water, with little tendency to form flakes or to curdle.

Feb. 12. Urine very scanty, of a brightish yellow colour; coagulates strongly by heat in the more usual curdlike manner. He has been evidently declining for some days; his cough more troublesome, the expectoration puriform, and for some days there have been symptoms of inflammatory affection in the chest. Purging frequent; dejections watery. He died on the 14th.

Sectio Cadaveris.—Feb. 15th.

General œdema in the lower extremities, though not tense; skin sallow, not jaundiced. About a pint and a half of turbid serum was effused into the left cavity of the thorax; and the pleura both of the lung and the ribs was covered with flakes of coagulable matter, evidently the product of recent inflammation. The lung itself firmer and more red than natural. The right side of the chest nearly free from disease; the lung on that side remarkably healthy. The heart rather flaccid, as if but little called into action. The liver pale, inclined to granulation in its appearance, but not enlarged, nor materially firmer than natural. The gall-bladder well supplied with bile; spleen rather pale coloured; pancreas natural, but grayish. The whole peritoneum appeared to have suffered from recent inflammatory action; a general gray opake appearance prevailed throughout, and a considerable quantity of clear straw-coloured serum was effused, from which much coagulable matter had separated in flakes adhering to different parts, and particularly gravitating towards the pelvis. On laying open the canal of the intestines, it appeared that throughout the whole considerable irritation had existed, and a great secretion of serous fluid, so that the small intestines in particular, had exactly the appearance of having been washed out with water till no vestige of mucus was left. The duodenum near the stomach rather firm and rough; the stomach healthy. KIDNEYS large, very dark on their upper surface, on the lower mottled with yellow; no elevated granulation to be seen externally, but many small yellow specks. Internally the substance was remarkably pale, and had assumed the appearance of a fatty substance, with some traces of granulated structure throughout: this however depended in part on a flaky opake matter thickly disseminated (Plate III. Fig. 4.); and this same appearance became very obvious, over the whole external surface after the kidney had been kept in pure water for a day or two; in fact, the general morbid state of the kidney approached very much to that observed in the last Case, except that the flakes of opake matter were less numerous and defined, and the general structure was more inclined to granulation.

———

In this case we have another decided instance of anasarca with coagulable urine connected with disorganization of the kidneys. The long continuance of the symptoms before the patient became the subject of treatment, the very scanty secretion of urine and its coagulable nature, and the comparative freedom from disease either in the thorax or the liver, led me from the first moment I saw him to anticipate that he would not recover: and the belief that the kidneys would be found the marked seat of disease, induced me to pay attention to the progress of the symptoms, though the case was not under my own care. The result fully justified my expectations: and the peritoneal inflammation and more acute pleuritic attack which appeared to hasten his dissolution, afford but fresh proofs of the disposition which exists in this disease to severe inflammatory affection of different structures, but more particularly of the serous membranes.—I thought it probable that dissection would have shown some peculiarity in the structure of the kidneys, to which we might have ascribed the modification which the albumen in the urine seemed to have undergone, judging from the peculiar manner in which it coagulated. In this, however, I was disappointed: the kidneys appeared to be in the less advanced stage of that granulated change of which the case of Peacock has afforded one variety in its early stage; and of which the case of King, and that which I shall next relate, afford more confirmed examples.

CASE VI.

MARY ANN RICHARDSON, a middle-aged woman, was admitted November 8th, 1826, with anasarca: she had been two or three times in the hospital during the last two years with renewed attacks of the same disease, and had gone out relieved. She was now, as I understood,—for I did not see her,—in the most hopeless and advanced state of disease. The effusion somewhat diminished under moderate depletion, followed by the use of squill pill and the gray oxide of mercury, which remedy was continued for ten days without affecting her mouth. On the evening of the 21st she became rather suddenly worse, complaining of great difficulty of drawing her breath; and although assistance was immediately obtained, she died in a few minutes.

SECTIO CADAVERIS.

Lungs tolerably healthy in structure; but it was found that the pulmonary artery was completely blocked up by a coagulum of fibrin of firm texture. The heart was not particularly large.

On examining the abdomen it was found, that the vena portæ and its large branches going into the liver, were obstructed likewise with coagulum nearly separated from the red particles; and the splenic vein was in the same condition. The liver itself very healthy in colour and consistency, except that it bore a little of the speckled appearance resulting from a difference in the colour of the acini and the connecting substance. The gall-bladder contained some greenish bile: spleen healthy.

The KIDNEYS afforded very fine specimens of the confirmed granulated change. Of one I procured a very exact drawing; the other was injected carefully with coloured size; but they approached so exactly to the kidneys depicted in Plate I., that I did not think it necessary to have them engraved. They were rather large and bulky; the granulation was seen

externally over every part of the surface, even before the tunic was removed. The granular bodies were small, of a yellow colour, and the surrounding substance more pink. On cutting longitudinally through the
kidney, it was seen that the whole cortical substance was composed of the
same altered structure, and the striated arrangement near the surface was
almost lost. With respect to the kidney which was injected,—red size was
first thrown into the artery, and this passed with tolerable facility so as to
fill the whole pelvis; when the red injection had run completely, yellow
size was thrown into the vein. On examining this kidney externally, a
mottled surface was seen, in which the ground-work was a pink and a
whitish yellow colour nearly in equal parts; and in this were seen frequent
spots of the red injection as large as moderate sized pins' heads: and besides this, the yellow injection was seen filling the beautiful star-like vessels
which ramified quite superficially. On making an incision longitudinally,
the cortical substance presented a confused and indistinct congeries of
points of red injection and of yellow injection, with much fatty-looking
matter which had not been injected. Around the outer part of the tubular
portions the yellow vessels were very numerous, converging towards the
centre, and a few penetrated at least two-thirds of the whole depth of the
mammillary processes. The lower portion of the tubular part contained
the converging vessels filled with red injection, and these were seen opening on the points of the mammillæ.

CASE VII.

ELIZABETH STEWART, aged about 40. This woman, who appeared to have been exposed
to the difficulties and temptations of the lower classes, had for eight years been subject
to slight attacks of dropsy; during which time she had twice been in the London Hospital labouring under this disease, and had received relief. She ascribed her present
attack to great exposure about a year ago, having walked in the rain from Deal to
Gravesend without afterwards putting off her wet clothes. She was admitted into
Guy's in October 1826, greatly swollen with anasarca, the serum running from her
legs: she passed but little urine, and her breathing was greatly oppressed. She first particularly attracted my attention November 25th. At that time she had been taking the
Pil. Scillæ cum Hydrargyro till her mouth was very sore, combined with other diuretics:
all her symptoms were greatly improved; the swelling had nearly subsided. Urine
increased to nearly three pints in the twenty-four hours; pretty clear and natural in
appearance: but from the history she gave of herself, her pallid cachectic appearance,

and the soft unnatural feel of her flesh, I was led to suspect this might be one of those cases in which the urine would coagulate, and probably the kidneys prove diseased. Accordingly, on the application of heat to the urine I found that it *coagulated very considerably:* and she stated that for the last six months she had experienced a good deal of pain and uneasiness in her loins.

The improvement she had experienced was but temporary. In about a week the urine again became most exceedingly scanty; the quantity varied much. On the 10th of December I found it to be scanty and clear, but *coagulating by heat, becoming first milky and then loaded with a great number of flakes.* She spoke very decidedly as to feeling at all times *a pain, weight, and weakness across her loins.* There was after this time frequent evidence of inflammatory action going on within the chest, and of effusion into the cavities, which led to several changes in the medicine, and to the application of blisters.—Jan. 2nd. She did not pass above an ounce of urine in the night. On the 3rd there were about four ounces, coagulating freely; and on this Dr. Bostock was so kind as to make some experiments.

Jan. 13th. She has been growing decidedly worse for the last three days: before that time she had been so much better as to be sitting up the greater part of the day. She is now confined to her bed, can scarcely lie on either side: her abdomen begins to swell, and her hands are œdematous; she has a frequent dry cough; her face is puffy. Urine scanty, and she complains of pain all round the lower part of the body.

17th. Evidently sinking, complaining much of pain passing through from the chest to the back; sits nearly erect; coughs, and expectorates a tough mucus slightly tinged with blood.—She died on the following morning.

SECTIO CADAVERIS.

We were not permitted to examine the chest. In the abdomen three or four pints of clear serum were effused. The liver was slightly lobulated in its appearance, and the acute margin rounded; the peritoneal coat a little thickened. The substance of the liver rather increased; the acini light-coloured, not projecting the least; the intervening substance of a brighter red than natural. Gall-bladder rather small, but containing well coloured bile. KIDNEYS small, rather lobulated, of a semicartilaginous hardness, completely granulated; the small whitish or yellow granules projecting with red intervening spaces, so as to form a scabrous surface, both appearing and feeling rough. On making a longitudinal section, the kidney cut with the resistance of a schirrous gland; the tubular part was drawn much nearer to the surface than is natural; the cortical part indistinctly granulated throughout, of a grayish drab mixed with purple (Plate III. Fig. 1 and 2.).

Although we were not permitted to examine the chest, there is little doubt from the symptoms, that the pleura had in this case been attacked by pretty active inflammation a few days before death, and not the least doubt that very extensive effusion had latterly taken place into the cavities of the chest.

CASE VIII.

WILLIAM BONHAM, æt. 55, a large man of florid complexion, living as a carter in the service of a cheesemonger, was admitted into Guy's Hospital, December 13th. A married man, habitually taking a good deal of spirits, stated to have enjoyed till within two or three years a good state of health, except that about eleven years ago he suffered from severe inflammation of the chest. For the last two or three years he has experienced occasional pain in his back and loins, and has been subject to complaints which he has considered gravel, passing his water frequently and in rather deficient quantities. For nearly a year he has been much out of health from an attack of gout, and great shortness of breath. About two months ago, after much exposure to cold and wet, his legs first began to swell. At the time of his admission his legs and thighs and scrotum were most enormously swollen. Anasarca extended over his whole body, both the abdomen and the back; his left hand was also puffed up by the effusion into the cellular membrane.

15th. Urine of a deep yellow colour, clear, and *coagulating in a very marked manner by heat*, assuming a white curdled form.

He derived great relief from the means employed, for a day or two, but then his cough increased; he was obliged to be raised very much in bed; his urine became more scanty, but was quite clear.—He sunk and died on the sixth day after his admission.

SECTIO CADAVERIS.

The lungs adhered almost universally; and in those parts of the cavity where this was not the case, serum had collected. The lungs themselves were œdematous in a high degree. The heart remarkably enlarged; on the left side it was very thick and strong; on the anterior surface was one of those opake, white, superficial patches which are frequently observed; the valves all perfectly healthy. The liver was rather hard and solid, but not diseased in structure. The spleen was soft; pancreas and intestines healthy. The bladder contained a few drams of urine. The KIDNEYS were very small, and hard in consistence, feeling almost cartilaginous; their prevailing colour was purplish; on their external surface they were distinctly granulated in texture; and on making a longitudinal section the same

-96-

was perceptible throughout: it was remarkable that the cortical portion was exceedingly thin, so that the distance between the termination of the tubular part and the external surface was much less than in the healthy organ. In this respect, as indeed in most others, the kidneys agreed very exactly with a drawing which was made for me from the kidney of a dropsical patient about two years ago; and likewise with the kidney of the last patient, which is most accurately depicted in Plate III. Fig. 1 and 2; the only difference being, as far as I could discover, that in the kidneys from which the engraving is taken, the granular appearance was rather more marked, owing to the less general prevalence of the purple colour.

In this case we again distinctly trace the existence of a highly diseased condition of the kidney, coupled with the secretion of albuminous urine. The enlarged state of the heart would seem to bespeak some cause of obstruction to the circulation through the system beyond what we discovered, nor will I venture to say what share this might have had in giving rise to the dropsy.

CASE IX.

—— SMITH, a married woman, who keeps a mangle, of a pallid countenance, marked with the small-pox; she has lived a very irregular life, and has drunk beer and spirits to great excess. I first saw her, and only casually, December the 3rd, three days before her death. A great variety of treatment had been adopted with care and perseverance: amongst the rest she had been put completely under the influence of mercury used in combination with squills, but nothing had afforded her more than very temporary relief. The account she gave me of her complaints was,— that thirteen weeks ago, without any cause of which she knew, a general swelling came on over her whole body and limbs, and had continued more or less ever since; she had never before experienced the same disease; for the last three days she had found the greatest difficulty in assuming the horizontal posture, and during the last night could not lie down at all: her countenance was somewhat bloated, her legs completely œdematous; her left arm, on which she had supported her weight, greatly swollen; she denied having any particular pain, except occasionally a *little across her loins*. Urine rather less than eight ounces in twenty-four hours, when first passed it was clear, but of a *dingy brown* colour; it became turbid on cooling, grew clear on the application of a gentle heat, and by raising the temperature nearly to the boiling point, *it coagulated in a very marked degree*, so that it put on the appearance of thick treacle-posset. My friend Dr. Prout was so obliging as to examine a portion of this urine, and he considered it a variety not very common; its specific gravity was about 1021; it contained a large proportion of albuminous matter partaking of the character of that of the serum of the blood, and it likewise deposited the lithate of ammonia. No particular change took place in the symptoms, except their gradual increase, and she died on the 6th.

As I felt quite convinced that this was a case in which the kidney had undergone alteration in its structure, I made every endeavour to procure the examination, which was with some difficulty granted on the following day, when it was performed by the assistance of my friend Dr. Hodgkin, and Mr. Wright of Rotherithe, who had seen the patient in an earlier stage of the disease.

Sectio Cadaveris.—Dec. 7th.

The lungs were compressed by the serum effused into the chest, but in other respects were perfectly healthy and crepitant; the heart quite healthy, both in its general structure and in its valves; a very large quantity of serum, not less than three pints, in each cavity of the chest, perfectly limpid in the right, rather turbid in the left; about one ounce in the pericardium. The liver appeared externally quite healthy, and the gall-bladder contained good bile in sufficient quantity. On cutting into the liver, although the structure was not deranged, yet towards the thinner parts it was more firm than in perfect health, and a little more pale. The pancreas, of healthy structure and colour, but rather hard. The internal lining of the stomach towards the pylorus a little vascular. The duodenum was likewise remarkably vascular, so that the folds of the mucous membrane looked like turgid red lines crossing the internal surface in different directions; the other abdominal viscera were healthy.

The KIDNEYS presented most decidedly the granulated structure; this was somewhat marked externally, the lighter points of the granulation being smaller than I have often observed; and on cutting into the substance, it was seen that the natural structure was destroyed throughout the whole cortical part, which was mottled as in the two last cases I have described; but this morbid structure appeared in its most advanced stage around the tubular parts. I could not obtain permission to have a drawing made of these kidneys; but I regret this the less, as the gentlemen who were present, both of them observed the fact, as likewise the comparatively slight derangement of the liver.

CASE X.

MARY CASTLE, æt. 39, was admitted into Guy's Hospital, December 27th, 1826. Has been subject to cough and dyspnœa for eight years, but more severely for the last four years, after having suffered from an intermittent fever. She has been three times in different hospitals, affected with anasarcous swellings : the present aggravation of her symptoms took place about a month before her admission. Her legs and thighs were swollen to the greatest excess; the cellular membrane of the abdomen was also tense with serum, and there was decided fluctuation from fluid in the cavity. The countenance exceedingly purple and bloated; the lips, nose and tongue, purple; eyes suffused and prominent; and the dyspnœa so great that she lay down with the utmost difficulty. The urine very scanty, not above six ounces in twenty-four hours; *coagulating decidedly*, though not to the extent I have often observed.

In the progress of this disease some alleviation was occasionally procured, but no very material amendment at any time took place. The urine always continued very scanty; sometimes it was tolerably clear, at other times it became turbid on cooling; at other times it bore the dingy colour which usually denotes the presence of blood: almost always the urine retained its coagulable property; but in general this was limited to a dense deposit of brownish flakes, the whole fluid not becoming milky or curdled. On one or two occasions diuretics had the effect of increasing the urine to a pint and a half and two pints in the twenty-four hours; but although benefit was generally derived at first from each new combination, yet after a very short time it lost its power. The *vinum colchici* was occasionally combined with purgatives with advantage; indeed purgatives always gave relief. The infusion of juniper berries with the acetate of potash was given as a drink, and the infusion of broom tops with preparations of squill: but decidedly the most relief was derived from the solution of the supertartrate of potash, and at the same time small doses of digitalis in powder.—She died on the 17th of February.

SECTIO CADAVERIS.—Feb. 19th.

There was but little effusion into the cavity of the chest, but the lungs adhered very considerably in some parts to the pleura costalis. The membrane lining the bronchial tubes was injected and vascular, and the tubes themselves appeared dilated; the substance of the lungs was healthy, but they were in a state of œdema. The heart was remarkably pale and flaccid, and there was very little difference in the thickness of the parietes of the two ventricles; a small quantity of serum more than natural had collected in the pericardium. The abdomen contained several pints of serum. The liver was mottled, showing the yellow acini in a red ground :

-99-

but although this was very strongly marked, yet the liver was neither hard nor tuberculated in its structure; but on the contrary, was smooth and not very firm in its consistence; the gall-bladder was full of bile. The KID-NEYS were contracted and hard, and on removing their tunic the surface was scabrous; but the projecting roughness was of a pretty uniform gray purplish colour, and the same was observable on making a section.

In this case it appears that the cause of the effusion was somewhat complicated. No doubt the condition of the lungs and the obstruction produced by the chronic bronchial disease had a large share in producing the symptoms we have observed: still, however, the condition of the kidneys so nearly according with that of others in cases where the urine has possessed similar qualities, leads us in this fresh instance to mark the connection between the obvious morbid state of the organ and its very deficient powers of healthy action.

CASE XI.

HENRY IZOD, æt. 25, was a Smithfield drover, and a man of very irregular habits. He had long been accustomed to get intoxicated with porter, but had only taken spirits to excess, for the last year, during which time he had generally lodged at a public-house, and had been much exposed in his work to the inclemency of the weather; seldom wearing a hat, never changing his clothes when wet, and being almost daily intoxicated: he had frequently suffered from cough, particularly in the winter. He had not enjoyed good health for two or three years; and on one occasion about a year ago had an attack of dropsical swelling; he had been nearly well again till the beginning of October, about seven weeks before his death, when after drinking and exposure he became swollen all over. He was under the successive care of two very judicious physicians. He took squills, digitalis, and other diuretics, and a state of salivation was kept up for some days. I never saw him but once, (about five days before his death,) at which time his swellings were reported to be considerably diminished; but he passed very little water, and not being able to obtain any I did not examine its qualities: he was in an exceedingly low and reduced state, his mouth still very sore.—He died on the 23rd.

SECTIO CADAVERIS.

As this was a case in which, though the habits of the man were those which are supposed to give rise to chronic hepatic disease and consequent dropsy, I saw no evidence of such disease either in the appearance, or in the other symptoms; and as the effusion had come on in the last instance rather rapidly, and the patient had not seemed to bear mercury well, I was very desirous of ascertaining the relative state of disease in the liver and the kidneys; and accordingly obtained permission to examine the body on the 25th, which I did at the late residence of the patient, with the assistance of my zealous friend Dr. Hodgkin.

The legs œdematous; slight œdema of the abdomen, about three pints of clear straw-coloured serum effused into the cavity of the abdomen; about an equal quantity in the two cavities of the chest. The lungs were not closely contracted, as if long compressed by a fluid, but were tolerably healthy in their first appearance; the whole, however, somewhat œdematous, and the upper lobe on each side rather condensed and red, as from some degree of chronic inflammation. Near the apex of each lung was a contraction or cicatrix, and within that a small portion of white gritty matter.—The heart was rather large, but in its structure healthy.—The liver was of the most natural liver-coloured red. I should have said that I never saw this organ in a more healthy state; but on very careful inspection the acini appeared lighter than the ground, and somewhat more so than natural. The spleen small, but natural. The stomach was rather loaded with mucus, and the inner coat grayish. Intestines healthy both internally and externally.—KIDNEYS most decidedly diseased; they did not feel so firm as natural, were almost white in external appearance, rather large and lobulated, without any signs of granulation, and only showing a few star-like vessels distributed on the surface; otherwise of nearly one even surface, and on most minute inspection no mark of structure as usually seen on the surface of the healthy kidney was discoverable. On making a complete longitudinal section, the same gray-white colour pervaded all the cortical part, with little sign of natural structure; the faint appearance which did exist, preserved those marks of lines proceeding towards the surface, which are often more evident in the healthy kidney. The tubular part was also faintly coloured. An external view and a section were drawn with great care, and from them the engravings of Plate IV. Fig. 1. and 2. were executed. The other kidney was injected,—the arteries with red, the veins with yellow size. The injection ran freely from the arteries into the pelvis of the kidney; the general structure did not seem greatly deranged. (Plate IV. Fig. 4. and 5.) After that part of the kidney which had not been injected had undergone maceration in spring water for about a fortnight, it showed a number of white opake specks over its whole surface. (Plate IV. Fig. 3.)

———

This then was a case of general anasarca, connected with most decidedly diseased appearance of the kidney, and scarcely any other organic lesion; but it was not ascertained what had been the condition of the urine.

[While the proof of this page was before me for correction (April 4th) the following case occurred.]

CASE XII.

—— GALLOWAY, æt. 22, a watch-case maker by trade, was admitted on the 7th of March, 1827, into Guy's Hospital. He was in a state of general anasarca. It appeared that for the last year or two he had been intemperate in his habits, being often intoxicated with spirits, particularly with gin. About the month of November last, while under the action of mercury for syphilitic disease, he got wet, and soon after this began to show signs of dropsical effusion. A little before Christmas he was admitted into one of the hospitals of the metropolis, and was treated with mercurials for his anasarcous affection; he left the hospital, however, but slightly relieved. When admitted into Guy's his mouth was still very sore with mercury; he was swollen generally, his countenance was pallid and bloated, and his legs distended with œdema. His urine was scanty, and of *a slightly dingy colour, coagulating decidedly by heat.* Various remedies were employed, but with little effect: he became the subject of seizures of an epileptic character, which returned several times during the last three or four days of his life; and very decided symptoms of inflammatory affection of the chest, with cough and a quick sharp pulse, came on.—He died upon the 2nd of April.

SECTIO CADAVERIS.

On both sides of the chest were well marked signs of recent inflammation of the pleura. A few ounces of serum were effused, in which gelatinous coagula and shreds of fibrin were floating; and both the pleura of the lungs and of the ribs were covered in parts with thin layers of a recent false membrane, presenting a rough and rather reticulated surface. The substance of the lung did not appear altogether to have escaped the effects of inflammation; but the injury done was slight, and every part admitted air. The bronchial tubes were of a more chocolate colour, from venous congestion, than natural. The pericardium contained about two ounces of clear fluid. The heart was quite healthy in the structure of all its valves, but the parietes of the left ventricle were decidedly thickened. The aorta was quite natural. The liver was a perfect specimen of the healthy organ, without the slightest tendency to hardness or to granulation. The gall-bladder rather small, filled with healthy bile of the usual bright yellow colour. The spleen healthy. The pancreas a little loaded with blood. The stomach and small intestines perfectly healthy. The colon internally speckled with gray, but otherwise not diseased. The KIDNEYS disorganized throughout, smooth in their external texture, rather lobulated, of a pale yellow colour, with a few superficial vessels; and on being examined internally, the same gray yellow colour pervading the whole cortical part, with some more opake yellow spots irregularly intermixed. The tubular structure pale and indistinct; in a word, approaching more to the condition of the kidneys mentioned in the last case, than any others I have examined.

Here then we have another illustrative example of this most fatal disease. The short history would appear to be, that the kidneys became deranged, perhaps disorganized, by the abuse of spirituous liquors; that in this state the combination of circumstances which gave rise to suppressed perspiration had confirmed the disease; and in its progress, not only anasarca had shown itself, but the pleura had become inflamed, and the head had suffered. To what extent or in what way the head had been implicated, we had no opportunity of ascertaining by inspection; but there could be little doubt that some serious mischief had lately taken place. My diagnosis in this case had been formed entirely from the nature of the urine, and the absence of all symptoms indicative of other organs being diseased; while the general leucophlegmatic aspect of the patient, and the history of the disease, strongly confirmed my judgement.

CASE XIII.

THOMAS DRUDGET, æt. 37, was admitted under my care into Guy's Hospital on the 7th of December 1826. He was a carman, in the habit of drinking a little, while in his work, but by no means an intemperate man, coming home very regularly, and

always passing his evenings with his family.   About a fortnight before his admission
he was attacked with sickness at the stomach, and shortness of breath; purging then
came on, and vomiting: about nine days before admission his face and legs began to
swell.   The urine had been deficient in quantity the whole time.   He complained
much of tenderness at the pit of the stomach.   Pulse 72, of good strength.   Tongue
white; the œdema was by no means great; his face looked a little puffy, and his
legs were so far swollen that he could not button the knees of his small-clothes.

Applicentur Cucurbitulæ cruentæ Scrob. Cordis et detrahatur sanguis ad f℥xiv.
Habeat Pulv. Rhei cum Hydrargyri Submuriat. gr. xv. statim.
Mist. Magnesiæ cum Magnes. Sulph. ʒj et Tinct. Camphor. comp. fʒſs ter die.

8th. Bowels free: urine about three quarters of a pint in twenty-four hours; *coagulates.*   The anasarca by no means considerable, and the symptoms altogether so
mild as to excite no particular alarm; he is walking about in the ward, and says he
does not feel inclined to remain in bed.

℞ Potassæ Supertartratis ℥j,
Aquæ puræ f℥x. fiat Mistura quotidie sumenda.

9th. Urine not quite one pint; thinks his swelling rather increased; some feeling
of oppression at the chest.   He now says that two or three days before his admission
he had felt some pain in the loins.   Two dejections.

Applicentur Cucurb. cruent. lumbis, et detrahatur sanguinis f℥xij.
Repetatur Mistura.

10th. Felt much relieved from the weight at the chest by the cupping; legs remain
unaltered.   Pulse 68, of good strength.   Urine rather turbid, about a pint and a half;
coagulates, but not so much as before.

Repetatur Mistura.

11th.   Detrahatur sanguinis f℥xij e regione lumborum ope Cucurb. cruent.
Habeat Infusi Lini ℔jſs pro potu quotidie.

℞ Jalapæ Radicis gr. x,
Potassæ Supertartratis Əj,
Capsici Baccarum gr. j.
Fiat Pulvis quotidie sumendus si opus fuerit.

12th. Urine one pint and a half, dingy as from very slight admixture of blood,
coagulates: five stools from the powder, watery, without pain; swelling not relieved.

Adde Potassæ Nitratis Əijſs Infuso Lini quotidie.
Rep. Pulvis pro re nata.

13th. Face rather more swollen; legs diminished; urine about the same quantity, clear, but rather high coloured. Pulse 72.

14th. Feels much better, the swelling less. Urine about the same quantity.

15th. Pulse 72, legs diminished. Urine same quantity, and does not coagulate, but a slight permanent frothy scum remains after boiling.

17th. He was walking about the ward; said that his water was rather increased and his body less swollen: but he did not speak quite so cheerfully of his progress as he had done the day before.

> Rep. Pulvis ex Jalapa et Potassæ Supertart. alternis auroris,
> et Repetantur Medicamenta.

Towards the evening he complained to some of the patients that his head ached: he slept apparently as usual, which was always with an inclination to snore; he went two or three times to the water-closet about six or seven o'clock, for which he had to walk half the length of a pretty long ward. About eight o'clock it was observed that he lay in bed making a very singular noise, and on going to him he was in a state of profound apoplectic stertor. Mr. Stocker was immediately called; took away twenty ounces of blood from the temporal artery, gave him ten grains of calomel, and a colocynth injection. He had one or two fresh attacks, accompanied with so much convulsion that he could scarcely be held in bed. I saw him at eleven o'clock. Pulse about 96, sharp with a jerk; he lay on his back perfectly insensible, with some inclination to convulsion of the arms, and a convulsive mode of blowing his saliva from his mouth. Pupils rather contracted, particularly the left.

> Mittatur sanguis ad f℥xvj. Olei Tiglii ♏ ij. Enema catharticum.
> Applicetur Emplastrum Cantharidis Nuchæ.

Twelve o'clock: The pulse a good deal lowered just after the bleeding; no dejection. One o'clock: Pulse risen again.

> Applicentur Cucurbitulæ cruent. regioni hepatis et detrahatur sanguis ad f℥xvj.
> Repetatur Enema.

He died at nine o'clock.

Sectio Cadaveris.

General serous effusion under the integuments, from which the scalp itself had not escaped. About six ounces of clear serum in the left cavity of the chest, and less in the right; about one ounce of serum in the pericardium. Lungs healthy, except some apparently old and sluggish tubercles, two or three in number, at the apex of each upper lobe. Heart healthy. Liver rather soft, but not strikingly so; quite natural in struc-

ture throughout.   Gall-bladder healthy.   Spleen soft.   Stomach and intestines healthy.   Arteries and veins perfectly sound and healthy: the
lower part of aorta and cava were particularly examined.   KIDNEYS very
pale and rather soft; discovered externally nothing but the natural structure rather more marked than usual, but internally was plainly to be traced
a motley granulation very small and faint in its colour and markings.

On opening the head no morbid appearance was observable in the
membranes; the convolutions of the hemispheres were obviously flattened,
as is generally the case when any quantity of fluid is effused within; and
on slicing off the superior portion and laying open the ventricles, we
found them all completely filled with a clot of blood and serum, apparently
separated from the effused blood.   The right crus cerebri was lacerated,
soft, and full of dark bloody spots.   It was evidently from this part that
the blood found in the ventricles had been effused.   The left crus and the
portion of brain immediately between the crura was in a similar state with
the right crus, but to a much less degree.   There were two or three small
coagula in the right thalamus, but they appeared to be quite detached.
There was a very small spot of the same character in the corpora quadri-
gemina; the rest of the brain and cerebellum were quite healthy.

In this case the kidney, though most decidedly differing from that organ
in its healthy condition, was, as might be expected from the very recent
date of the disease, by no means so marked by morbid appearance as in
most of the other cases of coagulable urine which I have examined.   It may
be considered the incipient and perfectly curable stage of this formidable
disease; and I have no doubt that but for the accidental rupture of the
vessel in the brain, this man might, for a time at least, have recovered
perfectly, to all appearance.   My treatment was directed in the first place
to take off from that general plethoric state of the system, which had been
induced by the deficient secretion of urine.   This I endeavoured to accomplish by abstracting blood and by free purging; and I hoped, by taking
blood locally, more effectually to reduce the irritation of the kidneys themselves.   At the same time I wished to urge the kidneys gently to the performance of their secretion; and for this purpose I preferred diluted solutions of diuretic salts, in the employment of which I should certainly
have been more active, had I not conceived that I was fast gaining ground;
and had I not wished to obtain my object without irritating the kidneys

so much as to produce hæmaturia, which I have so often seen accompany this disease.

In the examination of this patient, the circumstance of the effusion of blood having taken place into the ventricles is somewhat unusual, inasmuch as by far the greater number of cases where blood has been effused show the coagulum embedded in the substance of the brain; and though approaching very near to the ventricle, not entering it. The peculiar convulsive character of the apoplectic seizure is also worthy of remark as connected with lesion in the structure of the crus cerebri.

CASE XIV.

LEONARD EVANS, a Welshman of remarkably stout frame: about ten or twelve years ago said to have been the strongest man out of 1400 in Deptford dockyard; has enjoyed much good health till about two years ago, when he had the syphilitic disease; but this was completely subdued. His occupation of late has been one which has exposed him very much to alternations of heat and cold,—being a journeyman currier; in some part of which business he has often been exposed to cold, when in a state of most profuse perspiration; but his habits have been very sober and steady throughout life. The day before his attack,—about ten days before his admission into Guy's Hospital,—he had been employed in washing skins; his feet were very wet: he found the swelling coming on about six o'clock the same evening, and he continued to swell till the time of his coming into the Hospital, under my care, Nov. 15th. He was at that time labouring under general anasarca to a great extent. Urine very scanty. He had taken very little medicine.

Sumat Extract. Elaterii gr. ſs sexta quaque hora.

18th. The swelling rather diminishes.

Extract. Elaterii gr. j bis quotidie.

19th. The pills have purged him very often, with much pain before they act, and much sickness. Pulse 80, full. Urine rather increased: today he first observed the dark-brown tinge in the urine, which is now very obvious, being a mixture of the red particles; *coagulates by heat.*

Rep. Extractum Elaterii mane quotidie.

20th. Urine three pints and a half in twelve hours, which is nearly six times as much as he had passed before; slightly coagulable; turbid, with red particles: feels altogether much relieved: one very copious watery and fæculent dejection.

Sumat Infus. Spartii scoparii ℔ij quotidie.

Habeat pulverem ex Jalapæ Radice et Potassæ Supertart. alternis auroris.

F

21st. Swelling a good deal reduced; urine in sixteen hours six pints and a half, of a high brandy colour; does not coagulate.

Repetantur Medicamenta.

24th. Urine six pints from 8 o'clock last night to 8 o'clock this morning, lighter-coloured; scarcely coagulates.

27th. Urine still contains some red particles, and is copious, but does not coagulate; swellings diminish daily.

Extr. Conii gr. v, ter die.
Repetantur Medicamenta.

Dec. 1st. Complains of a pain under his jaw, but the œdematous swellings are nearly gone, except a little on the instep. Urine four pints, coagulates, and contains much blood, looking quite red; three stools yesterday from the powder. Pulse 84, of good strength.

Mittatur sanguis ad f℥x. Rep. Infusum et Pulvis.

2nd. Blood not buffed, but a firm and large coagulum, quite elastic, like a mould of jelly, and of florid colour. Urine about four pints, very red, with a great quantity of ropy mucus deposited at the bottom. Œdema much subsided. Bowels not yet opened by the powder.

Mittatur sanguis ad f℥x.

℞ Antimonii tartarizati gr. ½,
　　Opii purificati gr. ij,
　　Theriacæ q. s.

Fiant Pilulæ ij, quarum sumat unam bis quotidie.
Omitt. Infus. Spartii; habeat Haustum Sennæ pro re nata.

3rd. Blood with thin buff; complains of a sore throat; reports the urine which has been thrown away to be of the same colour as yesterday. He is walking about, and appears much improved upon the whole.

Liniment. Ammoniæ gutturi infricandum.
Repetantur Medicamenta.

4th. Urine decidedly less red, but less copious; about two pints, mucous matter at the bottom diminished; it coagulates much more sparingly: throat relieved; he looks rather pallid; tongue moist and clear; pulse moderate.

5th. The whole of yesterday afternoon he seemed well,—was walking about the ward, and seemed comfortable: he slept soundly, but this morning at seven o'clock suddenly complained of a great difficulty of swallowing and breathing, and constriction at his throat and chest. Fourteen ounces of blood were taken from his arm, sixteen leeches were applied to his throat, and an emetic was administered; but all was unavailing,—and at about eleven o'clock he expired: the blood was highly buffed. I was informed that the urine passed since I saw him was somewhat further improved in appearance.

As I felt assured that this was a case in which neither the general circulation through disease of the heart, nor the biliary secretion through disease of the liver had any direct influence in the production of the Anasarca, but could not doubt that the kidney was more immediately the seat of the derangement,—I was very desirous of obtaining an examination, to ascertain whether any change had taken place in that organ, which could betray itself to the eye ; and this was at length granted, at the late residence of the patient, about sixty hours after death.

Sectio Cadaveris.

No sign of effusion of serum into the cellular membrane of the integuments ; muscles of the body unusually strong; limbs rigid. Lungs rather gorged with blood ; otherwise in structure quite healthy. Heart and pericardium quite healthy. In the cavity of the chest on each side about four ounces of fluid ; in the right cavity the serum of a red colour, the lung adhering by old adhesion on the front part, and there was great congestion of blood in the back part by subsidence after death.

The liver rather gorged with blood, but perfectly healthy in structure. Spleen so soft that when the tunic was lacerated, the substance of the viscus flowed out of a chocolate colour. Stomach and intestines healthy ; no effusion of serum into the cavity. The bladder contained about three quarters of a pint of clear and yellow urine, which was not coagulable, or at least yielded only the slightest flaky coagulum ; but some mucus had subsided to the bottom. The KIDNEYS presented a very curious appearance ; they were easily slipped out of their investing membrane, were large, and less firm than they often are, of the darkest chocolate colour, interspersed with a few white points, and a great number nearly black; and this, with a little tinge of red in parts, gave the appearance of a polished fine-grained porphyry or greenstone. On cutting longitudinally into the kidney, this structure and these colours were found to pervade the whole cortical part ; but the natural striated appearance was not lost, and the external part of each mass of tubuli was peculiarly dark ; the whole mammillary processes were also of a dark colour. On being cut through and left for some time, a very considerable quantity of blood oozed from the kidney, showing a most unusual accumulation in the organ ; and indeed it seemed to be from this cause that the peculiar appearance and colour arose; the very dark spots being the effect of blood either extravasated or in vessels greatly gorged. I had an opportunity of procuring very faithful drawings of the kidney. (Plate V.)—We next examined the epiglottis; and this we found to be thickened by an œdematous effusion beneath the membrane on its upper side : it was bent into the form of a penthouse with a sharp angle ; and the lower surface was also thickened, and presented a doubtful appearance of superficial ulceration. When the epiglottis was cut into, a considerable quantity of serous fluid was easily squeezed out; and on the whole the opening was much contracted, and the epiglottis completely disqualified for performing its natural valvular functions.

There could then be no doubt of the nature of the attack under which the patient sunk so rapidly: inflammation of the epiglottis had been followed by œdema of that part which had produced suffocation.

In this case we have the most unequivocal proof of the derangement of the kidney being connected with the extensive and sudden occurrence of anasarca :—there could indeed be no doubt of this, from the first moment that I had an opportunity of seeing the patient. The coagulable urine, —and that urine already containing the red particles of the blood in large abundance,—led me from the beginning to form my opinion as to the seat of the disease. Moreover, dissection showed no other adequate cause for the dropsical affection : and as during life no suspicion could be entertained that either the liver, the intestines, the heart, or the lungs were diseased, so the examination showed all these organs to be in a state of perfect health. I feel that it may be matter of doubt how far the employment of diuretics during such diseased tendency may have been instrumental in producing the peculiar appearance of the kidneys ; but it is to be remembered that the particular symptom, the hæmaturia, which appears so immediately connected with this morbid state, has been observed to occur in a greater or less degree under all modes of treatment, and even before any treatment has been adopted in the sudden anasarca, and therefore we cannot in fairness ascribe the morbid appearance of the kidney to the remedies,—or at all events we must admit a certain high degree of disease to have existed in that organ from the commencement of the symptoms ; but whether to the extent discovered in this case after death or not, we can never determine. The symptom of hæmaturia was evidently on its decline when the accident occurred which led to a fatal termination; and it was my intention in this case, as in the case of Fish, (to be related hereafter,) to have had recourse to local bleeding by cupping from the loins, as soon as the excessive general action had been sufficiently subdued: and very possibly if the sudden affection of the epiglottis had not come on, the disease in this case would for a time at least have completely yielded, as the symptom of anasarca had already totally disappeared, under the treatment adopted.

CASE XV.

WILLIAM RODERICK, æt. 45, was admitted under my care into Guy's Hospital, on the 29th of March, 1826. A man of large stature, by trade a house-carpenter, much accustomed to drinking spirits. Three weeks before Christmas,—about four months previous to his admission,—he first found himself out of health: at that time he says that he experienced much pain in the right side near to the situation of the liver, accompanied by occasional rigors and cough, and he lay always on the right side. All these symptoms have subsided by the use of medicines, and he now lies well on either side. He is universally swollen with anasarca in a most unusual degree; particularly the legs, thighs, abdomen, and back as high up as the shoulders. He can scarcely bend his knees the least, and his hands are puffy: it appears that the left arm is more swollen than the right; but this may be casual. Countenance pallid. Bowels regular. Urine scanty and high coloured. Pulse 84, regular, of tolerable strength. Tongue rather dry.

Sumat Pilul. Scillæ cum Hydrarg. Oxyd. ciner. iij. et Digitalis fol. contrit. gr. j. omni nocte.—Habeat Infusum Juniperi pro potu.

March 30th. Bowels not sufficiently open. Urine one-third of a pint in twenty-four hours, turbid on standing; but on the application of heat becomes for a few moments perfectly transparent, and then *coagulates* in a most marked degree, so as to form one curdled white mass.

R Jalapæ Radicis gr. x,
Potassæ Supertartrat. Əj. Fiat pulvis statim sumendus.

31st. Œdema rather increased: urine in appearance and quantity nearly the same.

R Aceti Scillæ ♏ xx,
Spirit. Ætheris nitric. ♏ xx,
Liquoris Ammoniæ Acetatis fʒvj,
Aquæ Menthæ viridis fʒvj;
Misce fiat Haustus quarta quaque hora sumendus.
Pil. Scillæ cum Hydrag. Oxyd. ciner. iij. omni nocte.

April 3rd. He has taken his medicines regularly; the swelling of the legs has much subsided. Pulse 88, rather weak.

Habeat Olei Ricini f℥vj statim.

5th.   ℞ Oxymellis Scillæ f℥ij,
               Potassæ Supertartratis contritæ ℥iij;
Misce sumat cochleare medium ter quotidie.
Repetantur Haustus et Pilulæ.

7th. Urine the same in quantity, clear, brownish. Bowels confined.

Pulv. Jalap. cum Potass. Supertart. ℈fs. cras mane, et repetatur pro re nata.
Repetantur etiam Medicamenta.

14th. A blush of red over the right thigh and the pubes. Anasarca generally increased. Bowels inclined to be costive; he feels relief when they act.

         ℞ Extracti Elaterii gr. ½,
           Potass. Supertartrat. gr. iij,
           Zingib. Radicis contritæ gr. j;
Misce fiat pulvis statim sumendus, et Repet. quarta quaque hora ad sedes.
Repetantur Medicamenta.

15th. The powder produced much vomiting, but no stools.

         ℞ Extracti Elaterii gr. ¼,
           Potass. Supertartrat. gr. v,
           Zingib. Radicis contrit. gr. j;
Misce fiat pulvis statim sumendus.
Repetantur Medicamenta.

17th. He was much purged and vomited by the powder; stools watery. Much better in the afternoon; but the relief was only temporary, and he is nearly in the same state as before.

Repetatur Pulv. Elaterii cras mane, et continuantur Medicamenta.

19th. Again felt much relief from the powder, which produced vomiting, and was followed by many watery stools; the œdema was diminished, but it has returned.

24th.   Opii gr. j omni nocte, et continuantur Medicamenta.

28th. Rather improved. He has passed more urine, but it is still very coagulable by heat.

May 1st.   ℞ Cambogiæ Gummi-resinæ contritæ gr. x,
         Potassæ Supertartratis gr. xx,
         Zingib. Radicis contritæ gr. ij,
         Syrup. Zingiberis quantum sufficiat: fiat Bolus statim sumendus.
Habeat Mistur. Camphoræ fȝix cum Liqu. Ammon. Acet. fȝiij et Tincturæ
Digitalis ♏ x ter die.

5th. On examining the state of the chest by means of the stethoscope, it was found
to be resonant where the external œdema admitted of the examination. There was a
general sonorous rattle throughout the lungs; little impulse in the heart's action; the
sound not loud but clear.

     Sumat Extract. Elaterii gr. ¼ cum Potass. Supertartrat. gr. iv, sexta quaque
     hora ad sedes; et Opii gr. j omni nocte.

8th. Upon the whole there had been little progress towards improvement, all the
symptoms remaining very nearly as at the time of admission six weeks ago.

                ℞ Potassæ Supertartrat. ȝfs,
                  Aquæ destillat. fȝx;
        Fiat Mistura mane quotidie sumenda.

10th.   Rep. Mistura bis quotidie.

12th. The swelling in general is slightly diminished. Urine decidedly increased;
still coagulates by heat, but not so completely as before. Several watery dejections.

15th. Continues to pass more urine: the medicine still acts gently upon his bowels.

19th. Swelling is decidedly diminished. Urine increased to two pints, remains
coagulable by heat. Bowels relaxed, several watery stools.

22nd. Hands much less swollen; thighs as before: the medicine still acts freely on
the bowels. Urine unaltered in its quality.

               ℞ Pulv. Uvæ Ursi ℈j,
                Pulv. Conii gr. iij;
       Fiat Pulvis ter die sumendus. Repetatur Mistura.

26th. Anasarca diminished. Urine nearly the same.

      Repetatur Pulvis et sumat Misturam bis quotidie.

29th. Urine not so coagulable. Feels himself better; still considerably swollen.

June 2nd. Urine much increased, nearly three pints. The knee joints can be bent,
and the anasarca of the whole body is much diminished. Urine scarcely the least
coagulable. Bowels bound.

     Sumat Potass. Supertart. ȝvj; ex Aquæ puræ fȝxv bis die.
     Repetatur Pulvis.

5th. The swellings subside gradually and regularly ; the urine increases. He complains of the taste of the medicine.

Adde Syrupi simplicis f℥j Misturæ ; et continuatur Pulvis.

9th. Urine six pints in twenty-four hours, *does not coagulate.* Bowels freely open.

26th. Urine of a dark olive colour, turbid, and of ammoniacal odour. Coagulates very slightly.

July 3. The urine, which had become quite clear for three or four days, is now again brown and turbid, and deposits a white sediment, which sticks to the vessel : odour ammoniacal, scarcely the least coagulable by heat.

The urine became again clear in a few days. He continued the same remedies uninterruptedly to the end of July, when he was completely cured, having been detained a few days by a slight feverish attack.

————

In this patient the extent of the anasarca and the coagulable quality of the urine were both of them more remarkable than I ever before observed. After his admission under my care, no symptoms at any time induced me to consider the liver in the least implicated in the disease. The account, however, which he gave of his previous symptoms,—the pain in the right side, and the difficulty of lying on the left,—induced me to employ for some time a mild form of mercury in moderate doses, combined with the squill. I did not perceive any advantage to arise from this remedy during the period of nearly a month, for which time it was continued ; nor did the other remedies which were from time to time added, produce any permanent good effects : and if at any time relief were experienced during the continuance of this plan, it was only when on the 24th of April he took a grain of opium at bed-time ; or when active purgatives, more particularly elaterium, produced watery evacuations. The elaterium, however, distressed him much, and its good effects appeared but temporary. At the expiration of six weeks very little ground had been gained. I then resolved to give a full trial to the supertartrate of potash ; and the good effects were almost instantaneous, in increasing the secretion of the kidneys, and in producing absorption of the effused fluid : still, however, the coagulable quality of the urine in a great degree remained, and my impression that the unhealthy and irritated state of the kidneys themselves was probably the great source of the anasarca, led me to adopt the use of the uva ursi and the conium. This was about a fortnight after the supertartrate of potash had been commenced ; and although there were some very unequivocal marks of irritation subsisting in the kidneys, all this subsided, and there was no occasion to change the remedy till the cure was apparently complete.

He remained quite well for four months, when being exposed to wet and cold his legs began to swell; and one month after, on the 11th of December, he was again admitted into the hospital. At this time his legs were greatly swollen, hard, and decidedly œdematous. Urine *coagulated strongly by heat*. Pulse 80, of good strength. Resp. 24, with occasional cough, particularly when lying. Since his present illness has had irregular cold shivering fits every two or three nights; denies having any pain either with or without pressure; no palpitation or beating of the heart.

Applicentur Cucurbitulæ cruentæ Lumbis et detrahatur sanguis ad f℥xij.

Sumat Infus. Lini ℔ij quotidie.

12. The cupping performed by mistake across the chest, has relieved the cough a good deal. Urine two pints in fifteen hours; moderately high coloured, with a flocculent sediment.

13th. Urine more clear in colour, three pints in fourteen hours. Two stools from an opening powder; but it made him sick.

14th. Urine almost the same in quantity, scarcely becomes clouded by heat.

Habeat Pulv. ex Jalapa et Potassæ Supertartrate mane quotidie si opus fuerit.

15th. Urine rather less; coagulates more. Two stools this morning without sickness or griping. Takes ℔ij of the infusion of linseed every day.

Adde Sodæ Subcarbonatis ʒj Infuso Lini quotidie.

20th. Urine nearly two pints, clear, rendered very slightly turbid by heat. Pulse 84. Bowels opened six or seven times from every powder.

Pulv. Rhei cum Hydrargyri Submuriate gr. xv cras mane.

25th. Swelling increased. Urine one pint, coagulates. Bowels not well opened. Pulse rather sharp.

Mittatur sanguis ad f℥xij. Repetatur Infusum Lini.

26th. Urine one pint; coagulates by heat. Blood firmly coagulated and buffed.

℞ Potassæ Supertart. ℥ſs,
   Aquæ destillatæ f℥x,
   Syrup. simpl. f℥j : fiat mistura quotidie sumenda.
Habeat Haust. Sennæ pro re nata.

27th. Urine about the same in quantity, has a slight cloud in it; coagulates by heat. He did not begin his supertartrate of potash till this morning.

28th. Urine two pints; coagulates less, but becomes cloudy : two stools. Pulse 80, of good strength.

29th. Four tolerably healthy stools passed with a good deal of urine; two pints saved. Pulse 96. He finds the swelling increase towards night.

31st. Urine does not coagulate.

January 1st. The swelling has a tendency to increase. Urine four pints in forty-eight hours; coagulates. Pulse active. Bowels freely open.

> Mittatur sanguis ad f℥x.
> Opii grſs bis die. Repetatur Mistura.

2nd. Much relieved in every respect. Urine three pints in sixteen hours; two stools; swelling diminished.

3rd. Urine three pints in sixteen hours; does not coagulate, but becomes rather milky by heat. He passed a good night, feels much more comfortable, and is less swollen. Pulse 72, rather weak. He says he is not at all thirsty, and avoids drinking as much as he can.

4th. Better in all respects. Urine in same quantity; does not coagulate at all.

5th. Pulse 88, moderate. Urine the same; does not coagulate: swellings diminished.

6th. Pulse 88, rather more sharp, but he thinks himself improving; always finds the left leg and thigh swell most. Urine one pint and a half, in the slightest possible degree milky by heat: one stool. He takes daily about one pint and a half of the mixture of supertartrate of potash.

7th. Urine *not in the least degree coagulable;* two pints in sixteen hours; other urine passed with three stools. Pulse 84, rather weak; swelling much diminished, very little œdema remains except in the left leg.—To have a mutton chop.

> Continuantur Medicamenta.

At this period of his disease, it appeared as if he were again rapidly approaching to a state of convalescence; but unfortunately, without any obvious cause, his disease took a less favourable turn ; his bowels became disordered; his urine in the course of two or three days became nearly as coagulable as ever: and in spite of a great variety of remedies, he still (April 5th) remains under my care, with all the symptoms of confirmed disorganization of the kidneys: a tendency to anasarcous effusion only moderated by the most constant attention, and a scanty flow of urine always decidedly coagulable, but varying a little from day to day.

CASE XVI.

MARY FITZGERALD, æt. about 30, was admitted under my care into Guy's Hospital, October 4th, 1826. Her usual employment was needle-work, and she had generally enjoyed good health. She considered herself quite well on going to-bed ten days ago, but when she rose on the following morning found her feet much swollen. Since that time the anasarcous swelling has extended over her whole body and face: her breath was very short at the time of admission, with frequent dry cough, particularly troublesome when in bed. Pulse 84, sharp: her general appearance bloated and leucophlegmatic. Urine scanty, *coagulating by heat.*

> Mittatur sanguis e brachio ad f℥x.
> ℞ Potassæ Supertart. ℥j,
> Aquæ destillat. ij℔ ;
> Fiat Mistur. quotidie sumenda.—Low diet.

5th. The blood has not separated very completely: the serum is quite transparent: face and legs less swollen; one dejection. Urine about a pint and a half; coagulates slightly, forming a permanent scum at the top when boiled. Cough very troublesome.

6th. Urine increased; swelling gradually subsiding.

9th. Urine copious. Bowels regular; swelling subsiding.

13th. Complains of an acute pain in the left side below the ribs, running backwards, which has now continued for forty-eight hours.

> Applicentur Cucurbitulæ cruentæ parti dolenti, et detrahatur sanguis ad f℥xij.
> Rep. Medicamenta.

16th. Swelling entirely gone. Pulse 80, of good strength. Urine copious. Skin perspirable. Bowels confined.

> Pulveris Jalapæ cum Potassæ Supertartrate ℈fs pro re nata.
> Repetatur Mistura Potassæ Supertartratis.

20th. Completely convalescent.—She went to the Convalescent ward, and was dismissed in a few days.

This was a very recent case of anasarca with albuminous urine. I employed general bleeding in the first instance, and then pursued the simple plan of saline diuretics and purgatives, because I had found such manifest advantage from the same plan in the first attack of this disease which RODERICK had experienced; the plan answered, I confess, beyond my most sanguine expectation.

CASE XVII.

FRANCIS FISH, æt. 26, was admitted under my care into Guy's Hospital, October 4th, 1826. He was a stout man, tall and well proportioned, who had been employed as a porter to a broker, and had often been occupied in beating feather-beds on the top of a house; and was consequently much exposed to changes from heat to cold. His general health had always been good; and according to his own account he had been a sober hard-working man, nor did his appearance lead to a contrary opinion.

About a month before his admission he felt feverish with headache; he took some remedy, which he believes was mercurial; was afterwards exposed to the air, and thinks he caught cold by that means. The night after the exposure or the same night he began to swell, and this he first observed in the legs and the scrotum; the swelling went on increasing; and at the time of his admission he was greatly swollen in every part, particularly his thighs and legs; and the cellular tissue of the abdomen was quite filled with fluid, as was that of the scrotum. Pulse 110, rather sharp: bowels relaxed: slight cough. I could not learn the quantity of the urine passed; but what I saw was very high coloured, *coagulating* by exposure to heat more completely than I have almost ever seen; becoming nearly one white curdlike mass. There was nothing either in the countenance or the symptoms which pointed out the least hepatic derangement.

Mittatur sanguis ad f℥x.—Low diet.

5th. Blood neither cupped nor buffed, serum milky. Urine one pint and a quarter, of a turbid yellow sandlike colour. Bowels not open. Pulse 80, of good strength: swelling unaltered.

℞ Potassæ Supertartratis ℥j,

Aquæ puræ ℔ij.

Misce et sumat quotidie pro potu.

6th. Reports that he has passed considerably more urine: one lax stool. Anasarca slightly diminished. Pulse 96, rather sharp.

9th. Urine nine pints in the last forty-eight hours, besides some passed with his stools: four or five relaxed dejections daily. Urine high coloured, clear; coagulates much less, but still becomes milky on exposure to heat. Thighs reduced one inch and a half in circumference, the calf of the leg the same. Abdomen so much smaller that his waistband nearly meets. Pulse 80, natural.

11th. Urine high coloured: bowels open. He continues to improve.

13th. Very little œdema left in the thighs; legs also diminished. Urine five pints in twenty-four hours, besides what passed with stools; high coloured: scarcely in the slightest degree coagulable by heat. Pulse 80. Bowels costive.

Habeat Pulveris Jalapæ cum Potassæ Supertart. ʒſs statim.
Continuatur Mistura.

16th. Urine diminished, though still copious. Pulse 96. He speaks of a sense of uneasiness, though inconsiderable, in the loins.

Applicentur Cucurb. cruent. regioni Lumborum et detrahatur sanguis ad f℥x.
℞ Pulv. Uvæ Ursi gr. x,
Sodæ Subcarbon. gr. x,
Pulv. Conii gr. ij ; fiat pulvis ter die sumendus.
Repetatur Mistura.

20th. No swelling remains except at the ankles and insteps. Urine about four pints in twenty-four hours, high coloured; does not coagulate at all. Bowels rather confined. Perspires a good deal at night; appears weakened.

Repetatur Pulvis purgans et continuantur Medicamenta.—Middle diet.

23rd. Urine red-coloured from slight admixture of blood. Anasarca almost completely gone, very slight about the feet. Skin perspirable. Urine throws up a slight frothy scum on boiling, which remains ; four pints in seventeen hours.

Omittatur Pulvis ex Uva Ursi, Soda, et Conio ; et Rep. Mistura.

26th. Urine about five pints in twelve hours, rather less red: bowels inclined to be costive.
℞ Potass. Supertart. ℥ſs,
Aquæ puræ ℔j fiat Mistura quotidie sumenda.
Habeat Infusum Cascarillæ cum Tinct. Cascarillæ. ter die.
Haust. Sennæ mane quotidie.

30th. Pulse natural. Very slight swelling occasionally observed at the ankles. Urine five pints in fourteen hours, brownish. Complains of cough, but looks well.

Linctus Opiatus pro re nata, et Rep.

November 6th. No remains of œdema. Urine very copious, still of a dusky colour, coagulates considerably ; three pints in sixteen hours. Pulse 106, compressible. Still some cough.
℞ Potass. Supertart. ʒij.
Aquæ puræ ℔ſs fiat Mistura quotidie sumenda.
Applicetur Emplast. Cantharidis Lumbis, et Repetantur alia.

8th. The blister, which was only to be kept on till it rose and then immediately removed, remained on about ten hours, rose well, and discharged. Urine copious, of a dark colour, coagulable. No stool yesterday : has perspired freely.

Haust. Sennæ et Rep.

10th. Has been sick at the stomach. Slight tenderness at the pit of the stomach. Urine high coloured. Pulse quick.

> ℞ Antimonii tartarizati gr. ¼,
> Opii contriti gr. j,
> Theriacæ q. s.
> Fiat pilula bis quotidie sumenda.
> Decoct. Lini pro potu.
> Applicetur Cataplasma Lini lumbis.

13th. Complains of sickness and vomiting every morning between nine and ten o'clock: this does not return during the day, but he sometimes experiences slight nausea. Bowels costive. Urine as before. Tongue moist, rather red. The cataplasm is still applied; but he denies having any internal pain in the loins.

> Olei Ricini f℥ſs hora somni omni nocte
> Pil. Saponis cum Opio ter die.

16th. Much relieved; stomach is nearly well. Urine less brown, but still coagulates.

17th. Urine five pints in fourteen hours. He is still hoarse, and appears to be losing flesh; frequently complains of hunger.

> Sulph. Quininæ gr. j ter die.
> et Rep. Pil. Saponis cum Opio.

20th. Very slight coagulation in the urine.

> Rep. Sulph. Quininæ et Pil. Saponis cum Opio omni nocte.

24th. Urine four pints in fifteen hours. Pulse 100, moderate. Still coughs a little, but does not seem to suffer from it.

27th. Urine dingy, in sufficient quantity; still shows a slight flocculent coagulum on the application of heat.

> Julep. Acidi nitrici ℔ſs quotidie.

December 1st. Urine scarcely coagulates at all, still of a reddish colour. He complains of nothing but a frequent desire to pass his water.

3rd. Appears perfectly well. His urine of a natural colour as nearly as possible.— In a few days he left the hospital.

This was a case of anasarca in which there was not the slightest evidence of any internal organ except the kidney being deranged. The origin of the disease was pretty plainly traced to exposure to atmospheric changes; the cure was effected by a simple and nearly undeviating plan, in which I was led from experience to have placed some confidence. Moderate bleeding and a low diet, with the administration of saline diuretics, increased the daily flow of urine from a pint and a quarter to four pints and a half, before the plan had been five days adopted. The coagulable nature of the urine likewise diminished, and the swelling subsided rapidly. At the end of about ten days more, obvious symptoms of renal irritation showed themselves: which might indeed have arisen from the continuance of the diuretic treatment; but I was induced to view it rather as a natural variation of symptoms, seeing that in a great majority of the cases which I had lately witnessed, hæmaturia was present in a greater or less degree. The blister which was applied on the 6th, under a hope that the external irritation might produce a favourable change in the action of the kidneys, increased the irritation, and the stomach sympathized strongly. This temporary irritation yielded to demulcents and opium. The kidneys were still decidedly deranged in their action; the quantity of urine passed was rather in excess; and the loss of flesh, together with the unusual hunger experienced, gave some room for drawing an analogy between the present state of the disease and *diabetes insipidus*. I thought it probable that in this state of things, tonics combined with opiates might do much; the sulphate of quinine was used with advantage, but afterwards the nitric acid seemed to exert a still better influence.

In two months after his first admission he was so far cured as to have no evidence of disease remaining, and four months have now passed (April) without any recurrence of symptoms. I do not however feel at all sanguine that he will be free from relapse; for I see no reason to doubt that at one period his kidneys were in a condition exactly analogous to that of EVANS, and possibly, as in that case, the white granular deposit had already in some degree taken place.

CASE XVIII.

WILLIAM BROOKS, æt. 57, was admitted under my care into Guy's Hospital, October 25th, 1816. He was a sawyer, habitually healthy. About six weeks ago he perceived his ankles swell; and this has gradually increased: the whole thighs and scrotum are now œdematous; and this to such an extent, for the last fortnight, that he has been prevented from working. Slight tenderness at the pit of the stomach. Urine reported not very scanty. (Low diet.)

℞ Potassæ Supertartratis ℥j,
　　Aquæ puræ ℔ij.

Fiat Mistura pro potu.

Sumat Pulveris ex Jalapa et Potass. Supertartrate ℈j statim.

26th. Pulse 48, somewhat labouring; much pain in the forehead, particularly in the right temple; occasional giddiness: lies down well in bed. Urine one pint and a quarter, of a *dingy* colour, but clear; *coagulates by heat.*

27th. Urine much the same; complains of pain in the stomach and bowels: the bowels confined.

℞ Ol. Ricini f℥ſs,
　　Tinct. Rhei f℥ij,
　　Aquæ Menth. pip. f℥vj. M.

Fiat haustus statim sumendus.

29th. Repetatur Mistura pro potu.

30th. The drink disagrees with the stomach. Pulse 58. Urine one pint and a quarter.

Mittatur sanguis ad f℥viij.

℞ Liquoris Ammon. Acet. et Aquæ Menth. viridis āā f℥vj,
　　Spirit. Ætheris nitrici f℥ſs,
　　Acet. Scillæ ♏ xx,
　　Spir. Armoraciæ Comp. f℥ſs.

M. fiat haustus sexta quaque hora sumendus.

Habeat Pulveris Jalap. cum Potass. Supertartrate ℥ſs.

31st. Coagulum of blood small, not firm: serum turbid. Pulse 60. Urine unaltered; feels somewhat relieved.

November 3rd. Urine two pints and a half; colour more natural; coagulates much less: frequently complains of pain in the head with some noise and confusion. Pulse 72, strong. Bowels confined.

Applicetur Empl. Cantharidis Nuchæ.

Habeat Pulver. Jalap. cum Potass. Supertartrate ℈ij.

5th. A good deal oppressed, and complains of headache.

Rep. haustus tertia quaque hora.

6th. Still complains of noise in the head and deafness on the left side. Pulse 64, full; anasarca of limbs rather increased. Urine two pints in fourteen hours, clear, and of good colour.

Infus. Spartii scopar. pro potu, et repetantur Medicamenta.

8th. Has taken about one pint and a half of the infusion; considerably relieved;

rests better : head less painful. Urine quite clear, three pints in eighteen hours ; co-agulable, becoming milky by heat.

10th. Urine above four pints, healthy in appearance. Pulse 74, strong. Head much relieved, feels better, but the œdema remains. He mentioned to-day for the first time, that he has occasionally felt palpitation of the heart while at work, and the action of the heart seems to be labouring.

11th. Feels much relieved : takes his medicine every three hours, and from one pint to one pint and a half of the infusion daily. Urine abundant; coagulates less. Bowels regular.

13th. The thighs are reduced five inches in circumference. Urine four pints in sixteen hours, rather dingy.

17th. Continues to take the mixture every three hours, and a pint of the infusion daily : the œdema is subsiding. Urine about three pints and a half; coagulates much less, and is nearly natural in colour.

20th. Complains much of a short cough.

Linctus opiatus cum Vino Ipecacuanhæ pro re nata. Repetantur Medicamenta.

24th. By a mistake of the nurse he has been taking a grain of Calomel and half a grain of Opium, night and morning for the last three days; and I now find him completely salivated, although I had stated my resolution of giving him no mercury. He has passed very little urine for the last two days ; none during the last night : it coagulates as much as at first. Pulse 96, strong.

Habeat Julepi Acidi nitrici ℔fs cum Tinct. Opii fʒfs, pro Gargarismate.
Sumat Pulv. Jalap. cum Potassæ Supertartrate Əij statim, et Rep. Medicamenta.

25th. Urine one pint in eighteen hours, coagulates strongly : two or three stools.
27th. He has not resumed the infusion or the mixture. The swelling has not returned; but the urine is scanty and coagulable. Ptyalism subsiding.

Habeat Infusum Spartii scoparii pro potu.

28th. Urine about one pint and a half since last night with ropy sediment. He has only taken the infusion once.

Dec. 1st. Urine less than one pint in twenty-four hours. Pulse 96, small but rather sharp.

Infus. Juniper. cum Potass. Acet. ʒj, et Sp. Armoraciæ comp. fʒj, sexta quaque hora.
Fotus Papaveris regioni lumborum.

2nd. Rather improved in appearance and feelings. Urine still very scanty ; no swelling of the legs. Fomentation not used.

4th. Urine one pint in sixteen hours. Ptyalism not yet subsided.

5th. Two stools in the night. He was seized suddenly yesterday evening with

most violent pain in the loins, which still continues in some degree.   Urine about one
pint and a half; coagulates.   Cough constant, as from some obstruction about the
throat.

> Infricetur Liniment. Terebinthinæ Lumbis.
> Applicetur Emplast. Cantharidis Gutturi.
> Olei Ricini f℥fs cum Tinctura Opii ♏ vij statim, et Rep. Medicamenta.

6th. Blister not applied, but he feels better.

> Rep. Oleum Ricini cum Tinctura Opii, et Medicamenta alia.
> Applicetur Emplastrum.

7th. Improved.   Urine three quarters of a pint.   One stool.

> Rep. Ol. Ricini cum Tinctura Opii.

8th. Much improved in general health.   Urine three quarters of a pint, and forms
a copious flaky coagulum by heat.

> Infus. Lini pro potu, et Repetantur alia.

11th. Pulse 80, moderate.   He is quite recovered from the effects of the mercury.
Urine about one pint and a half, turbid, becomes clear by heat, and does not coagulate.
He takes about one pint of linseed tea daily.—(Mutton chop.)

15th. The urine saved, two pints and a half; and nearly an equal quantity is said to
have been passed with his dejections : it is clear, and coagulates a little.   Very slight
œdema may still be discovered about the instep.

> Adde Infuso Lini ℔j, Sodæ Subcarbon. ʒfs.
> Rep. Medicamenta.

18th. In the evening he felt much oppressed in his breathing, and said he almost
lost his senses.

> Mittatur sanguis ad f℥viij, et Rep. Medicamenta.

19th. The serum of the blood is turbid, and in large proportion : he felt relieved by
the loss of blood.   Pulse 72, rather labouring.   Urine about two pints and a half, perfectly clear, does not coagulate.   Complains of dulness in the head.

> Applicentur Cucurb. cruentæ inter scapulas, et detrahantur sanguinis f℥x.
> Rep. Medicamenta.

20th. A good deal relieved by cupping.   Pulse 84, rather labouring.   Urine two
pints and a half, quite clear.

> Rep. Medicamenta.

21st. Feels better.   Pulse 80, less labouring.   Urine light-coloured, but not quite
clear ; not coagulable : two pints saved, more has been passed.   Two dejections.

26th. Urine three pints in eighteen hours; *not the least coagulable.* Pulse 80, of good strength : appears quite well.

29th. (Middle diet.)

Jan. 1. Swelling returned a little at the ankles. Pulse 84, rather labouring. Urine three pints in eighteen hours; still does not coagulate. Appetite good, and in all other respects he appears well.

> Mittatur sanguis ad f$\mathfrak{Z}$x.
> Omit. Medicamenta, sed Rep. Oleum Ricini pro re nata.

2nd. Let rollers be applied to the legs. Serum of the blood milky.

5th. Urine not the least coagulable, clear, and in sufficient quantity. No complaint.

7th. Urine clear, light-yellow, two pints and a half since last night, not the least coagulable.

This was a case of anasarca with coagulable urine having all its characters well marked. There was no evidence either of hepatic disease or of derangement in the structure of the heart or lungs ; but the urine loaded with red particles seemed to bespeak decided renal affection. I attempted in this case to adopt the plan which had proved successful in the two last cases ; but the stomach would not bear the quantity of saline fluid, and I was obliged to have recourse to other diuretic combinations, which acted very favourably. It was necessary to pay attention to the bowels ; and symptoms of local congestion more particularly in the head, rendered it a matter of security at least to take away blood occasionally. I had purposely abstained from the employment of mercury ; and its accidental exhibition was undoubtedly attended by injurious consequences at the time, as will be immediately seen by a comparison of the reports just preceding the 20th of November, with those of the following days. How far it was ultimately beneficial or injurious, is still a matter well worthy of consideration. The fact that this was a successful case, is at least sufficiently important to induce us to hesitate in denying any salutary efficacy to the mercury. Although the improvement had begun in the coagulable quality of the urine before the mercury was taken by mistake, and that morbid state did manifestly increase greatly during the mercurial action; yet when the salivation subsided, his condition did not appear to be worse than it was before, and we find the symptoms yielding rather easily to the different diuretics which were then administered. In this stage of the disease, at the beginning of December, it appeared to me that he derived great relief from the use of the turpentine liniment rubbed morning and night upon his loins. It was not however till the 11th of December, when the sensible effects of the mercury had subsided, that the quantity of urine began to increase, and its tendency to coagulate gradually to cease.

CASE XIX.

Robert Spooner was admitted into Guy's Hospital, under the care of Dr. Back, November 29th, 1826, in a state of general anasarca; he was a stout-looking man, aged 50; and having been employed as a pewterer, was in that occupation a good deal in the habit of being exposed to the heat of fires. A fortnight before his admission he was apparently in perfect health; at that time he first found his legs to swell. After three days he began to take some pills and draughts, which he continued till his admission; and after taking them about eight days he found his mouth become sore; he observed his urine to be dingy and brown in colour about the same time. The quantity of urine has not increased; it is about a pint and a half in twenty-four hours, coagulating by heat. Pulse full.

> Mittatur sanguis ad f℥xvj.
> ℞ Pulv. Jalapæ gr. xx,
>   Hydrarg. Submuriat. gr. v. statim sumendus.
> Habeat Solutionis Potas. Supertartrat. ℔j quotidie.
> Pil. Scill. comp. gr. v cum Hydr. Oxyd. ciner. gr. ſs, omni nocte.

Nov. 30th. Bleeding relieved him. Urine not increased, but swelling diminished.

December 1. In the afternoon was seized with great dyspnœa, with a full throbbing pulse.

> Mittatur sanguis ad f℥xij.
> Sumat Pil. Conii gr. v cum Pulv. Digital. gr. j, quarta quaque hora ex Julepo Oxymellis.

Four hours afterwards, the symptoms being but little relieved and the blood highly buffed,

> Repetatur detractio sanguinis ad f℥xvj.

2nd. Much relieved by the last bleeding; the blood not buffed. To-day he appears much reduced in strength; breathes with great difficulty; looks pallid. Urine dingy, coagulating by heat.

> Pulver. Jalap. cum Hydrarg. Əj statim.
> Rep. Medicamenta.

3rd. Still complains of some difficulty of breathing. Pulse rather sharp. Urine of a lighter colour.

> Applicetur Emplast. Cantharidis Sterno.

4th. He seems improved, the swelling being diminished, as well as the difficulty in lying down. The urine rather more copious; still dingy; coagulates by heat, rising from the sides of the spoon in dense clouds. Pulse quick, and rather sharp.

5th. Urine of a florid blood colour. His countenance is pallid, and his face puffy.

> Repetantur Pulv. purgans, et Medicamenta alia.

8th. The œdema still remains, both in the face and the legs, and slightly in the hands. Pulse full and frequent; he feels, however, generally improved; passes more urine, and is less swollen.

9th. Urine more scanty than for three or four days; about thirteen ounces in twenty-four hours; reddish brown, from the admixture of red particles, some of which gradually subside to the bottom of the vessel; coagulates into a completely curdled fluid by heat. Complains of no pain.

> Sumat Pulv. Jalap. cum Calomel. gr. xv quotidie mane.
> Misturæ Potas. Supertartrat. ℔j quotidie.
> Pil. Scillæ cum Hydrarg. omni nocte.

12th. Urine about a pint and a half in twenty-four hours, very highly charged with red particles. He complains of a sense of load and oppression about the pit of the stomach. Pulse rather full and sharp, swelling much diminished. He has no pain on pressure of any part.

> Mittatur sanguis ad f℥xij.

14th. Swelling much diminished. Blood not buffed. Urine still dark coloured. Altogether greatly relieved, but complains of his mouth being sore.

15th. Much reduced in size. Urine of a dark red, very coagulable.

16th. Mouth very sore.

> Perstet in usu Misturæ; Habeat Pulv. Jalap. cum Potassæ Supertart. Əij mane
> quotidie, et Pilul. Scillæ comp. gr. xij cum Opii gr. j, omni nocte.

17th. Swelling much reduced. Pulse sharp.

25th. Mouth nearly well; swelling much subsided. Urine still very coagulable and dingy.

January 3rd. In all respects improved, passes a good quantity of urine; now scarcely dingy in its colour, and coagulating very slightly. Countenance still pallid and swollen. Pulse a little sharp.

7th. Urine nearly clear, of a slightly pink cast from a few red particles; scarcely coagulates, becoming rather milky by heat.

13th. Decidedly improving from day to day.

22nd. Urine of a dingy colour, coagulating slightly by heat; he appears nearly free from complaint.

February 7th. Left the Hospital nearly well: still however the legs were slightly œdematous, pitting on pressure, particularly along the shin bones. Urine in natural quantity, pale, of a dingy colour; having by no means the natural bright appearance. Pulse 96, sharp.

In this case the disease of which I have been speaking was marked by all its symptoms, and there can be no doubt that the inflammatory tendency, which is so strong a feature in the complaint, would have proved destructive, but for the active depletion which was put in force. Whether we are to ascribe the improvement which took place, both in the quantity and the quality of the urine, to the mercurial action induced, or to the continued exhibition of saline diuretics, it is no easy matter to decide.

CASE XX.

William Todd, æt. 28, a printer, was admitted into the Clinical ward of Guy's Hospital November 15th, 1826, under the care of Dr. Cholmeley, labouring under anasarca with some effusion into the abdomen. He stated that he had been out of employment for the last six months, and had been subjected to many privations both of food and clothing; for about a month had suffered from a cold, and for a fortnight past had found his legs and ankles swell without any pain; the swelling gradually became worse, and the week before his admission he observed his abdomen to swell towards the evening, and when he rose in the morning his head and face were swollen; at the same time a cough and difficulty of breathing, particularly on walking up stairs, came on, and tightness at the pit of the stomach. He complains of thirst, but has always had a good appetite: he makes but little urine, which is high coloured. Bowels regular. Pulse 72, small. Tongue natural. He says that he has never been in the habit of drinking either spirits or porter. The urine in this case was very scanty, and coagulated so as to look almost like water-gruel by exposure to heat. He was cupped at the pit of the stomach, and put upon the frequent use of the extract of elaterium, with the effect of purging him very freely. He took a combination of squills, mercury and opium, every night; he occasionally had recourse to combinations of jalap and gamboge, and various other purgatives. He took the infusion of juniper-berries for drink, and sometimes small doses of digitalis in the form of powder or of tincture. Under this treatment at first the urine increased, and shortly even exceeded the natural quantity; but it became of a dark coffee colour, frequently depositing a considerable brown sediment.

December 8th. Leeches applied to his temples. On the 12th eight ounces of blood were taken by cupping from the neck, and on the 14th the same quantity from the arm. The progress made was very slow, and from the first he constantly complained of severe headache. At the beginning of January his mouth had become completely affected by mercury, given in the form of calomel combined with conium and opium.

January 2nd. Feels very unwell, complains much of headache; his mouth is sore, the glands of the neck swollen; the countenance pallid; his ankles swell towards evening. Urine very high coloured, with a copious brown sediment. Pulse 102, with considerable action. He is thirsty.

> Habeat Julep. Potassæ Acetat. ter die.
> Omit. Hydr. Submuriat.

3rd. Mouth and gums very sore; cheeks swollen. Headache; bowels inclined to be costive. Pulse 96, soft.

> Infus. Rosæ cum Magnes. Sulphat. ter die.
> R Extr. Hyoscyami gr. v,
>   Pulveris Ipecac. gr. j ;
> Fiant Pilulæ ij ter quotidie sumendæ.

4th. Face swollen; mouth sore. Pulse 116 : one scanty dejection. Urine very dark, with coffee ground sediment.

> Applicetur Emplastrum Cantharidis Nuchæ.
> Gargar. Argenti Nitrat.
> Rep. Medicamenta.

5th. No dejection. Face swollen; mouth very sore. Urine the same : much headache.

> Olei Ricini fʒj statim.

6th. Much salivation; four or five dejections.

7th. Face continues swollen. Mouth very sore. No dejection; skin hot. Urine less turbid.

> Sumat Spir. Æther. nitr. ℳxxx, ex Julepo Ammoniæ Acetat. sexta quaque hora.
>   Pulver. Ipecacuanhæ comp. gr. x omni nocte.
>   Gargar. Acidi nitrici.
> Pulv. Jalap. comp. ʒj statim.

9th. Pulse very quick; looks pale. Urine still has a thick brown deposit; two bilious dejections; spits very much. Legs do not swell; face still swollen.

-129-

℞ Decoct. Uvæ Ursi,
　　　Infus. Rosæ, āā, f℥j ;
Misce, fiat haustus ter die sumendus.
　　　Pulver. Jalap. comp. ʒj, alternis auroris.

16th. The flow of saliva diminished, but he cannot yet put out his tongue. One pale dejection. Urine lighter coloured, increased in quantity. Pulse 90, with considerable action; gets no sleep at night. He continued this form of medicine, with occasional purgatives, till the 24th, with little alteration ; the urine being always dingy, and the face inclined to swell. He was then put upon the use of small doses of nitric acid ; leeches were applied two or three times to his temples with the effect of relieving the headache, and at the same time the combination of compound extract of colocynth with a grain of ipecacuanha, was given two or three times a day, to keep up a regular action on the bowels.

February 9th. Feels rather better : bowels open. Tongue whitish. Pulse 90, sharp. Urine six pints in the twenty-four hours, clear and without sediment. As there had been manifest deficiency in the secretion of the skin, the warm bath was tried two or three times, but it increased the tendency to headache.

19th. Much headache. Tongue rather white, but moist. Pulse 106, sharp ; one dejection, deficient in bile. Urine about five pints, lighter in colour.

　　　Pil. Hydrarg. gr. v omni nocte, et Rep. Medicamenta.

24th. The legs still swell towards night; the face a little swollen. Urine with slight deposit. One copious dejection.

℞ Pulv. Conii gr. iij,
　　— Uvæ Ursi Əj, ter die.
　　Omitt. Pilul. Hydrarg.

The exact period at which the urine ceased to be coagulable, I cannot with certainty mention, but about this time the fact was observed ; and while continuing the use of this form of remedy, a seton having also been inserted into his neck, and a mixture with the balsam of Peru added to his other medicines, he gradually became better. On the 9th of March he was cupped between the shoulders to twelve ounces, and on the 15th lost the same quantity of blood by cupping from the loins.

March 29th. Urine of good colour, quite clear, without any deposit. He feels tolerably well : one scanty clay-coloured dejection ; no swelling of the legs.

30th. Two darker coloured figured dejections; feels pretty well : appetite indifferent. Urine copious, of good colour.

April 4th. He left the Clinical ward, and was sent in a comparatively healthy state into another ward, but still complained much of headache, and his countenance was pallid. His urine apparently natural in all respects.

12th. At this time he is apparently free from complaint, except a slight occasional headache and a little tendency to quickness of pulse. He remains in the Hospital only because the seton in his neck is troublesome.

CASE XXI.

Eliza Plume, a single woman æt. 18, was admitted into the Clinical ward of Guy's Hospital, January 18th, 1827, affected with anasarca, more particularly showing itself in the legs, but likewise in the arms and face. She had at the same time some swelling of the abdomen, and a troublesome hard cough. Pulse sharp. Tongue whitish. Bowels natural. Urine in tolerable quantity. She had never menstruated. It appears that her complaint first came on after exposure to cold and wet, about four months previously to her admission, the swelling beginning in the feet and legs, and gradually extending.

Applicentur Cucurbitulæ cruentæ Scrobiculo Cordis, et detrahatur sanguis ad f℥xiv.

℞ Pilul. Scillæ comp. gr. iv,
Hydrarg. Oxyd. cinerei gr. ſs,
Pulver. fol. Digitalis gr. j,
Extracti Conii gr. iv.

Contunde ut fiant pilulæ ter quotidie sumendæ.

Habeat Mistur. Camphoræ, cum Liquore Ammoniæ Acetat. singul. dosib. pilularum.

She continued the use of these medicines, with the addition of ten drops of the tincture of digitalis to each dose of the mixture and half a grain of opium at bed-time, till the 5th of February. It was not till after she had been ten days in the Hospital that any examination was made of her urine: it was then found to be moderate in quantity, dingy in colour, and coagulable by the application of heat. On the whole, amendment took place under this plan of treatment; slight changes occurred, and on one occasion the urine was observed not to coagulate by heat. Once or twice moderate bleedings were had recourse to when the pulse was sharp. After the 5th of February the mercury was discontinued. About this time the urine did not coagulate, and was increased to four pints in twenty-four hours. On the 17th of February the urine still coagulated decidedly by heat.

℞ Pulveris Conii gr. iij,
Pulveris Uvæ Ursi ℈j.

Fiat pulvis ter die sumendus.

February 27th. Feels much the same. Urine less copious, rather lighter coloured. Tongue white as usual. Pulse 100. Bowels open.

℞ Liquor. Antimonii tartarizat. fʒj, sexta quaque hora, ex Julepo Menthæ.

28th. Eyes nearly concealed by œdema of the eyelids. Pulse 88, rather sharp; perspires pretty freely.

March 5th. The tartarized antimony occasionally makes her sick.

Infricetur Linimentum Terebinth. abdomini, et Rep. Medicamenta.

7th.   Admoveatur Emplast. Picis Burgund. lumbis.

12th. Legs somewhat œdematous; right arm very much so. Pulse 96, sharp. Urine in quantity as usual, coagulates by heat and becomes like almond emulsion. The skin not generally perspirable.

Mist. Balsam. Peruvian. quarta quaque hora.
Continuatur Linimentum.

14th. Rather more swelling about the legs and abdomen.

Applicentur Cucurb. cruent. regioni Lumbor. et detrahantur sanguinis fℨxij.

15th. Limbs much less swollen; feels more comfortable. One liquid dejection. Urine unaltered.

26th. Right arm nearly returned to its natural size.

Pilul. Aloes cum Myrrh. gr. x, omni nocte.

27th. Increased flow of tears with œdema of eyelids ; face also a little swollen.

Applicentur Cucurb. cruentæ nuchæ, et detrahatur sanguis ad fℨxiv.
℞ Infus. Sennæ fℨiſs,
Potas. Tartar. ʒij.
Fiat Haustus semel vel bis quotidie sumendus.

28th. Some relief from the cupping. Eyelids much more comfortable, but still œdematous. Three dejections.

℞ Pil. Scillæ Comp. gr. x,
Extracti Hyoscyam. gr. iv, omni nocte.
Repetatur Haustus.

29th. All œdema gone from the eyelids. Urine in usual quantity. Pulse 104. Bowels open ;—feels better.

April 4th. Legs still a little swollen. Bowels open ; and she feels comfortable.

Misturæ Potas. Supertart. ℔bjſs, quotidie,
Rep. Pilul. omni nocte.

14th. Feels comfortably, and continues to pass a tolerably natural quantity of urine; it is of a light whey-colour, but slightly dingy; becomes milky on the application of heat, and forms a great quantity of white flakes. Legs still swollen, and rather hard; her face has a tendency to swell, and her pulse is quick.

This case still remains under treatment, and I mention it chiefly as being one of those to which Dr. Bostock has referred in his Observations on the State of the Urine. The disease had already existed four months before her admission; and although the symptoms of anasarca have always been mild, they have not yielded in a satisfactory manner. She is indeed greatly improved; but as long as the urine remains in so morbid a condition, we cannot but feel the daily probability of relapse. It is not unlikely that could the flow of the catamenia be regularly established, this might have a favourable effect in the disease.

CASE XXII.

In the month of February in the present year, when I was speaking to one of the physicians' pupils to the Hospital on the subject of albuminous urine, and was wishing to show the difference between the action of heat on this and on healthy urine, I requested him to bring me a specimen of the ordinary fluid from any of the patients around,—To my surprise the specimen he brought *coagulated most decidedly by heat.* This led me immediately to examine the patient: he was a boy of the name of HOBSON, about 14 years of age, who had been for three years the subject of a most manifest enlargement of the liver, the bulk of which now distended his abdomen; and its margin was distinctly to be felt below the umbilicus, and extending far towards the left side. His general aspect was pallid and unhealthy, and there was evidence of some chronic disease of the heart, the origin of which could be traced to rheumatism, of which he had experienced a very severe and protracted attack when ten years of age. On questioning him more particularly, it appeared that he had formerly, when a patient in another Hospital, passed blood in his urine, and had experienced some pain occasionally in his loins. The urine was now perfectly clear, and rather light coloured, but nothing could be more marked than its property of coagulating. I did not hesitate to predict that we should find some obvious organic change in the kidney, connected with this morbid condition of its secretion. Towards the middle of March he had rheumatic swellings in the joints; the urine became very dingy, apparently from the admixture of red particles; and a short time afterwards, symptoms of inflammation of the heart and of the pleura came on,—and he died. As I could not be present at the examination, I requested most particularly that the kidneys, the heart, and a part of the liver might be preserved for my inspection; which was done: so that I was enabled to have excellent drawings made of them all;—and I am obliged to Dr. Hodgkin for the following particular account of the appearances.

Sectio Cadaveris.—March 25th.

"The body exhibited no signs of puberty. The head was not opened. The pleura on the right side was adherent, especially laterally and towards the lower part, by means of a false membrane of rather recent date; it was soft and rather bloody, with somewhat of a honeycomb appearance. At the upper part and between the lobes the inflammation appeared to have been still more recent. There was some bloody serous effusion, but nothing puriform. The adhesions on the left were equally general, but much slighter; on this side also they seemed to have been of different ages. The substance of the lungs was free from adventitious deposit, was not more bloody than usual, and if a little too firm in some parts, the cells were somewhat dilated in others. The heart was a little enlarged; there was very little serous effusion into the pericardium, but both of the secreting surfaces of this membrane were doubled by an adventitious layer of about the thickness of an old shilling, having considerable firmness, and a very remarkable hirsute or scabrous surface, somewhat like that of an ox tongue. There were besides bridles of adhesion of about an inch in length, but slender and scabrous. The valves were healthy, and the parietes of their natural thickness. There was a small quantity of straw-coloured clear serum in the peritoneal cavity, and some traces of recent inflammation on the convex surface of the liver, and old adhesion between the omentum, liver, and spleen. The omentum was contracted and drawn upwards. There was nothing remarkable in the mucous membrane of the stomach or of the greater part of the upper portion of the small intestines; but that of the ilium, though free from ulceration or follicular disease, was minutely injected and of a purple colour, and was readily separated from the subjacent coats. That of the colon was nearly in the same state. The surface of the liver was generally smooth, but there were one or two unusual depressions in it. This organ was so large as nearly to reach to the crista of the ilium, and to the left it extended even beyond the spleen, which it overhung. About where the left lobe usually terminates there was a pretty deep notch, beyond which the substance of the liver was continued by a portion equal in size to the left lobe in its ordinary state. The liver was of a light yellowish colour throughout. The posterior part was firm and almost cartilaginous, having a peculiar translucency, and an unnatural uniformity of structure with little or no appearance of acini. In the neighbourhood of the indurated parts the acini were small, but in the greater part of the liver they were much enlarged; and though themselves indurated, were but feebly connected together. The gall-bladder was pretty full of light-green bile. The spleen was about three times its usual size, but of pretty healthy structure. The pancreas was large, white, firm, or even hard. The KIDNEYS were complete specimens of a white mottling degeneration. The deposit which chiefly affected the cortical part, was collected in large granulations."—To this minute statement of the dissection, I may add, that this kidney approached a good deal in external appearance to that of SALLAWAY (Case III.); but on minute inspection it was obvious that the whole was strewed with, or even composed of opake yellow bodies: and on macerating the kidney for a few days, this became still more evident,—so that the appearance of the macerated kidney differed very little from that of RICHARDSON (Case VI.), in which case the granulated condition was remarkably illustrated.

CASE XXIII.

WILLIAM HUNTER, æt. 47, was admitted into Guy's Hospital March 7, 1827, labouring under general anasarcous swelling. On the 14th my attention was first drawn to him when he was greatly swollen, more particularly his legs, and lay with difficulty on his left side. His face was puffy and pallid, his urine scanty, very dingy in colour and *coagulable* by heat. By trade he was a tailor; and although he said that he had always been temperate, and had indeed refrained from drinking because he had observed for the last two years that his water was often very scanty, and therefore feared some bad consequence from drinking much, yet he acknowledged that he had frequently taken a pot of porter and two or three glasses of rum in a day, and that occasionally he took gin instead of rum, with a view of promoting the flow of urine. He said he had occasionally experienced pain in his loins, and his bowels were habitually costive, but he had never observed any thing peculiar in his evacuations, nor had he ever been in the least jaundiced. He was first taken ill two days after Christmas, having been in difficulties in his business about that time and exposed much to wet. The first symptom he observed was the swelling of his legs, which increased so much that he was unable to walk or bend his knees; his hands, and more particularly his left hand, swelled very much.—He had taken medicine before his admission, and said that for about a fortnight his gums were rendered sore by the medicine he took;—he had derived no benefit from the treatment adopted.—When he came into the Hospital, it was understood that he had suffered from a fit, which had left one side much weaker than the other; and after he had been in the house about three weeks he had two fits somewhat of an epileptic character, which greatly impaired his mental powers. Blisters being applied between his shoulders, and a seton inserted in his neck, his reason returned after some days. The chief remedies employed with a view to his dropsical affection were mercurials, the action of which was maintained till his death. The swelling was decidedly reduced, and the urine for the few last days of his life was so little coagulable, that nothing of the kind was traced except in the frothy scum which was produced by boiling and remained after cooling; but he seemed to decline under the influence of mercury, and died on the 20th of April.

SECTIO CADAVERIS.—April 21st, 1827.

In the cavity of the chest a very considerable quantity of serum was effused,—at least four or five pints, of a light straw colour. The right lung adhered by rather long and not very recent adhesions to the pleura costalis. On the surface of the upper lobe several puckered parts were observed, beneath which, in one or two parts a gritty earthy deposit was found. In the lower lobe an abscess had formed with defined parietes, as from a single suppurating tubercle; yet the pus which it contained was of a greener colour than generally seen in tubercles, and in other respects seemed to differ from it. The whole substance of the lung was compressed by the effused fluid. The left lung was attached by slighter adhesions to the pleura costalis; in its substance not diseased, but in some parts considerably compressed by the fluid in the cavity, in other parts very œdematous. The heart firm in its structure; the left ventricle particularly thick and firm, and the columnæ carneæ thick and hard. The valves perfectly healthy. The aorta large. The quantity of serum in the pericardium was not precisely ascertained, owing to its making its escape; but there was evidently more than natural; the cellular substance towards the apex of the heart was filled with œdematous effusion, and the whole of both portions of the pericardium covered with a thin coating of coagulable matter, forming a villous membrane easily detached. The liver in its first appearance healthy, except from some part of the peritoneum being thickened by old inflammation: on narrow inspection it became obvious that the whole organ was composed of acini rather larger and more pale than natural, held together by the red connecting substance. The gall-bladder was moderately full of a very imperfect bile, of a turbid orange or saffron colour. The intestines appeared healthy; the bladder was full of urine of a light straw colour, which did not coagulate by heat; but when boiled in a spoon formed a permanent scum upon the surface. The KIDNEYS were both of them decidedly diseased, the whole cortical part presenting the granulated structure of which I have so often spoken; it was by no means in its most advanced state. The kidneys were of a natural size, rather flaccid, but tough to the feel, the granulated texture was not strongly, yet quite distinctly, marked on their surface. In the pelvis of the right kidney, which was considerably the smaller of the two, a great number, not less than a couple of hundred of exceedingly minute calculi like millet seeds, of a yellow colour, were found. The brain was unusually free from vascularity, looking externally blanched, and this appearance was very remarkable at the base. The ventricles rather distended with fluid; and the membrane lining the ventricles, more particularly the right, was rendered rough by very minute villi, as from some process of inflammation, not unlike what occurs on the pericardium.

In this case we again observe an illustration of many circumstances attending anasarca with coagulable urine :—the slight derangement of the liver, the marked disease of the kidneys, and the tendency to insidious inflammatory affection of the serous membranes, betrayed not only in the pericardium but in the lining membrane of the ventricles of the brain.

CASE XV.

(Continued from page 42.)

January 9th. Awoke last night about 12 o'clock with vomiting and purging, but it subsided in a few hours.

10th. The same attack returned during the last night, and the purging continues. Urine much diminished, coagulating strongly.

> Omit. Mist. Potassæ Supertart.
> Sumat Pulveris Opii gfs bis die, et
> Confect. Opiat. gr. vj ex Mist. Camphor. sexta quaque hora.

12th. Much purged yesterday, but more quiet to-day. Pulse weak, swelling considerably diminished. Urine high coloured and yellow, very coagulable.

In the further progress of this case several changes were made in the remedies employed. On the 29th he was bled, on account of an increased sharpness observable in the pulse, though he always denied having any local pain; the blood was highly cupped and buffed; he felt somewhat relieved, but no alteration was made in the quantity or quality of the urine. The nausea which he often experienced, suggested to me the probability that relief would be derived from a free evacuation of the stomach, and accordingly he took emetics two or three days in succession, but with no particular relief. The *Uva Ursi* proved equally inefficacious. I again returned to the use of the mixture of supertartrate of potash, and the soap and opium pill twice a day; and under these remedies about the first week of February the urine again lost in some degree its coagulable property, and there appeared to be some improvement in his symptoms generally :—but this change, like the rest, was only for a time.

February 14th. One stool. Urine about one pint and a half; still coagulates.

> Habeat Infusi Spartii scoparii ℔jfs quotidie
> ℞ Oxymellis Scillæ f℥ij,
>   Potassæ Supertartrat. contritæ ℥iij.
> Misce sumat Cochl. min. ij pro re nata.

16th. Urine about two pints, coagulates. Three stools. Pulse 76, soft and natural.
17th. Urine not increased; coagulates. Swelling remains nearly the same, feels comfortable because the bowels are freely open.

> Adde Acidi nitrici f℥fs ad ℔ij Infusi Spartii.
> Extracti Conii gr. v, quarta quaque hora.
> Rep. Electuarium Scillæ.

22nd. Pulse 96, rather sharp. Swelling increased. Three or four stools.
25th. Pulse 84. Swelling increases. Urine as before; coagulates.

> Applicentur Cucurbitulæ cruentæ Lumbis, et detrahatur sanguis ad f℥xij.

26th. The swelling increases. Urine as before; coagulates. Pulse 84.

> ℞ Potassæ Supertart. ℥fs,
>   Aquæ puræ f℥x. M. sit pro potu.
>   Rep. Electuarium Scillæ.
>   Infricetur Linimentum Terebinthinæ abdomini nocte maneque.

This form of medicine with the addition of a little of the balsam of Peru was continued for above three weeks, and at first appeared attended with some abatement of the swelling and improvement in the condition of the urine;—there was however no material change. He continued anasarcous to a high degree, and seemed to be losing ground in general health; and I at length determined to induce mercurial action on the system; for which purpose I ordered a few grains of the gray oxide of mercury to be given every night combined with squills on the 19th of March, and this was continued till the 30th; when no effect being produced, I ordered a drachm of the mercurial ointment to be rubbed-in every night. This was continued for three nights; when his mouth becoming sore, a scruple was rubbed-in every other night. I continued at the same time the occasional use of saline and other purgatives. The mercury was altogether relinquished on the 10th. The effect was to reduce the swelling; but not in any considerable degree to increase the flow of urine,—for a short time it seemed to become less coagulable, but after a time was more coagulable than ever. His strength now began evidently to fail: he sometimes complained of shortness of breath and cough, but even within five days of his death was able to lie flat on either side without coughing. He sunk gradually, and died on the 30th of April.

Sectio Cadaveris.—April 30th, 1827.

The cavity of the chest contained a pint or two of clear serum: but the lungs were very healthy, and did not appear even to be compressed by the fluid; they were somewhat œdematous. The pericardium contained about four ounces of limpid serum; the whole of its surface, both that attached to the heart and the loose portion, was completely covered with a rough coating of fibrin, in some parts assuming a completely honeycomb appearance, in others formed into projecting points, in others into raised ridges and lines. In some parts the coating was pretty firmly attached, in others it was easily removed by the back of the scalpel; there were no adhesions between the two surfaces of the pericardium. The heart itself was rather large, the valvular structure perfect. The internal lining of the aorta had several patches of incipient ossification. The liver was perfectly healthy, rather soft in its texture. The gall-bladder rather distended with bile, diluted by the mucus of the gall-bladder, and containing four or five biliary calculi from the size of a very small chesnut to that of a pea. The stomach had its internal surface covered with vessels of a brownish colour; in other respects healthy. The duodenum was rough, with enlarged mucous follicles. The small intestines in several parts showed marks of turgescence, and the edges of the valvulæ conniventes in some parts were rough, with an appearance somewhat resembling abrasion of the surface, to which the fæces had communicated a stain. The colon healthy. The pancreas and spleen healthy, but the latter rather firm and fleshy. The KIDNEYS were the seat of very decided disease. The right was small and misshapen, with projecting parts of a lighter colour: its tunic thickened very much, and so firmly attached that it was with great difficulty the kidney could

be separated from the surrounding fatty matter. The left kidney was large
completely disorganized. throughout: it had not much of the granulate
appearance, but was of one light yellow colour throughout, with some spot
of more opake yellow, differing very little in appearance from the kidney
of Hugh Thomas (Case V.).

The former part of this case was printed off as it at present stand
(p. 37 to 42.), before any such alarming change had taken place in th
condition of this patient as to threaten a speedy dissolution; and the fata
conclusion, with the appearances presented after death, too plainly poin
out the correctness of the views I had entertained, and confirm in my min
the position which I have been trying to establish. We have in this cas
likewise another instance of the proneness of the serous membranes unde
such circumstances to run into a state of inflammation, and a fresh warning
of the difficulty with which the inflammation of the pericardium is disco
vered; for except from the appearance of the inflamed surface, I am totall
at a loss to say at what period the pericardium in this case became inflamed
He always denied most positively any pain; he used to assert day after da
that he had none; for, being well aware of the risk of inflammation, I wa
never unmindful of it. Till within the last ten days he never complaine
of cough or shortness of breath; and probably this was the time when th
more recent inflammation came on, though I was inclined to consider thes
symptoms rather the result of effusion taking place into the cavities, tha
of any inflammatory process.

SOME GENERAL REMARKS ON THE FOREGOING CASES.

FROM the observations which I have made, I have been led to believe that there may be several forms of disease to which the kidney becomes liable in the progress of dropsical affection: I have even thought that the organic derangements which have already presented themselves to my notice, will authorise the establishment of three varieties, if not of three completely separate forms, of diseased structure, generally attended by a decidedly albuminous character of the urine.—In the *first*, a state of degeneracy seems to exist, which from its appearance might be regarded as marking little more than simple debility of the organ. In this case the kidney loses its usual firmness, becomes of a yellow mottled appearance externally; and when a section is made, nearly the same yellow colour slightly tinged with gray is seen to pervade the whole of the cortical part, and the tubular portions are of a lighter colour than natural. The size of the kidney is not materially altered, nor is there any obvious morbid deposit to be discovered. (Plate II. Fig. 4.) This state of the organ is sometimes connected with a cachectic condition of body, attended with chronic disease, where no dropsical effusion has taken place either into the cellular membrane or into the cavities of the body; I have found it in a case of diarrhœa and phthisis, and in a case of ovarian tumour. In the former it was connected with slight and almost doubtful coagulation of the urine by heat; in the latter I had omitted to examine the state of the urine. I also met with nearly the same condition of the kidney, with some opake yellow deposits interspersed through the structure, in the case of a man who died exhausted with diarrhœa brought on by hardships and intemperance, and in whose case the secretion of urine was very deficient, but whether coagulable or not I had no opportunity of ascertaining. When this disease has gone to its utmost, it has appeared to terminate by producing a more decided alteration in the structure; some portions becoming consolidated, so as to admit of very partial circulation; in which state the surface has assumed a somewhat tuberculated appearance, the gentle projections of which were paler than the rest, and scarcely received any of the injection which was thrown in by the arteries. (Plate II. Fig. 1. 2. and 3.) In this more advanced stage, if it be the same disease, dropsy has existed, and the urine has been coagulable (SALLAWAY, Case III.).

The *second* form of diseased kidney is one in which the whole cortical part is converted into a granulated texture, and where there appears to be a copious morbid interstitial deposit of an opake white substance. This in its earliest stage produces externally, when the tunic is taken off, only an increase of the natural fine mottled appearance given by the healthy structure of the kidney; or under particular circumstances, gives the appearance of fine grains of sand sprinkled more abundantly on some parts than others. (Plate V. Fig. 3.) On making a longitudinal section, a slight appearance of the same kind is discovered internally, and the kidney is generally rather deficient in its natural firmness. After the disease has continued for some time, the deposited matter becomes more abundant, and is seen in innumerable specks of no definite form thickly strewed on the surface; and on cutting into the kidney these specks are found distributed in a more or less regular manner throughout the whole cortical substance, no longer presenting a doubtful appearance, but most manifest to the eye without any preparation (Plate III. Fig. 3.); and other cases less advanced, requiring maceration in simple spring water for a few days to render them more obvious. (Plate IV. Fig. 3.) When this disease has gone on for a very considerable time, the granulated texture begins to show itself externally, in frequent slight uneven projections on the surface of the kidney; so that the morbid state is readily perceived even before the tunic is removed. The kidney is generally rather larger than natural; sometimes it is increased very much, but at other times it is little above the natural dimensions, (Plate I.) Occasionally I have seen (HOBSON, p. 59.) the kidney assume a good deal of the tuberous appearance observed in the advanced stage of the first disease, as shown in the representation of SALLAWAY's kidney (Plate II.): but then it has been manifest even by simple inspection, but much more so after maceration, that the whole is made up of small opake deposits. It is evident from the case of HOBSON, that this state of kidney attended also with highly coagulable urine may exist without any marked appearance of anasarca.

The *third* form of disease is where the kidney is quite rough and scabrous to the touch externally, and is seen to rise in numerous projections not much exceeding a large pin's head, yellow, red, and purplish. The form of the kidney is often inclined to be lobulated, the feel is hard, and on making an incision the texture is found approaching to semicartilaginous firmness, giving great resistance to the knife. The tubular portions are observed to be drawn near to the surface of the kidney : it appears in short like a contraction of every part of the organ, with less interstitial deposit than in the last variety. This form of disease existed in a case from which I had a drawing executed about three years ago, it also existed in BONHAM (p. 22.); and a most decidedly marked instance of it may be found in STEWART (Plate III. Fig. 1. and 2.), where however the kidney was of a lighter colour than in the other cases, which were more of a purplish gray tinge. I believe the case of SMITH (p. 23.) belonged to the same. In most of these cases the urine has been highly coagulable by heat, at times forming a large curdled deposit, though in one case (CASTLES) where an approach to this appearance was found on the outside of the kidney, but with marked structural change in the liver, and with confirmed bronchial congestion, only a dense bran-like deposit of a brown colour was produced by the application of heat.

Although I hazard a conjecture as to the existence of these three different forms of disease, I am by no means confident of the correctness of this view. On the contrary it may be that the first form of *degeneracy* to which I refer never goes much beyond the first stage ; and that all the other cases, including SALLAWAY, together with the second series, and the third, are to be considered only as modifications, and more or less advanced states of one and the same disease.

I have sometimes felt doubtful whether the cases of PEACOCK and THOMAS (Plate III. Fig. 3. and 4.) were to be viewed as the more early stages of the decidedly granulated kidney, (KING, BEAVER, and RICHARDSON,) or whether the opake flaky deposit which they exhibited in their structure might be considered altogether another form of disease. I think however, from the appearance, that the former is probably the case; and although KING dated his disease from a less remote period than either PEACOCK or THOMAS, yet there is no reason that the disease should not have made either a more insidious, or a more rapid progress, in his case than in that of the others.

Besides these three forms of disease, passing almost into each other and usually attended with decidedly coagulable urine, there are two other deranged conditions of the kidneys in which the coagulation is sometimes observable, but in a very subordinate degree, and often though observable on one day is quite lost on another. One of these morbid states consists in a preternatural softness of the organ ; the other in the blocking up of the tubular structure by small portions of a white deposit bearing the appearance of small concretions. In the former a corresponding loss of firmness has been observed in the structure of the liver, and the spleen and the parietes of the heart, the action of which organ had been observed during life to be deficient in force. In the other cases, besides the obstructed state of the uriniferous tubes, the whole structure of the kidney has been somewhat deranged, the cortical portion firmer than natural, and the tubular part has lost the regular convergency of the vessels, so that they have assumed a waved direction.—It is by no means improbable that we shall hereafter find many other sources of renal irritation to be connected with an analogous state of the urine.

OBSERVATIONS ON THE TREATMENT.

In the foregoing statements it has been my great object to establish the fact, that certain dropsical affections depend more on the derangement of the kidneys themselves than has generally been supposed ; and that the albuminous nature of the urine frequently points out the particular cases in which these organs are the seat of disease. I wish that I were now able to add any thing completely satisfactory to myself with regard to the mode of treating these diseases of the kidney. It will be very obvious from a review of the cases I have cited, that they sometimes present difficulties so formidable as to defy the ordinary means of cure ; indeed I am inclined to doubt whether it be possible, after the decided organic change has taken a firm hold on the kidney, to effect a cure, or even to give such relief as may enable the patient to pursue for a few years the occupations of life ; where, however, the mischief is less rooted, we may undoubtedly do much. In the treatment of the disease, as it occurs in sudden attacks of anasarca from intemperance and exposure, in its early stages, and before organic changes have taken place, we have two distinct indications to fulfil ;—we have to restore the healthy action of the kidney, and we have to guard continually against those dangerous secondary consequences which may destroy the patient at any period of the disease.

The two great sources of casual danger will be found in inflammatory affections, more particularly of the serous, sometimes of the mucous membranes, and in the effusion of blood or serum into the brain, and the consequent occurrence of apoplexy. Of these secondary or casual dangers we have illustrative examples in many of the cases which have been stated above. Out of seventeen dissections, we have found ten or eleven betraying inflammation of the pleura, generally old, but sometimes of more recent date. We have found three instances in which the patients had suffered decided attacks of inflammation in the pericardium shortly before death ; and in two of these cases we had proof of some previous affection of the same kind. In one only were the signs of inflammation in the peritoneum well marked. Five out of the seventeen had altogether escaped inflammatory affections of the serous membranes ; and one of these died with inflammation of the epiglottis. Thus then we have proof of the frequency of these attacks ; and at the same time it is obvious that they form no essential part of the disease, since in several of the best marked cases there has been no reason whatsoever to suspect inflammation during life, and no traces of its existence have been discovered after death. With regard to the cerebral affections coming on in the progress of these diseases, we find in the cases above related both apoplexy and epilepsy to have occurred ; and a very well marked instance of the former was witnessed in a patient of the name of MACGUIRE, in the Clinical ward in 1825. Whatever mode of treatment is adopted must therefore have a reference to these impending dangers ; and hence it is that in the early stages of the disease it will generally be indispensably necessary to have recourse to active depletion, even as a preventive measure ; but still more should we be ready at every stage of the complaint to combat the first symptoms of inflammation on the one hand, or of cerebral congestion on the other, by the free abstraction of blood the moment we have our fears awakened. And here it is well to remark, that the approach and progress of inflammatory affection of the chest in these cases are peculiarly insidious : for the attention is apt to be drawn off by the marked hydropic tendency ; and we are led to ascribe many of the symptoms,— such as the slight cough, the dyspnœa, and the difficulty of lying down, —to effusion rather than inflammation ; and this the more because the pulse throughout the disease is often marked by a preternatural sharpness and frequency. Thus although in the case of HOBSON the inflammation of the pericardium was confidently predicted, it was but suspected in KING, and was altogether concealed from observation in RODERICK. When the inflammatory attack comes on early in the disease, it is often overcome by very free depletion, as was decidedly the case with SPOONER; but in the more advanced stages of the disease, the patient bears the depletion so ill as necessarily in some degree to check its employment. Bleeding is also a most important remedy with a view of restoring the healthy action of the kidneys; that is, with the view of removing what appears to be the chief source, if not of the disease itself, at least of many of its most alarming symptoms. There is reason to believe that a state of great congestion, perhaps an actual process of slow inflammation, exists in various internal organs, and particularly in the kidneys, where it probably lays the foundation for their future disorganization. The appearance exhibited on the examination of EVANS (Plate V.) gave most striking evidence of this circumstance, had there been any room to doubt the fact after the very frequent occurrence of hæmaturia in the other cases I have related. In a great many instances the abstraction of blood generally has been productive of speedy good effects; and in other cases it has seemed to me, that by drawing blood locally by cupping from the loins much good has been effected.

Purgatives generally act well; the Elaterium in the case of EVANS evidently gave much relief; and all the saline laxatives which unite a certain degree of diuretic power are decidedly useful. Amongst these I have found the Supertartrate of Potash the most efficacious; and the best mode of exhibiting it when the stomach will admit, is by directing the patient to take a large draught of a mixture containing more of the salt than the water will dissolve, the first thing in the morning: and it will be seen that in some cases I have almost trusted entirely to this remedy. Where the stomach will not bear this mode of administering purgatives, the combination of Jalap, Supertartrate of Potash, and a little Ginger repeated from time to time, answers well, or even frequent doses of Castor Oil have been very useful.

The diuretic remedy which I have generally used, has been the Squill in its different forms: but it has always acted best when given in combination with Hyoscyamus, or when a grain of Opium has been prescribed once or twice a day. Indeed I cannot but consider this an important part of the treatment, with a view to diminish the irritation of the kidneys, as well as to allay the general disturbance which must necessarily result to the constitution, from the circulation of blood which has been so imperfectly acted upon by these organs. Digitalis has in some instances been cautiously administered with temporary advantage, and seems by its power of checking the circulation to be well adapted to those cases where the pulse is sharp, as frequently occurs throughout the whole progress of this disease. In the case of PLUME, Digitalis acted well: in the treatment of THOMAS it entirely failed. Under certain circumstances, more particularly when the more inflammatory stage of the disease has subsided, Turpentine employed in the mode of friction, and the Peruvian balsam administered internally, have seemed decidedly useful.

One of the most important questions in the treatment of this class of dropsies, is the propriety of employing Mercury. It is consistent with the most successful treatment of many forms of inflammatory disease, that we should have recourse to the valuable combination of Calomel with Opium; and it is consistent with what is generally deemed good practice, that by the cautious use of mercury we should endeavour to produce more healthy action, and to promote absorption when there is reason to believe that disease has left any chronic morbid action tending to produce unhealthy deposit in glandular structures. Still however, the cases which have proved most successful in my own practice, have generally been those in which I have rigidly abstained from the use of mercury. In some cases I have seen the good effects of other remedies entirely interrupted by the mercurial action; and I have likewise seen several instances in which the cure, when mercurials have formed part of the plan, has been protracted to a great length; and a great many in which the full action of mercury has not prevented the regular progress of the disease, and its fatal termination. Yet I have undoubtedly seen well marked cases of this disease with decidedly coagulable urine, when taken early, in which the free use of mercury to complete ptyalism has not prevented the patients from deriving great, perhaps even perfect relief, from the remedies with which it was combined,—these remedies having been bleeding, purging, and diuretics. Independently of the very great doubt which exists as to the advantage to be derived from mercury, there is one circumstance which most materially limits our power of employing it, and that is the violence and rapidity with which the ptyalism often comes on, and the great difficulty which is frequently experienced in restraining its effects: for when the cellular membrane is in the peculiar state of anasarca induced by this disease, the gums and cheeks are not capable of supporting the process of ulceration, and often pass into a state of gangrene.

In those cases where, as in BONHAM and STEWART, the kidney, besides apparently having some morbid deposit, has become preternaturally hard, we can only employ palliative remedies: and if we could ascertain by well marked symptoms the existence of this state, probably the great advantage we should gain from the knowledge, would be in its restraining us from adopting those more active remedies, which would be apt to wear out the powers of life, without affording any permanent relief to the organs affected.

Where, as in a case to which I have only referred, we have a flaccid, watery and dissolved state of the kidney, I can point out no diagnostic symptoms by which it can be discovered, except such as show general debility of circulation and feebleness in the structure of the heart; for probably the feeble condition of the two organs may often be found coexistent. If this be the case, it is not improbable that Tonics will be the most appropriate remedies. In one or two cases of anasarca which I have lately had under my care, where from the feeble but extensive beat of the heart I was led to suppose that a feeble state of that organ existed, a combination of Sulphate of Quinine with Squill, effectually restored the patient. And occasionally we find anasarca even with coagulable urine so marked by debility, that tonics and steel give decided relief; probably it is as a tonic that the Uva Ursi is sometimes useful.

OBSERVATIONS ON THE CHEMICAL PROPERTIES OF THE URINE IN THE
FOREGOING CASES. By JOHN BOSTOCK, M.D.

Upper Bedford Place, April 24th, 1827.

DEAR SIR,

I PROPOSE in this letter to give you some account of the experiments which
I have performed on the various specimens of morbid urine which I have
received from you, for the purpose of illustrating your pathological observations.

The number of specimens upon which I shall remark are twenty-eight.
There were six obtained from the patient RODERICK, the respective dates
of which were Dec. 26th, Jan. 12th, two on Jan. 31st, April 14th and 18th;
these I shall designate by consecutive numbers; five from PLUME, received
on Feb. 1st, two on the 19th, March 1st, and April 14th; two from HOBSON,
on the 13th and 15th of March; two from THOMAS, Jan. 12th and 22nd;
two from WEST*, March 7th and April 14th; and two from HUNTER, on
March 14th and April 22nd, which I shall designate in the same manner;
and a single specimen from each of the following cases:—STEWART, received Jan. 4th; SALLAWAY, Jan. 8th; CASTLE, the 15th; SPOONER,
the 26th; DAVIES†, the 31st; ALCORNE‡, Feb. 27th; GALLOWAY,
March 15th; OPIE§, April 14th, and TODD on the same day.

1. With respect to the quantity of matter dissolved or suspended in the
urine; this I found, in most of the cases which I examined, to be below the
average. The greatest specific gravity which I have found in any of the
specimens, occurred in the case of ALCORNE; it was 1·032. In the six specimens from RODERICK it was 1·024, 1·029, 1·022, 1·024, 1·022, and 1·017;
four of the specimens from PLUME were 1·022, 1·021, 1·021, and 1·015;

* A sailor, æt. 56, admitted into Guy's Hospital, 28th Feb. 1827, with anasarca which had already existed
for five months. Urine copious, light coloured, highly coagulable. Pulse from 85 to 100, sharp. He has
been bled twice, and the blood has been buffed. He has chiefly been treated by diuretics and opiates, and
some tonics; mercury has been avoided. He still remains under treatment.

† A case of anasarca after recovery from ague, which was admitted into Guy's Hospital, Nov. 29th, nine
days after its first appearance; the urine coagulating by heat in numerous small flakes. He left the house
much relieved.

‡ A young woman, æt. 26, who had suffered several attacks of anasarca, and at length died with
evidence of inflammation and effusion in the chest; the urine coagulating freely by heat. It was impossible
to obtain any examination after death.

§ A carter, æt. 23, attacked with anasarca and ascites on April 4th, the day of his admission into Guy's
Hospital on account of diarrhœa. He has since had ten quarts of serum taken from the abdomen, and still
remains under treatment.

CASTLE was 1·019; STEWART, SPOONER, and DAVIES, was each 1·016; SALLAWAY and THOMAS, 1·014; WEST, 1·015 and 1·012; TODD, OPIE, and HUNTER (No. 2), were 1·012. The two specimens from HOBSON were 1·011 and 1·010; GALLOWAY, 1·008; and HUNTER (No. 1), 1·006. The average of these twenty-six cases is 1·017. The specific gravity of the urine even in a state of health, and in the same individuals, differs so much at different times, according to the period it has been retained in the bladder, and from a variety of other circumstances, that a great number of observations are necessary to enable us to draw any general conclusions upon the subject; but my experiments are sufficiently numerous to warrant the conclusion, that the specific gravity of dropsical urine which coagulates is less than that of urine in the healthy condition of the system.

2. Urine which has a lower specific gravity than ordinary, may be considered under three points of view: either as natural urine, merely in a state of dilution; as having a deficiency in the proportion of some of its ingredients; or, together with this deficiency, as containing some extraneous substance. My experiments lead me to conclude, that the specimens of urine which you have sent me were all of them in the third condition, being deficient in some of the natural constituents, yet at the same time containing a quantity of extraneous matter. The circumstance which was originally noticed by Cruickshanks, and afterwards more particularly attended to by Dr. Blackall, as occurring in certain species of dropsy, of the urine coagulating in a greater or less degree by heat, must be ascribed to the presence of albumen, as this is the only proximate principle with which we are acquainted that possesses this property. But it still remains for us to inquire, whether the albumen in dropsical urine is precisely similar to the albumen in the serum of the blood, or in the white of the egg. Upon this point I think it may be asserted, that in certain cases the albumen in dropsical urine possesses every property of the albumen of the blood; the urine coagulates by the application of heat in the same manner with diluted serum, and is similarly affected by chemical re-agents. If such urine be exposed to the heat of boiling water, and still more if we add to it the solution of the bichloride of mercury, muriatic acid, a strong infusion of tan, or, according to Dr. Prout's process, the ferro-prussiate of potash, and if the fluid is afterwards heated, the albumen, even when it exists in minute quantity, separates in the form of dense flakes, leaving the urine nearly transparent.

There are, however, certain cases in which, although the quantity of extraneous animal matter is very considerable, as indicated by the specific gravity and by the effects of heat and of chemical re-agents, yet still the complete separation of it cannot be effected. The fluid is rendered thick and viscid; but no distinct coagulum forms in it, nor can it be separated by passing the fluid through a filter: in some cases the albuminous matter remains suspended for an indefinite period; in others it is very slowly deposited in the form of a flocculent cloud. Some of the specimens of urine after the application of heat very much resembled a solution of jelly; and I found that after the bichloride of mercury had acted upon it, the more complete separation of the albumen was effected by the application of a strong infusion of tan. Yet I do not consider this as a proof of the presence of jelly in the urine, because the operation of heat upon it did not correspond to what we know takes place with respect to this proximate principle: nor did the urine in these cases resemble a fluid which contained mucus; so that I am disposed to regard these peculiar effects to depend rather upon some change or modification in the nature of the albumen, than upon the admixture of any other proximate principle. With respect to the state of the albumen in the cases under examination, if we arrange them according to the degree in which the application of heat or of chemical re-agents had the effect of separating the albuminous matter, they will stand in about the following order. In RODERICK (No. 3), in CASTLE, SPOONER, DAVIES, ALCORNE, WEST (Nos. 1 and 2), and in GALLOWAY, the separation was nearly complete. In RODERICK (Nos. 1 and 4), in STEWART, SALLAWAY, PLUME (Nos. 1 and 4), and in HOBSON (Nos. 1 and 2), the separation took place slowly, and the precipitate always remained soft; while in RODERICK (Nos. 2, 5 and 6), in PLUME (Nos. 2 and 3), in THOMAS (Nos. 1 and 2), and in OPIE, the fluid never became clear, owing to the imperfect separation of the albumen. It appears that the state of the albumen, with respect to its disposition to separate from the fluid, bears no exact ratio to its specific gravity. The urine of ALCORNE and of GALLOWAY, the first having the greatest, and the second nearly the least specific gravity, agreeing in this respect.

The state of the urine, with respect to the presence of uncombined acid or alkali, will have some effect upon the separation of the albumen, as produced by the application of heat. This indeed I found to be the case in the urine of RODERICK (No. 5), which indicated an excess of alkali. When heated without addition, it was converted into a uniform coagulum, which could scarcely have been distinguished by the eye from the serum of the blood; but when the alkali was saturated with acetic acid, a tendency to separation took place, although still in a very imperfect degree. The urine of HUNTER (No. 2), was also alkalescent; and when simply heated, did manifest any tendency to coagulation; but after the neutralization of the alkali, a small quantity of a soft coagulum was thrown down. But the deficiency of acid or the presence of alkali, although separately or conjointly they may produce some effect, cannot be considered the principal cause. In the case of RODERICK (No. 6), the coagulum produced was more considerable than in No. 5, and showed at least as little tendency to separation, although in the former case the urine was not alkaline. In the urine of THOMAS and of OPIE, where the separation of the albumen was very imperfect, the fluid appeared to be rather more than usually acid, and had even that sourish smell, especially when heated, which is occasionally met with in dropsical urine, and which appears to depend upon the presence of acetic acid. I may further remark, that in the natural albuminous fluids which are characterized by their property of coagulating, we always meet with an excess of alkali. With respect to the acid or alkaline state of the different specimens of urine which I examined, those of THOMAS, of HUNTER (No. 1), and of OPIE, seemed to contain the greatest quantity of uncombined acid: those of SPOONER, of RODERICK (No. 6), of WEST (Nos. 1 and 2), and of PLUME (No. 5), were nearly neutral; while RODERICK (No. 5), HUNTER (No. 2), and TODD, were decidedly alkaline.

The next point is to ascertain in what quantity the albumen exists, and what proportion it bears to the urea and the salts, which are found in healthy urine. For this purpose the urine was evaporated to a thick extract; this was digested in alcohol, by which the urea was removed from it, and the residue was afterwards digested in water, by which the greatest part of the salts was dissolved. Another method which I adopted was to separate the albumen by heat, or by heat in conjunction with the bichloride of mercury, and to estimate its quantity by comparing the specific gravity of the urine before and after the process; the fluid was then evaporated, and the extract examined in the usual manner. By these means I obtained results which, although by no means perfectly accurate, were sufficiently so for the object in view. The most correct chemists differ so much in their account of what may be considered as the quantity of solid contents in healthy urine, depending upon the variation which actually takes place in this respect, that our estimates can only be regarded as indicating a general average. We find the same uncertainty, depending probably upon the same cause, in the proportion which the urea and the salts bear to each other. My own experiments would lead me to conclude that the average quantity of the urea, as separated from the salts by alcohol, composes about two-thirds of the extract; and supposing the whole to amount to 6 per cent of the weight of the urine, it will give us 4 per cent of urea, and 2 of the salts.

I must now inquire how far the composition of some of the specimens of urine agreed with the above proportion. In the first specimen of RODERICK's urine which I examined, the amount of the albumen when completely dried was equal to about two-fifths of the whole of the solid contents; after an interval of seventeen days, the urine of the same patient was again examined; its specific gravity was now increased from 1·024 to 1·029, and the albumen was very nearly double the weight of the urea: in this latter case the albumen was soft, and separated very slowly from the fluid. In the case of STEWART, where the specific gravity of the urine was 1·016 or 4·2 per cent, the albumen was only about 1 per cent, or one-fourth of the whole of the solid contents. The specimens of RODERICK's urine (Nos. 3 and 4), deserve attention, as having been voided the one before, and the other after bleeding. The specific gravity of the first was 1·022; the quantity of albumen was not large, but it separated completely by coagulation, leaving the fluid clear, and holding in solution a considerable quantity of urea. After bleeding, the specific gravity was increased to 1·024; the urine was turbid, there was a copious deposition of the earthy phosphates, while the albumen seemed to be in less quantity and was only imperfectly separated by the chemical reagents.

I had likewise an opportunity of examining the urine of PLUME before and after bleeding. In the first case the specific gravity was 1·021, equivalent to about 4·5 per cent of solid contents; by adding the bichloride of mercury and exposing it to heat, a copious precipitate was produced, but it did not separate from the fluid, nor was it completely removed by filtration; by this operation the specific gravity was reduced to 1·007, indicating 3·3 per cent of albumen, or nearly two-thirds of the whole. The urine of the same patient after bleeding had the specific gravity of 1·015; and after the separation of the albumen it was reduced to 1·005, indicating 4 per cent of extract, and 2·5 of albumen. In this case therefore bleeding had the effect of diminishing the total amount of the solid contents, without much affecting the proportion of the ingredients. After an interval of ten days, I received another specimen of this patient's urine; the specific gravity was as at first 1·021, but the quantity of albumen was now very much diminished, amounting to no more than about 1·25 per cent of the weight of the fluid. The urine which exhibited the lowest specific gravity of any of the specimens which came under my observation, except that from GALLOWAY, was HOBSON's, of which I had two specimens. They were very nearly similar in all respects, the specific gravity of the one being 1·010, of the other 1·011. But although the total amount of the solid contents was so small, the proportion of albumen was very considerable, being nearly double the amount of the urea and the salts taken together. In this case although the total amount of solid contents was only about 3 per cent, nearly 2 per cent of this appeared to be albumen. In the urine of GALLOWAY however, which contained not much more than 2 per cent in the whole, the albumen constituted not much more than ½ per cent. That of ALCORNE on the other hand, the specific gravity of which was the greatest of any that I examined, indicating 8·5 per cent of solid contents, had 5·5 per cent, or nearly two-thirds of the whole of albumen ; while the urine of PLUME (No. 5), which agreed with that of ALCORNE in its specific gravity, had exactly the same proportion of albumen with that of GALLOWAY. Without going further into the detail of individual cases, I may state as the result of my experiments generally, that the quantity of albumen in the urine bore no exact relation to the total amount of its solid contents, or to that of the urea in particular.

3. I may appear to be encroaching upon your province, if I offer any remarks upon the inferences which may be drawn from the presence of this albuminous matter in the urine ; but as my remarks will principally refer to the chemical nature of the fluid, you will perhaps think them not altogether out of place. It is commonly said that the presence of albumen in the urine is a morbid occurrence, and it has even been supposed to be a pathognomonic symptom of a certain state of the constitution, or still more to be an indication of the existence of certain specific diseases. The first of these positions may be literally true, if we regard the albumen as existing in a state which is coagulable by heat; but it must be admitted on the other hand, that an albuminous state of the urine is produced by such a variety of circumstances, and many of them of so trifling a nature, as to render it almost a constant occurrence. In a great majority of cases it may be detected in the urine of persons in apparent health, by means of the appropriate tests. In my own person I have very seldom found the fluid to be entirely free from it, and I have observed it to be increased to

a considerable amount by the slightest causes. But although the substance which is here present in the urine may be characterized generally as albumen, yet it is to be regarded as albumen in a modified state, because mere heat will detect albumen in the state in which it exists in the white of the egg in much smaller quantity, than in some specimens of urine where heat has no action upon it. I have also found certain states of the urine where heat had no effect, but where muriatic acid threw down a precipitate; and again, where muriatic acid had no effect, but where the albumen was detected by the bichloride of mercury, or the ferro-prussiate of potash. How far these different states of the albuminous matter in urine indicate different stages of diseased action, so as to throw any light upon the nature of the symptoms, I will not decide; but I think it is a subject which deserves to be further examined.

4. Among the miscellaneous circumstances which I shall notice, is the peculiar colour which the urine often assumes in its morbid state. Instead of the orange or citron colour of healthy urine, it is sometimes brown, straw-coloured, or of a reddish hue. With respect to the straw colour it is, I think, generally connected with the presence of albumen, or rather with the deficiency of urea, and I am inclined to think that the brown colour indicates an excess of saline matter. In the case of OPIE, the urine was very decidedly browner than ordinary, and the proportion of the muriatic salts to the urea appeared to be larger than ordinary. The other cases in which this brown colour was the most marked were SALLOWAY and CASTLE. The straw colour was the most apparent in the urine of PLUME, WEST and GALLOWAY, and also was perceptible in that of RODERICK before bleeding: HOBSON afforded the best example of the reddish tinge of the urine; in this case there was indeed a deposition of the pink sediment, but the colour of the fluid remained after the deposition, as if depending on some other cause. Some of the specimens of urine which I examined deposited a copious white sediment upon the bottom and sides of the vessel; this was particularly the case with the urine of RODERICK after bleeding, and with that of CASTLE, THOMAS, and GALLOWAY, and in a slight degree with SPOONER. It will appear, from these observations, that I was not able to trace any connection between the deposition of the white or pink sediment and the albuminous state of the urine.

I have observed a considerable difference in the tendency to decomposition in the different kinds of urine. The albuminous urine frequently acquired an acidulous odour very similar to that of sour milk, and it was certainly less disposed to become putrid than in ordinary cases. This, however, I am disposed to think was the case with dropsical urine generally, which may depend upon its containing a smaller proportion of urea.

There are two of the specimens of urine which may deserve particular notice, as having been voided while the system was under the operation of mercury. This was the case with the fifth specimen of RODERICK's urine, received on the 14th of April. It was of the usual colour, although rather of a light shade, somewhat opake, and by standing for thirty-six hours it threw down a copious white flaky precipitate. Its specific gravity was 1·022, it had an acrid penetrating odour, and indicated a considerable excess of alkali. On the 18th I received from you another specimen from the same patient (No. 6), the properties of which were considerably different. It was now of a dingy light straw colour, somewhat opake, and contained a number of small flakes which gradually subsided. Its specific gravity was 1·017, and it was very slightly acid; in forty-eight hours it had thrown down a copious white precipitate, which seemed to consist principally of the earthy phosphates, and after an interval of five days it indicated a slight excess of alkali.

The other case to which I referred was that of HUNTER. The first specimen I received on the 14th of March; its characters at that time were as follows: it was brownish, slightly opake, specific gravity not more than 1·006, it was unusually acid, and had a sourish smell; a very copious precipitate was produced by boiling, but it did not separate very completely from the fluid. On the 2nd of April I received the second specimen, after the patient had undergone a mercurial salivation; the urine was now of a dingy straw colour, rather opake, specific gravity 1·012, decidedly alkaline. Boiling without addition produced no effect upon it, but by adding acetic acid in sufficient quantity to neutralize the alkali, a small quantity of a soft coagulum was produced, which slowly subsided. It may be well worth observing how far an alkalescent state of the urine is the usual consequence of mercurial action upon the system.

I am, dear Sir, most truly your's,

J. BOSTOCK.

- 156 -

Upper Bedford Place, May 28th, 1827.

My Dear Sir,

Since the date of my last letter I have received from you three additional specimens of urine, the leading properties of which I will briefly state to you.—The first was received on the 16th of April, and, as you informed me, was procured from a Dispensary patient under the care of Dr. Hodgkin, named William Elsely. It had been exposed to heat before it was sent to me, and was converted into what appeared a uniform soft solid, very similar to the serum of the blood. On the following day there was some tendency to separation, and upon throwing the whole upon a filter, a quantity of a light straw-coloured fluid passed through; the albumen when dried, appeared to exist in the proportion of about 5·6 per cent.

The next specimen, sent on the 24th of April, which was from the same patient, was of a light straw colour, and had the specific gravity of 1·012. It was converted by heat into a soft solid, from which the coagulum slowly separated; after filtration the fluid had the specific gravity of 1·010. The total amount of solid contents in this urine was 3·2 per cent, of which the greatest part was albumen.

The third specimen, received on the same day with the last, was one which had been sent to you by Dr. Alderson; it was light-coloured, and had the specific gravity of 1·014. Upon the application of heat a precipitate was separated in small quantity, but of a dense consistence, leaving the fluid perfectly clear and bright. The specific gravity of the urine was reduced by boiling to 1·012, so that the total amount of the solid contents may be estimated at 3·7 per cent, and the albumen at 2 per cent.

I have received from you at different times specimens of the crassamentum and serum of some of the dropsical patients whose urine I examined. With respect to the former substance, the only remark that I have to make is, that it was, in most of the cases, covered with a thick buffy coat, and was generally of a firm consistence. The appearance of the serum was more varied; it was occasionally turbid, and upon standing for twenty-four hours a white creamy substance rose to the surface, but I could not detect any proper oily matter in it. On exposing it to heat, it coagulated in the ordinary manner, except that the coagulum seemed to contain an unusual number of cells and that a greater quantity of serosity separated from it. I think I may venture to say, that the serum generally in these cases contained less albumen than in health, although I am not able to state precisely the amount of this difference.

The serosity which drained from the coagulated albumen, on being evaporated, was found to consist in part of an animal matter, possessing
peculiar properties, which seemed to approach to those of the urea ; it was
partially soluble in alcohol, and was acted upon in a somewhat similar
manner by nitric acid. These phænomena were particularly noticed in
the serosity of RODERICK and of WEST*.

I must apologize for sending you so imperfect an account of this substance, which I am aware can be of little value, except so far as it may
induce others to examine the subject with more attention.

I am, my dear Sir, very truly your's,

J. BOSTOCK.

June 4th, 1827.

I have to give you the account of one more specimen of dropsical urine,
which you sent me on the 2nd of June. It was opake and muddy, and by
standing twenty-four hours deposited a considerable quantity of a white
flaky sediment, but no precipitate adhered to the sides of the glass. It
had a putrescent odour, and was strongly alkaline; its specific gravity
was 1·012. The usual reagents indicated a large quantity of albumen ;
and by boiling it was converted into a uniform soft solid, which showed
no tendency to separation after standing for thirty-six hours, and from
which only a small quantity of a colourless fluid drained off, the whole
presenting an appearance which could not have been distinguished by the
eye from the coagulum of serum, and the separation of the serosity. I
was prevented by an accident from ascertaining the exact proportion of
the albumen to the other contents of this urine ; but I may state in general
terms, that the quantity of urea was very small, so that nearly the whole of
the animal matter may be regarded as albumen, nearly in the same state
in which it exists in the serum of the blood.

At the same time you sent me a portion of crassamentum and of serum
from the same patient. The crassamentum was buffed and cupped in a
very remarkable degree, indeed so much so that I shall attempt to give an
accurate idea of it by stating the following particulars. The clot was 2·4
inches in diameter, and 1·1 in thickness : the buffed part of the surface

* A substance slightly analogous to urea was discovered by Dr. Prout in a specimen of serum of the
blood, which I sent to him in November last, taken from a patient labouring under partial suppression of
urine from an inflammatory attack in the kidneys, in which the urine was coagulable and mixed with blood ;
and in many respects this case illustrated the source of that anasarca of which I have been treating.—R. B.

was so much contracted, as to be only 1·8 inch in diameter : it was depressed ·5 inch at its centre, and was between ·1 and ·2 inch in thickness at its edge ; it was almost perfectly white, and the passage from the white to the red part was with scarcely any intermediate gradation. I am well aware that the appearance of the clot depends much upon the mode in which it flows from the vessel, and upon the cup into which it is received ; but I apprehend that, making every allowance for these circumstances, the blood in question will be admitted to exhibit, in a very remarkable degree, those appearances which are ordinarily ascribed to the inflammatory action of the system, in whatever we may conceive this to exist.

The serum was also worthy of attention as taken in connection with the state of the other fluids. Its specific gravity was almost exactly the same with that of the urine, being no more than 1·013, which I believe to be lower than had ever occurred to me in the numerous experiments which I have made upon this substance. In conformity with this circumstance, I found that upon exposing it to the heat of boiling water, it was converted into a mass so soft as not to bear cutting with a knife, having a consistence scarcely as dense as that of the coagulated urine from the same patient. We have here, therefore, an example of the blood exhibiting a very great deficiency of albumen, at the same time that we observe the mode in which it passes off from the system by means of the kidney, while this organ has its appropriate office of secreting urea nearly suspended.—I regret that I did not attend particularly to the specific gravity of the other specimens of dropsical serum which you sent me : from some incidental remarks in my notes, I suspect that its specific gravity would have been found lower than ordinary ; but it is a circumstance which I shall be anxious to ascertain when any opportunity occurs.　　　　　　　　　　J. Bostock.

———

The above specimens of urine and blood were procured from Sarah Sutton, æt. 25, who has been under my care about a fortnight : a woman of intemperate habits attacked with anasarca about two months before I saw her, and who has very lately become the subject of ascites. The quantity of urine which she passes is very small, but she is at present improving under the employment of small bleedings and gentle diuretics. At some future time I shall report the progress and termination of this case : it has all the appearance of being completely analogous to those I have been recording.

-159-

CASE XXIV.

The following letter, which refers to the patient of whose urine Dr. Bostock has made mention in page 83, came to me just as the present sheet was in the press.

" MY DEAR FRIEND,

" WILLIAM ELSELY,—a specimen of whose urine I some time ago (April 16th) brought to thee as some of the most coagulable which I had ever met with,—became my patient at the London Dispensary on the 22nd of March last. He was a large and rather corpulent man, about 50 years of age, of a lymphatic temperament. He had at one period of his life indulged not very sparingly in drink; but his habits in this respect were reported to have improved of late. His occupation as a dealer in Spitalfields Market exposed him greatly to wet and cold. In the course of the winter he contracted the catarrh for which he came under my care. He had besides some anasarca; but as even his legs were never very much swollen, this symptom, if my recollection serves me, had not much attracted his attention. He was ordered a mucilaginous mixture with Nitrate of Potass and Tincture of Hyoscyamus, and a pill of Conium and Ipecacuanha at night. These with an occasional aperient he continued to take for about ten days. His catarrhal symptoms abated, but the anasarca remained unaltered. I believe that it was about this time that I first discovered that this patient's urine was coagulable. He then took ten grains of Squill pill with two grains of Digitalis at night, and ten drops of the Tincture of Squills were added to his mixture. He also used *chien dent* tea as a common drink, which considerably increased the flow of urine. His bowels were kept open, not relaxed, by compound Jalap powder. He continued on this plan without any other alteration than the addition of a very small quantity of Blue pill, (which was never allowed to produce any effect on the mouth,) for nearly three weeks. His urine still continued coagulable, but not to so remarkable a degree as in the specimens which I brought to thee. The anasarca was very much reduced, but the patient felt himself weak; I believe however that he implicitly attended to my directions, though he felt the loss of the porter which he had been in the habit of taking. He was allowed a dessert-spoonful of gin in the dog's-grass tea. His bowels became disturbed, and the abdomen rather tender: I had him bled to eight ounces: discontinued the dog's-grass tea and the mixture, and gave him five grains of the Hydrarg. cum Creta, and five grains of Dover's powder, with one grain of powdered Digitalis. The tenderness of the abdomen continuing, I ordered him a mixture of turpentine and ammoniacal liniment, which afforded him prompt and permanent relief. He appeared on the 3rd of this present month to be in most respects better, but the urine was still very coagulable. I then ordered him ten drops of the Liquor Potassæ with six drops of tincture of Opium in infusion of Gentian. From this time his urine improved in character, and the man found himself better. He requested leave to take his half-pint of porter in the middle of the day, to which I consented, at the same time continuing to warn him of the fatal nature of his complaint. His bowels required occasional aloetic pills. On the 14th instant he felt some little giddiness of head, which the recollection of the termination of DRUDGET's case, under thy care in Guy's, induced me immediately to combat by cupping. This for the time completely relieved him from the symptom: his legs at this time were scarcely sensibly œdematous. On the 17th he came to the Dispensary, and appeared to be doing well. On the 19th he was attacked with symptoms which, from the description given to me, appear to have been decidedly apoplectic. He lay for several hours motionless and in a state of insensibility, of which I had no intimation till after his death, which occurred on the morning of the 20th. The next day I applied for permission to inspect the body, which not being granted till the afternoon, I took advantage of the following morning."

SECTIO CADAVERIS.—May 22nd, 1827.

" Though only about forty-eight hours had elapsed, decomposition had made most rapid progress. Finding the body in this state, I made no attempt to open the head. On opening the chest a quantity of gas escaped: there was a little sanious fluid in this cavity. The right pleura was nearly or altogether free from adhesion: in the left the adhesion was pretty extensive, but old. The lungs like the rest of the body were far advanced in decomposition, excepting cadaveric infiltration they appeared quite free from adventitious deposit, but were perhaps a little emphysematous. The heart rather large, and very soft and flaccid; but I suspect this to have been part of the general change. The valves were healthy: some little earthy deposit was observable at the commencement of the aorta. From the abdomen gas also escaped; the collection of fluid in this cavity was very moderate. In the state in which the body was, I could observe no marks of inflammation, nor have I any thing to remark respecting the mucous membrane of the intestinal canal. The liver appeared to have been quite healthy. The spleen large, of a very dark colour, and, as might be expected, very soft. The KIDNEYS were both extraordinarily large; and decomposition having developed gas in their very substance, they were crepitant on pressure like a portion of lung. Though soft and very lacerable, and also containing a good deal of blood, it was very evident both to myself and to Dr. Millar, (who was kind enough to assist me,) that the cortical part was the seat of a pretty abundant quantity of the light co-

loured motley deposit, which thou and I have now so often had the opportunity of noticing together.

"If thou canst make any thing of the very rough scratch which I now
send, it is quite at thy service.

Thine truly,

THOMAS HODGKIN."

It is totally unnecessary to comment upon this case : it connects itself
immediately with those which have gone before, and stands completely in
confirmation of all which I have advanced. It presents us with another
instance of disorganized kidney discovered by the coagulable character of
the urine,—another instance of the probable effect of the abuse of spirituous liquors in inducing disease of the kidney while the liver retains its
healthy structure,—another instance pointing to cold, wet, and repressed
perspiration, as exciting causes of the anasarcous symptoms in this particular form of dropsy,—another instance of the difficulty of overcoming
the disease,—and another instance to warn us of the danger there is of
apoplectic symptoms instantaneously supervening, even when our fears in
that respect have begun to be allayed.

The other specimen of coagulable urine referred to in page 83, was
brought to me by Dr. James Alderson, who procured it from a patient
who had experienced slight œdema in his ankles as far back as July 1826,
but in whom the swelling of the legs had increased during the last three
weeks so as to lead him to seek for medical assistance. The anasarca has
in this case greatly diminished under complete abstinence from spirituous
liquors ; the use of five grains of the compound squill pill twice a-day ; the
daily employment of an infusion of Dog's-grass (*Triticum repens*) ; and a
gentle purgative twice a-week. The patient has likewise twice been bled,
once by the lancet and once by cupping. The urine has been for some
weeks increased to five pints daily ; the legs are much less œdematous :
but the character of the urine is in no way improved.

ON SOME
MORBID APPEARANCES
OF
THE ABSORBENT GLANDS
AND
SPLEEN.

BY DR. HODGKIN.

PRESENTED
BY DR. R. LEE.

READ JANUARY 10TH AND 24TH, 1832.

THE morbid alterations of structure which I am about to describe are probably familiar to many practical morbid anatomists, since they can scarcely have failed to have fallen under their observation in the course of cadaveric inspection. They have not, as far as I am aware, been made the subject of special attention, on which account I am induced to bring forward a few cases in which they have occurred to myself, trusting that I shall at least escape severe or general censure, even though a sentence or two should be produced from some existing work, couched in such concise but expressive language, as to render needless the longer details with which I shall trespass on the time of my hearers.

CASE I.

November 2, 1826. Joseph Sinnott, a child of about nine years of age, in Lazarus's ward, under the care of J. Morgan. His brother, his constant companion with whom he had habitually slept, died of phthisis a few months previously; he was much reduced by an illness of about nine months, during which time he had been subject to pain in the back, extending round to the abdomen. On his admission his belly was much distended with ascites. He had also effusion into the prepuce and scrotum. On the latter was a large ulcer induced by a puncture made to evacuate the fluid.

Head.—There was a considerable quantity of serous effusion under the arachnoid and within the ventricles. There were a few opake spots in the arachnoid, but this membrane was in other respects healthy. The pia mater appeared remarkably thin and free from vessels. The substance of the brain was generally soft and flabby, but no local morbid change was observable.

Chest.—The pleura on the right side had contracted many strong and old adhesions, in addition to which there were extensive marks of recent pleuritis. On the left the pleura was nearly or quite free from adhesion, but there was some fluid effused into

the cavity. There was some little trace of a tubercular cicatrix at the summit of the right lung, but the
substance of both lungs was generally light and crepitant, with a very few exceedingly small tubercles
scattered through them.

The mucous membrane exhibited an excess of vascularity ; the bronchial glands were greatly enlarged
and much indurated.

The heart appeared quite healthy.

Abdomen.—There was extensive recent inflammation of the peritoneum, in the cavity of which there
was a copious sero-purulent effusion, and the viscera
were universally overlayed with a very soft light
yellow coagulum, too feeble to effect their union,
though evidently having a tendency to do so. The
mucous membrane of the stomach and intestines was
generally pale and of its ordinary appearance, but in
some few spots it was softened and readily separated
itself from the subjacent coat. The contents of the
intestines were copious and of an unhealthy character,
overcharged with bile. The mesenteric glands were
generally enlarged, but one or two very considerably so,
equalling in size a pigeon's egg, of semi-cartilaginous
hardness and streaked with black matter. The substance of the liver was generally natural, but contained
a few tubercles somewhat larger than peas, white,
semi-cartilaginous, and of an uneven surface. The

-165-

pancreas was firmer than usual, more particularly at its head, which was somewhat enlarged. The spleen was large and contained numerous tubercles. The absorbent glands about both the two last-mentioned organs were much enlarged. Both kidneys were mottled with a light colour, but were free from induration. A continuous chain of much enlarged indurated absorbent glands of a light colour accompanied the aorta throughout its course, closely adherent to the bodies of the vertebræ, and extended along the sides of the iliac vessels as far as they could be traced in the pelvis. None of these vessels had been sufficiently compressed to occasion the coagulation of the contained fluids. The coats of the thoracic duct, which was large, were perfectly transparent and healthy.

CASE II.

September 24, 1828. Ellenborough King, aged ten years, was admitted into Luke's ward on the 6th of August, 1828, under the care of Dr. Bright. He was the youngest of six children, of whom the first five were reported to be all healthy. This child had also been healthy till about thirteen months ago, when his strength, flesh, and healthy appearance began to fail. He was at that time living in the west of England. A tumour was observed in the left hypochondrium in the situation of the spleen, the glandulæ concatenatæ on the right side were observed to be considerably enlarged, but under the treatment employed, these tumours, as well as that in the situation of the spleen, were at times very considerably reduced in size.

It does not appear that he was ever subject to hæmorrhage, nor till very lately to dropsical effusion; his appetite was generally good. After his admission into the hospital the tumour on the left side was observed to extend considerably below the left hypochondrium, but was reported not to be so large as it had formerly been. The glands on the left side of the neck were swollen, as well as those on the right, the abdomen was somewhat distended, and there was considerable œdema of the scrotum.

The head was not opened.

The glands in the neck had assumed the form of large smooth ovoid masses, connected together merely by loose cellular membrane and minute vessels : when cut into they exhibited a firm cartilaginous structure of a light colour and very feeble vascularity, but with no appearance of softening or suppuration. Glands similarly affected accompanied the vessels into the chest, where the bronchial and mediastinal glands were in the same state and greatly enlarged. There were some old pleuritic adhesions. The substance of the lungs was generally healthy. There was a good deal of clear serum in the pericardium, but this membrane, as well as the heart, was quite healthy.

In the peritoneal cavity there was a considerable

quantity of clear straw-coloured serum mixed with extensive, recent thin diaphanous films. The mucous membrane of the stomach and intestines was tolerably healthy.

The mesenteric glands were but slightly enlarged, and but little if at all indurated; but those accompanying the aorta, the splenic artery, and the iliacs were in the same state as the glands of the neck.

The liver contained no tubercles, and its structure was quite healthy. The pancreas was rather firm, and the glands situated along its upper edge, were, as before stated, greatly enlarged. The spleen was enlarged to at least four times its natural size, its surface was mammillated, and its structure thickly sprinkled with tubercles, presenting the same structure as the enlarged glands already described.

CASE III.

BY H. PEACOCK, ESQ.

November 28, 1829. William Burrows, aged about thirty years. He was admitted into Naaman's ward on the 26th of September, 1829, under Mr. J. Morgan, for ulcers of a scrofulous character in the axilla and neck, accompanied with general cachexia; he had previously been a patient in Samaritan's ward with secondary symptoms of syphilis, and was supposed to have taken large quantities of mercury.

About four months before his death, which occurred on the 27th of November, abdominal dropsy made its appearance.

The body was extremely emaciated, some ragged excavated ulcers were situated about the right axilla and thorax ; the ulceration extended beneath the neighbouring skin, and between the pectoral muscles. The muscles of the body were pale.

The head was not examined.

The left cavity of the chest contained about a pint of serum. The lung was rather œdematous, but otherwise healthy, with the exception of some puckering and apparently chalky deposit at its apex. The lung on the right side adhered closely to the walls of the cavity, the adhesions being firm and cellular. The lung resembled that of the left side, and was also slightly disorganized at its apex. The pericardium contained about an ounce of clear and straw-coloured fluid. The heart was small and flabby.

The abdomen contained about two pints of clear serum. The stomach and alimentary canal were much distended with flatus. The liver was of a shrunken irregular shape, and was connected to the diaphragm by a few firm adhesions. Its structure was indurated, pale, and thickly pervaded with a substance having a white, hard, tuberculous character which in some parts had the form of defined rounded masses of the size of large pin heads, but for the most part was diffused. Some sections exhibited parts apparently stained with a dark ecchymosis as if from extravasated blood.

From some portions of liver seen after the inspection by Dr. Hodgkin, it appeared to him that the liver was in that state in which the acini became dense, rounded, and of a light colour, resembling small tubercles, and are readily detached: a condition of liver which is almost peculiar to those who have laboured under a cachectic condition from mercury. The gall-bladder was small and filled with a dark coloured green bile. The pancreas was not diseased. The spleen had contracted several firm adhesions to the neighbouring peritoneum; it was enlarged to about twice its usual size, and was unusually firm. Sections exhibited its structure dense, rather dry, and of a dark red colour, but homogeneous. Dr. Hodgkin examined this spleen, a short time after its removal from the body, and found its substance generally pervaded by numerous minute translucent bodies somewhat resembling incipient miliary tubercles of the lung, but considerably smaller than these generally are.

The kidneys were pale, flabby, and slightly mottled.

A few small miliary tubercles were found in the peritoneum, about the inguinal region resembling those which have been noticed above in the liver. Some of the mesenteric glands were much enlarged and filled with a firm white deposit. The inguinal, lumbar, and aortic glands were similarly affected. The bronchial glands were in a similar state, and also extensively ossified (or loaded with earthy matter). The axillary glands were in a state of suppuration, and exposed by ulceration at the part. The thoracic duct presented nothing unusual.

CASE II.

January 8, 1830. Thomas Westcott, aged apparently about fifty years, by trade a carpenter, a patient of Dr. Addison in the Clinical Ward, admitted 30th of December, 1829. He was not at all wasted, but was rather plump than otherwise; he had a pale and peculiar, cachectic countenance, which, without minute description, may be suggested to the mind by comparing it to what is seen in some cases of confirmed disease of the spleen. The most remarkable feature in his case was the great enlargement of nearly, if not quite, all of the absorbent glands within reach of examination, but more especially in the axillæ and groins. Those at the side of the neck were scarcely less so. Most of these glands which were within reach, were of about the size of pigeon's eggs, a few somewhat larger, and others rather smaller. They were of a smooth rounded or ovoid figure, and were only moderately firm, rather than indurated. An enlargement was also to be felt in one epididymis. The abdomen was distended, but the substance of the parietes appeared thick, no distinct tumour could be felt in the region of the spleen, or in any other part of the abdomen.

The functions of the brain had been somewhat disturbed, and the left eye did not see so well as the right.

It did not appear that this patient had been liable to any particular exposure, nor could any circumstance be referred to as the exciting cause of his malady. His death took place very suddenly in the morning of the 8th, and the examination was made four hours and a half after.

The veins of the head and neck were turgid. There was no lividity of the face. There were some ecchymosed spots on one of the legs.

The arachnoid was remarkably thick and opake. On the surface of the right hemisphere there was a diffused light rose-red colour, occupying the space of about the size of a crown piece; it appeared to depend on infiltration of the pia mater. This membrane separated readily from the surface of the brain. No morbid appearance was discovered in the substance of the brain, and no undue quantity of fluid in the ventricles. The cerebellum seemed to be, proportionately, rather small.

The right optic nerve was rather smaller than its fellow.

The glands in the axillæ and neck, as might have been expected, were found prodigiously enlarged, the deepest seated being in general the largest. The cellular structure around these was loose and free from any morbid deposit. These glands were smooth and of a whitish colour externally, with a few small bloody spots. When cut into, their internal structure was likewise seen to be of a light, nearly white, colour with a few small interspersed vessels. They were of a soft consistence, which might be compared to that of a testicle. They possessed a slight translucence, and were nearly or quite uniform throughout, exhibiting no trace of partial softening or suppuration. Although in appearance and consistence these enlarged glands bore considerable resemblance to some fungoid tumours, they presented nothing of the encysted formation. The alteration in this case seemed to consist in an interstitial deposit from a morbid hypertrophy of the glandular structure itself, rather than on a new or adventitious growth. The glands in the groin presented precisely the **same** character as those just described; the same **may** also be said of those in the thorax **and** abdomen, the situation and extent of which **will be presently** stated.

-173-

The pleuræ were nearly, if not altogether, free from adhesions and effusion. There were a few ecchymosed spots on the posterior part of the right lung; both lungs were spongy and crepitant, but rather emphysematous, and of a light colour, from the small quantity of blood which they contained.

The bronchial tubes contained some thick mucus.

The pericardium was healthy. The heart was greatly enlarged, and the right cavities particularly dilated; but the left were also large and distended, with thickened parietes. The muscular structure however did not appear to be diseased. The blood in the heart was barely coagulated, resembling that recently drawn into a basin. The glands along the subclavian arteries and about the roots of the bronchi were much enlarged.

In the abdomen nothing particular was noticed about the peritoneum. The glands at the small curvature of the stomach, several in Glisson's capsule, and a large mass of them along the entire course of the abdominal aorta and iliac arteries were greatly enlarged. There was a marked difference in the mesenteric glands, which, though larger than is natural, were none of them of the prodigious size of those above mentioned; they were however of a light colour, and their increase of size evidently depended on an interstitial deposit similar to that of the other glands. One of the enlarged glands in the lumbar region had a good deal of superficial ecchymosis. The absorbent vessels connected with it were enlarged and distended with a bloody serum. A similar fluid less deeply tinged was found in the thoracic duct.

The liver was very large, pale, and slightly granular. The spleen was very greatly enlarged, being at least nine inches long, five broad, and proportionally thick; its colour was lighter and redder than is natural, and more firm and close. On cutting into it an almost infinite number of small white nearly opake spots were seen pervading its substance; they were of irregular figure, but a few appeared nearly circular. They appeared to depend on a deposit in the cellular structure of the organ. There were no tubercles in the spleen, but the spots just mentioned were perhaps a commencement of this kind of formation.

The pancreas was large and pale, but otherwise healthy. The mucous membrane of the stomach and bowels offered nothing remarkable.

CASE V.

Inspection of a middle aged man, who had latterly been a patient of Dr. Back. He had long been in bad health, and had been for some time a patient under Dr. Bright. His last most urgent symptoms were referrible to the chest. When in the hospital the former time, he was observed to have the glands of the neck, and more particularly those near the upper part of the thyroid cartilage, considerably enlarged.

The body was emaciated. The glands before mentioned were still much enlarged, those in the axillæ were not observed to be particularly so, those in the groins were somewhat so. The abdomen was distended.

The head was not examined.

The greater part of one lung was distended, solid and void of air, its texture was rather soft and readily lacerable. Its colour seemed to be the result of the acute white hepatization very deeply soiled with reddish brown. The other lung was far from healthy, but it was rather engorged and softened than hepatized, and still contained air. One, if not both, pleuræ exhibited traces of recent inflammation with little or no effusion.

Nothing remarkable is remembered to have been noticed in the heart or pericardium.

In the abdomen there was a large quantity of serum with little appearance of coagulable lymph. In the stomach the mucous membrane was not quite healthy, presenting some indications of chronic inflammation; it, as well as the intestines, contained unhealthy secretions. The liver was of remarkably large size, weighing upwards of seven pounds. Its form and the smoothness of its surface were little if at all altered. The colour was somewhat mottled with a mixture of darkish green and yellow. The acini were manifestly enlarged, and it was suspected that they had undergone the fatty degeneration; but on exposure to heat, it appeared to contain little, if any, greasy substance. The spleen was very large, its weight is not known, but it appeared to be four or five times the average size; its texture was rather more solid and compact than is natural; it contained no tubercles, but the cellular structure interspersed through the parenchyma was more conspicuous than is usual, in some parts appearing in the form of specks, in which it was soft and easily broken down. The absorbent glands accompanying the aorta were greatly enlarged, some equalling at least the size of a pullet's egg; some, but more especially those in the abdomen, were reddened by injected or ecchymosed blood. The receptaculum chyli and some of the larger lymphatic branches, contained blood mixed with dark and almost black coagula. The thoracic duct, which was large, was filled in the same manner.

CASE VI.

July 19, 1830. Thomas Black, aged about fifty years, admitted into Barnabas Ward on the 30th of June, 1830, under the care of Dr. Bright. He was affected with large tuberose swellings of considerable firmness on both sides of the neck, in both axillæ, and in both groins. His abdomen was greatly distended, he suffered from difficulty of breathing, and was pale and rather emaciated.

It appeared that, about two years before, he had laboured under fever. That, being exposed to cold, shortly after, he observed the glands swell on one side of the neck; not long after on the other side, and in succession, those in the situations above mentioned.

The body presented considerable lividity, especially the extremities on the left side. The left side of the neck, and the left axilla, presented the largest tumours.

The head was not examined.

The tumours evidently depended on greatly enlarged absorbent glands along the course of the carotid and axillary arteries. On raising the sternum they were found to extend along the subclavians and internal mammaries; they were also found, though in less number and size, along the aorta in the posterior mediastinum; but it did not appear that the bronchial glands were at all similarly affected. There was some appearance of recent pleuritis and serous effusion into the chest.

In the peritoneal cavity there was a large quantity

of yellow serum mixed with some flakes of lymph. A large and continued mass of nodulous glandular tumours surrounded the aorta and iliac arteries, but the mesenteric glands were very slightly affected. The omentum was corrugated. The liver was rather small, with an irregular and uneven surface, its colour was lighter than natural, and the acini were converted into rounded fleshy masses, without any very great change in the intervening cellular membrane. It also contained two or three white tubercles, which resembled fungoid tubercles of the liver, and were situated at the surface of the organ. The structure dependent on cysts was not demonstrable in them, but from their form it might be suspected. The spleen was of moderate size, and appeared to be quite free from any adventitious deposit, which is a fact worthy of remark, as in very many cases of glandular disease bearing resemblance to the present case, this organ has been affected, and generally tubercular. The pancreas was imbedded in the tumours, but appeared pretty healthy.

The kidneys were livid and congested.

The tumours which formed the most striking features in this case very nearly resembled each other in structure; there appeared to be merely a little difference in firmness; they were of various sizes, from that of a horse-bean to that of a hen's egg; they had a round or ovoid figure, and were invested by a thin membrane, pretty smooth externally, and connected to the loose and apparently healthy cellular membrane which surrounded the tumours; the other surface intimately adhered to the structure of the tumour.   This texture was apparently pretty uniform throughout, and was pale and slightly translucent, and could not be said to evince traces of the mode of formation dependent on cysts; they shewed no disposition to suppuration or softening; some, when just taken from the body, were of a semi-cartilaginous hardness, but became considerably softer after a little maceration.

The aorta appeared to be a little compressed by the tumours.

This patient had an old reducible hernia on the right side, on which side there appeared to be hydrocele also.

It may be observed that notwithstanding some differences in structure, to be noticed hereafter, all these cases agree in the remarkable enlargement of the absorbent glands accompanying the larger arteries; namely, the glandulæ concatenatæ in the neck, the axillary and inguinal glands, and those accompanying the aorta in the thorax and abdomen. That as far as could be ascertained from observation, or from what could be collected from the history of the cases, this enlargement of the glands appeared to be a primitive affection of those bodies, rather than the result of an irritation propagated to them from some ulcerated surface or other inflamed texture through the medium of their inferent vessels, and that although, in some instances, the glands so enlarged may contain a little concrete inorganizable matter, such as is known to result from what is called scrofulous inflammation, it is obvious that this circumstance is not an essential character, but rather an accidental concomitant to the idiopathic interstitial enlargement of the absorbent glandular structure throughout the body. That unless the word inflammation be allowed to have a more indefinite and loose meaning than is generally assigned to it, this affection of the glands can scarcely be attributed to that cause, since they are unattended with pain, heat, and other ordinary symptoms of inflammation, and are not necessarily accompanied by any alteration in the cellular or other surrounding structures, and do not shew any disposition to go on to the production of pus or any other acknowledged product of inflammation except where, as in the cases above alluded to, inflammation may have supervened as an accidental affection of the hypertrophied structure. Nor can the enlargement in question, with any better reason, be attributed to the formation of any of those adventitious structures, the production of which I have already had occasion to describe, and have referred to the type of compound adventitious serous cysts. Notwithstanding the different characters which this enlargement may present, it appears nearly in all cases to consist of a pretty uniform texture throughout, and this rather to be the consequence of a general increase of every part of the gland, than of a new structure developed within it, and pushing the original structure aside, as when ordinary tuberculous matter is deposited in these bodies. At the same time it must be admitted that the new material by which the enlargement is effected, presents various degrees of organizability, which in some instances is extremely slight, and appears incompetent to maintain the vitality of the affected gland. In such cases the new structure will generally become opake, soften, or break down, and acting as a foreign irritating body, excite irritation and lead to the formation of abscess. The case of William Burrows, (No. III.,) and also that of a native of Owhyhee, who died in Guy's Hospital with extensive abscess in the axilla, are, I believe, to be considered of this kind.

The remarkable appearance of blood in the thoracic duct and some of the absorbents, observed in the case of Thomas Westcott, (No. IV.,) although it sufficiently attracted my attention to induce me to have a drawing immediately made, was only regarded as an accidental occurrence; but the recurrence of the same phenomenon to a much more considerable and striking extent in the recent case, (No. V.,) induces me to suppose that it is intimately connected with this glandular disease. It may also be observed that in the last-mentioned case the enlarged glands from which the lymphatic vessels containing blood proceeded, were particularly loaded with blood; and if my recollection does not deceive me, a tendency to the same state was present in the case of Westcott, although it escaped notice in the record of the inspection.

Another circumstance which has arrested my attention, in conjunction with this affection of the absorbent glands, is the state of the spleen which, with one exception in all the cases that I have had the opportunity of examining, has been found more or less diseased, and in some thickly pervaded with defined bodies of various sizes, in structure resembling that of the diseased glands. We might, from this circumstance, be induced to suspect that these bodies in the spleen, like the enlarged glands themselves, are the result of the morbid enlargement of a pre-existing structure, an idea which may derive some support from the fact, that although in human spleens no glandular structure is distinguishable, in those of some inferior animals a multitude of minute bodies exist which appear to be of that nature. Malpighi indeed considered the acini or granulations in the spleen to be glands. In one instance it may be remarked that although the glandular derangement had advanced very far, the depositions in the spleen were extremely minute, assuming the appearance of miliary tubercles. Hence, we may conclude that if, as I conceive to be the case, there be a close connection between the derangement of the glands and that of the spleen, the latter is a posterior effect, and on this account may not always have been produced, when that of the glands or some other disease

-183-

carried off the patient. In other instances, the spleen, although much enlarged, contained no regular defined bodies, although the white cellular structure was very evident in increased quantity pervading the dense and enlarged mass of the organ. In such cases it might still be doubted whether, had the patient's life been protracted, the deposits in question might not ultimately have taken place, yet I am inclined to believe the contrary, and to suspect that either the previous derangement of the structure of the organ or the greater age of the patients may have opposed their production. I mention this effect of age merely as a suspicion or idea, founded on the fact that I have very rarely, if ever, met with any kind of tubercles, excepting those of malignant character, in the spleens of adults, whilst they have been by no means unfrequent in a far less number of spleens of children and young persons which it has fallen to my lot to examine. The only exceptions which I can call to mind, as having been furnished by my own observation, have been in the case of one or two foreigners from warm countries, on whom the change of climate may have had considerable effect.

Some further confirmation of my suspicion that a connection exists between the glandular derangement of which I have been speaking, and the state of the spleen, has occurred to me since the preceding observations were written. Whilst examining the unrivalled collection of pathological drawings made by my friend Dr. Carswell, I was struck with one representing a greatly enlarged spleen, loaded with large tubercles of a rounded figure and light colour. I immediately recognized it as a fine example of the affection I have been describing, and my suspicions were presently confirmed by the doctor's shewing me another fine drawing of the greatly enlarged glands of the neck, axillæ, and groins of the same subject.

The Doctor has favoured me with a copy of the case, and allowed me to place the drawings themselves before you.

CASE VII.

" Cancer Cerebriformis of the Lymphatic Glands, and of the Spleen.

" The delineations of this very remarkable case were taken from a man who died in the hospital St. Louis at Paris, in the month of April. Monsr. Lugol, one of the physicians of the hospital, and under whose care the patient was, has promised to give me the particulars of this case. I was told, however, that the patient, who was between thirty and forty years of age, stout made, and not lean, had been affected with swelling of the glands under the jaws, along both sides of the neck, in the axillæ and groins for between three and four months, from which he had suffered but little inconvenience, to which he had paid but little attention, and had employed no remedies. It was only a short time before he applied to be taken into the hospital that he felt a difficulty in swallowing, which rapidly increased, and for the last two or three days was such as to prevent him from taking any kind of food whatever. As his appetite had never been affected by the disease, he was, when he came to the St. Louis hospital, in a state of great suffering, not only from want of food and from debility, but from the idea that he was rendered incapable of satisfying the cravings of hunger, together with the prospect of inevitable death.

" He lived rather more than two days.

" *Inspection of the body.*—On each side of the neck were large groups of glands extending from the angle of the jaw down to the clavicle, where they were joined to another group, coming up from the axillæ and passing under the clavicle. The sub-maxillary and sublingual glands were greatly enlarged, and united with the other lymphatic glands, formed an almost continuous chain stretching along the border of the jaw, and uniting under the chin. These glands were of various sizes, some of them were not larger than a pea, while others were as large as a hen's egg; they were round, oval, or of an irregular form, particularly where they were united by a common capsule. A great many of them presented the colour which distinguishes them in the healthy state; others were of a yellowish tinge, with more or less redness and vascularity; whilst a few were of a deep red colour and highly vascular. The

greater number of them when pressed between the
fingers, felt pretty firm and somewhat elastic; those
that were red and vascular were softer. All of them
were enclosed in a thin but firm capsule, which contained a substance of the colour and consistence of
brain, and in which were distributed a considerable
number of blood-vessels. In the softest the vascularity was such as to give to the cerebriform matter
an appearance resembling a mixture of equal parts of
brain and blood. A similar state of the glands was
observed in both groins. The greater number of
them were as large as pigeons' eggs, and could be
followed passing upwards under Poupart's ligament,
surrounding the great blood-vessels, and terminating
in the diseased lymphatic and mesenteric glands. The
diseased appearances observed in the glands of the
groin are represented in No. 4—6. Fig. I; those of
the neck and axillæ No. 4. a. In No. 4—6 is seen
the appearance of the substance of which the glands
were formed; in one of them the vascularity of this
substance is seen to be very great, whilst in the other
the vessels are few in number, long, and slender. The
quantity of cerebriform matter is also seen to differ
considerably in each. Besides, in the lower figure
the lobulated structure which it presents is pretty
well marked. In Fig. III. two of the glands are
represented after having been injected. In the upper
one a large vein is seen coming out from it, and
arising from a great number of minute vessels, which
apparently are situated near the surface of the gland.
In the lower one, the corresponding artery is shewn,

dividing and subdividing into an immense number of extremely fine branches which are distributed throughout the substance of the gland.   No. 4. c. Fig. I. represents an enormous tumour formed by the lymphatic glands situated under the liver, duodenum, pancreas, and great blood-vessels of these parts.   It was as large as an adult's head, projecting forwards on a level with the convex surface of the liver, and carried before it the duodenum, pancreas, and gall-ducts, which passed over its anterior surface. Fig. II. represents a section of this tumour, which is seen to be formed of a great number of glands, some of which are as large as a small orange.   Like those of the neck and axillæ, they were composed of cerebriform matter, possessing a greater or less degree of vascularity.   In the centre of the tumour considerable hemorrhage had taken place, the centre of the hemorrhagic effusion was occupied by coagulated blood, and the circumference by layers of fibrine.   The vena cava and aorta passed through the tumour, and the former was nearly perforated by one of the diseased glands.

" No. 4. c. Represents the same pathological condition in the glands situated in the posterior fauces. The glands situated around the root of the tongue were so much enlarged as to shut up completely by their projecting upwards, backwards, and forwards, the posterior nares and superior aperture of the œsophagus.   I could not ascertain the precise state of the epiglottis, but it must to a certain

extent at least have been free, as it did not appear
that inspiration had been much impeded. The
amygdalæ, formed entirely of cerebriform matter,
presented a pale-yellow colour tinged here and there
with red specks, produced apparently from the rupture of minute blood-vessels. They have also lost
that characteristic appearance from which they derive their name, having become almost perfectly
smooth from the accumulation of the cerebriform
matter and the distention of their envelope.

" The spleen was the only organ apart from the
lymphatic glands which presented a similar, or indeed any, disease in this remarkable case. The external surface of this organ is shewn in No. 4. a.
Fig. I. Besides great increase of its bulk, it presented externally a great number of irregular elevations surrounded by redness and vascularity. When
divided longitudinally, Fig. II., it appeared to be
formed entirely of cerebriform matter and fine blood-
vessels ; hardly any trace of its natural structure being observable. It presented a lobulated structure ;
the lobules varying from the size of a small pea to
that of a large gooseberry ; these being again divided
and subdivided into smaller ones—the boundaries
of the lobules and the intersections of the latter were
the parts in which vascularity was greatest—it did
indeed appear as if the lobulated structure had been
the result of a vascular net-work so disposed as to
inclose and separate more or less completely portions of different sizes of the cerebriform matter. It

depended, however, in all likelihood, on the structure of the spleen, in the cells of which, or in the blood which they contain, the cerebriform matter was deposited or formed, whilst the blood-vessels which surrounded the lobules and ramified in their intersections arose from those which belong to the splenic cells.

" The body having been removed by inadvertence before I had time to examine the chest, I did not ascertain the state of the bronchial glands, but I was informed by one of the house-physicians that they were not diseased."

Although the Doctor has employed the term " cerebriform matter," which conveys a ready idea of the texture of the diseased glands, he will excuse my differing from him so far as to regard the affection in this case as distinct from cerebriform cancer. I feel the less difficulty in doing so, in the recollection that one of the cases of which I had given the details was, like Dr. Carswell's, considered as fungoid until a special and close inspection had detected the difference.

Besides the preceding cases, of which I have been enabled to obtain the inspections, I have met with other examples in the living subject which, as far as the glands were concerned, were evidently of the same character with those I have been describing. One of the most remarkable occurred in the person of a Jew, apparently between forty and fifty years of

age; the glands in the neck were prodigiously enlarged, forming smooth ovoid masses, unaccompanied
by inflammatory symptoms or thickening of the surrounding cellular structure. The glands in the axillæ
and groins were in the same state; in fact, in this
case, the enlargement was more considerable than in
any other that I have witnessed. His general health
was much impaired; I do not recollect that there
were any dropsical symptoms at the time I saw him.
I accidentally lost sight of him, but afterwards learnt
that he died about two months from the time of my
seeing him.

Another case occurred in a cachectic, rather emaciated child, who was brought, on one occasion only,
as an out-patient, to Guy's Hospital. The glands in
the neck, axillæ, and groins were considerably enlarged, and as far as I could judge were of the firm
character observed in the cases of Joseph Sinnott
and Ellenborough King, rather than the softer and
more fleshy character noticed in the glands of Westcott, Black, Case V, and as far as I could observe,
in that of the Jew just mentioned.

A pathological paper may perhaps be thought of
little value if unaccompanied by suggestions designed
to assist in the treatment, either curative or palliative;
on this head however I must confess that I have nothing to offer.

Most of the cases, it may be observed, were those

of patients in the hospital, where they had not sought admission until the disease had reached an advanced and hopeless stage. The Jew was the only individual whom I had an opportunity of treating myself, and him only for a short period, when his case had already become hopeless. The cascarilla and soda which were given with a view to improve his general health, and the iodine employed as the agent most likely to affect the glands, appeared to be productive of no advantage, on which account it is probable the patient withdrew himself from my observation. Were patients thus affected to come under my care in an earlier and less hopeless period of their malady, I think I should be inclined to endeavour as far as possible to increase the general vigour of the system, to enjoin, as far as consistent with this object, the utmost protection from the inclemencies and vicissitudes of the weather, to employ iodine externally, and to push the internal use of caustic potash as far as circumstances might render allowable. I mention this last part of the treatment in consequence of the strong commendation which Brandrish has bestowed on the use of this caustic alkali in absorbent glandular affections. The views which I have been induced to take respecting the functions of the absorbent vessels, would make me the more disposed to adopt it *.

---

* Shortly after the reading of this paper, I was favoured with the following communication from my friend G. O. Heming, of Kentish Town:—

98 DR. HODGKIN ON SOME MORBID APPEARANCES

Having been led to notice some morbid appearances in the spleen connected with the glandular disease of which I have been speaking, I take the opportunity, before quitting this organ, to advert to another morbid appearance presented by it. In the observations prefixed to the sixth section of the second part of the catalogue of Guy's Museum*, I have briefly noticed a derangement of structure met with in the spleen, which arrested my attention, rather from con-

DEAR SIR,

You will, I am sure, be pleased with the following extract from Malpighi.

Yours truly, G. O. Heming.

" In homine difficilius emergunt (speaking of the granules in the spleen): si tamen ex morbo universum glandularum genus turgeat, manifestiores redduntur, auctâ ipsarum magnitudine, ut in defunctâ puellâ observavi, in quâ lien globulis conspicuis racematim dispersis totus scatebat."

* " The preparations from 2000 to 2004 inclusive, although of but little pathological importance, possess some interest as specimens of a morbid appearance occasionally met with in the spleen, but which, so far as the author knows, has not been hitherto described or noticed. It consists of a partial or circumscribed degeneration of the structure which becomes preternaturally firm and dense, and of a light colour. The part thus affected may be easily mistaken for a tubercle, until close inspection has detected in it traces of the original structure of the organ. It is bounded by a defined line, and on the surface there is sometimes a slight depression where it is united to the healthy structure. In all the instances which the author has yet observed, the portion of spleen thus degenerated has been situated in a transverse direction. He has observed it principally, if not exclusively, in males, and he is inclined to consider it as the result of external injury."—Vid. Catalogue of the Museum of Guy's Hospital. Part II. Sect. 6.

sidering it as hitherto undescribed, than from having reason to attach any importance to it in conjunction with disease. The cases which I have since met with have not only thrown further light on its nature, but have shewn that it may become the cause of violent and even fatal symptoms. The partial induration of the spleen accompanied with loss of colour, and in general with a diminution of bulk, and having at first sight a good deal of the appearance of tubercle, seems to be only one of the stages in which this derangement of the spleen presents itself to our view. It appears to commence in a partial extravasation of blood, the character of which will perhaps be best conceived by stating it to be what would be called by some pathologists apoplexy of the spleen. This I had already conceived to be the case, and suspected that it arose from external violence. The case of Mary Hamblin, No. I., tends to confirm this suspicion : it is however by no means improbable that spontaneous or idiopathic apoplexies of the spleen may take place. Yet the general appearance of the lesion will, I believe, form a characteristic distinction between such cases and those in which external violence had been the cause.

When the effusion of blood is quite recent, the part affected is distinguished from the other parts of the organ, not only by its increased density, but by its deep venous hue. It does not remain long in this state, but soon begins to assume a brownish colour, the change generally taking place at the circumference, but sometimes at the centre. This change, the rationale of which is not easily given, is precisely similar to that which takes place in apoplexy of the lungs, in the transition of the red into one of the grey forms of induration of the lung from inflammation; in the coagula sometimes met with in the heart and vessels; in the layers of aneurismal tumours; and even in cerebral apoplexy.

The portion of spleen thus altered, although possessing little perceptible trace of organization, may yet retain its vitality, and remain a permanent structure, in which case its density increases, but its bulk contracts, and a thin semi-transparent boundary may be seen to separate the altered from the healthy structure of the organ; this I conceive to be occasioned by the former not participating in the constant variations of dimension to which the latter is liable. It was in this state that the derangement of which I am speaking first presented itself to my attention. (See 2d, 3d, and 4th Examples.)

Although, as I have remarked, the derangement in question, when arrived at this stage, may reamin quiescent for an indefinite length of time, and perhaps never throughout the life of the individual give rise to the slightest inconvenience; yet, it would seem to predispose the adjoining parts of the organ to derangement either from external force, or from unusual distension. In the 5th Example, this disturbance appears to be extremely slight, only amounting to a slight appearance of extravasation or apoplexy.

In the sixth case, that of Maria Lowther, the derangement in the structure of the spleen, in the neighbourhood of the indurated portion, was much more considerable, amounting to complete softening, accompanied by softening in the central part of the degenerated spot. It appeared pretty evident that this state of the spleen was the exciting cause of the severe peritonitis, in the same way that this inflammation is not unfrequently set up by disease in the appendix cæci from feculent concretions. It is also highly probable that some of the remarkable symptoms which attended this case, and excited the idea of phlebitis, were also dependent on what may be considered as the gangrenous softening of the substance of the spleen in contact with the indurated part. No light was thrown on the cause which excited this softening, but if my suspicions are correct as to external injury being the cause of the original derangement, it is likely that a repetition of this cause, may promote the secondary affection by producing a slight laceration on the surface of the indurated part. Although the sudden death of the patient who formed the subject of the seventh case was rather to be attributed to the heart than to the state of the spleen, yet I think we must principally ascribe to this latter cause, the symptoms under which this girl had laboured, and more especially those paroxysms which were regarded as occasioned by intermittent fever.

My enquiries in this case also did not succeed in leading to any information as to the mode in which the process of softening had been excited. It is possible that slight external violence may have been adequate to this effect. It may, however, be queried whether intermittent fever had not actually existed, in the cold stage of which the spleen being gorged may have sustained a partial laceration where its distension was restrained by the unyielding character of the previously degenerated portion. Be this as it may, there can be but little doubt that the occurrence of such paroxysms would either occasion such a dis-organization, or greatly aggravate it when once set up.

No. I.

May 3, 1831. Mary Hamblin, a patient of Dr. Bright's, in Charity Ward, admitted April 27th, 1831, in consequence of a state of mania, in which she was reported to have been a little more than a week. She was the mother of twins, whom she had suckled sixteen months, and being a spare and delicate woman, had been greatly reduced thereby. For some time before her admission she had complained of uneasiness in her head, and said she was afraid she should go out of her mind, as her mother and some others of her relations had done. Only an imperfect account could be obtained of her symptoms prior to admission, but it appeared probable that some restraint approaching to violence had been employed, since in a transient lucid interval which occurred whilst in the hospital, she expressed her satisfaction at not being likely to be again ill used. Whilst in the hospital she generally lay in a state of insensibility, almost amounting to coma, yet sometimes, in a state approaching to delirium, she would sing hymns, and try to get out of bed, but she was easily restrained. It did not appear that there was any erotic tendency in her delirium. She died six days after her admission.

Nothing remarkable was observed external to the dura mater. The vessels of the pia mater were less injected than is usual, more especially where forming the plexus choroides, which was nearly colourless. The arachnoid about the pons varolii was rather considerably but partially thickened. The substance of the brain offered nothing remarkable.

The pleuræ, lungs, pericardium, and heart were generally healthy.

The peritoneum appeared free from marks of either old or recent inflammation, and nothing remarkable was discovered in the mucous membrane of the alimentary canal.

The liver seemed healthy in form and texture, but

its convex surface was mottled with irregular spots and blotches of a yellowish colour, which suggested the idea that the organ had received some violence.

The spleen was of its natural size and generally of a healthy appearance, but it was irregularly mottled with spots of a deeper and darker venous hue, the central parts of some of which were of a lighter colour. Notwithstanding the irregularity of these spots, they imperfectly affected a transverse direction across the organ a little above its middle. On cutting into the spleen so as to pass through some of these spots, they were found to consist of portions of the substance of the spleen indurated by coagulated venous blood, like portions of lung in pulmonic apoplexy. Some of these masses were of a light colour internally, but with little or no softening. It seems highly probable, that these appearances in the liver and spleen, and which had in all probability nothing at all to do with the death of the patient, were the effects of some degree of injury produced by the means employed for restraint shortly after her attack.

The kidneys were not observed to offer any thing remarkable.

The uterus was of its natural size, but its lining membrane was of a deep red colour. The fallopian tubes were free from adhesions and appeared quite healthy. The ovaries were rather large, exhibited few cicatrices, and were remarkably smooth for those of a married female of her age. They were rather flabby.

EXAMPLE II.

Extract from the report of the Case of Daniel Patrick.

In the spleen, which was rather large, there was an irregularly shaped but circumscribed mass, rather larger than a hazle nut, of a structure which at first appeared to be tuberculous, but which proved to be dependent on a peculiar alteration of structure.

EXAMPLE III.

Extract from the report of the Case of J. Woodbridge.

The spleen was of moderate size; a defined portion of its structure was considerably indented, having about the firmness of liver a little indurated, the part so altered was of a light brown colour, approaching to that of new leather; the passage from this to the healthy part was abrupt, but there was no membranous separation between them. This derangement of structure did not appear to be attended with either increase or diminution of volume, so as to produce either depression or protuberance at the surface, although this was partially implicated.

-200-

EXAMPLE IV.

Extract from the report of the Case of William Hunter.

The spleen was of a moderate size; it had contracted some peritoneal adhesions, there were a few small semi-cartilaginous spots on its surface, and a circumscribed portion had undergone a peculiar degeneration, by which its texture was rendered solid and of a light brown colour. As in the three former cases in which this derangement has been already noticed, it appeared, on the surface of the organ, where a slight depression existed between the healthy and altered structure. A vessel of considerable size was seen passing through this part, which still retained some faint traces of its original structure.

EXAMPLE V.

Extract from the report of James Skelton.

The spleen was of moderate size, it was in its contracted state, and its structure was generally healthy, but deeply imbedded in its convex surface, there was a light yellowish brown well defined deposit. About some portion of the surface of this deposit, there was a little extravasation of blood, apparently of an apoplectic character.

CASE VI.

October 24th, 1829. " Maria Lowther, aged 17 years, admitted into the Clinical Ward on the 22d instant under the care of Dr. Bright. She had enjoyed but indifferent health for some time. About five weeks ago she suffered much from a whitlow on the forefinger, caused by the prick of a needle, her finger healed, but about a week after, she appeared to have a cold. She had cough, painful respiration, and frequent rigors, she complained of great pain in the bowels and head, particularly of the latter. An abscess now appeared under the axilla, but previously to its appearance she had suffered much from irritability; this abscess dispersed, but was immediately succeeded by another on the fore-arm, together with the reappearance of the one in the axilla. Her head at this period became more confused, she grew worse, and became delirious. Her legs were observed to be œdematous on the Monday or Tuesday previous to her admission, and general tenderness was complained of for the first time yesterday. For a week past her motions had appeared bloody, and epistaxis had taken place on two occasions. Soon after her admission she appeared in an exhausted state, her face pale and anxious, her eyes sunk, and there was exquisite tenderness to the touch throughout the body. The feet and legs were slightly œdematous, ecchymosed spots were formed on the hands and feet, there was an abscess in the axilla and another on the fore-arm. The abdomen was tumid as well as tender. At night the symptoms were aggravated, she became delirious during the night, and at the morning visit she was found in a dying state; death took place about half-past ten in the morning of the 23d."

The body was a little emaciated, the discolouration resembling purpura had almost entirely disappeared. The cuticle was raised both at the tip of the middle finger, and on one toe on the right side into two bullæ containing slightly purulent sanguinolent serum. The abscess in the axilla presented a cavity of about the size of a moderate orange, it was ragged internally, and of a dirty sanguinolent colour; one or more of the absorbent glands were nearly detached by the destruction of the surrounding cellular membrane.

Nothing remarkable was observed in the calvaria or membranes of the brain, except that the arachnoid was very transparent, and that there was rather an unusually small number of vessels visible in the pia mater. The substance of the brain was likewise healthy, except at the posterior part of the left hemisphere, where a portion of about an inch in diameter, occupying a part both of the cortical and medullary structure, was completely softened and broken down. It was slightly discoloured by blood imperfectly intermixed, it was not surrounded by any induration or distinct line of demarcation, but the softening was most considerable towards the centre.

Both pleuræ were healthy, with the exception of slight traces of recent inflammation at the lower part of the left lung. The substance of the lungs was likewise generally healthy, but at the posterior part of the left there were some traces of recent inflammation limited to a few lobules which were firmer and of a somewhat lighter colour than the surrounding structure, which was the seat of cadaveric infiltration. At the back part of the left lung there was some hepatization as well as cadaveric infiltration.

The pericardium was healthy, but contained about two ounces of straw coloured serum. There was a small opake white patch on the anterior surface of the heart. The organ itself was quite healthy, but contained a small quantity of blood which was imperfectly coagulated, except near the origin of the vessels where there was some coagulum prolonged into these vessels. A partial separation of the colouring matter had taken place.

The abdomen was somewhat distended, the peritoneum presented universal marks of inflammation, several convolutions of intestines were feebly glued together by tender and opake membranous flakes of lymph. There was considerable effusion of yellow colour mixed with flocculent particles of opake lymph, and presenting a sero-purulent character. The surface of the stomach in contact with the under surface of the liver was covered with a layer of yellow lymph. The peritoneal covering of the small intestines was easily detached from the muscular coat. The stomach and small intestines were distended with gas, their mucous membrane was generally healthy, but the patches of aggregate glands were rendered distinct by numerous minute blackish points. The mucous membrane of the colon was of a darkish grey colour, and was extremely irregular, which appeared to depend on lymph and other secretions becoming adherent to a number of small thickly scattered points. On scraping off this secretion, the subjacent surface presented either a smaller spot of very slight abrasion or a livid ecchymosis. This state had probably been preceded by suppressed mucous secretion. The liver was of large size, extending over the spleen to the left side, and passing down for some distance between it and the parietes. It was rather pale, but in other respects healthy, except that it presented spots of ecchymosis where it had been in contact with the spleen.

The spleen was rather large, and presented the following remarkable appearances: two portions rather more than an inch in breadth, placed transversely and occupying the whole of the shorter diameter of the spleen, were of a lightish yellow colour, they were of closer structure than the natural texture, and appeared to depend on a particular degeneration of a part of the organ itself. A process of softening had broken down the central parts of these portions, which were situated about an inch and a half from each other. The substance of the spleen in contact with these portions was of a deep livid colour and completely softened.

The pancreas was healthy. The kidneys were likewise healthy. The ovaries were of an elongated figure, full and plump, their surfaces presented numerous bright red points, their tunics white and dense, without any appearance of cicatrices. The vesicles of De Graaff generally clear and healthy, but a few, in one of the ovaries, were in the form of white opake semi-cartilaginous bodies. The intervening substance in both was pale, but unusually firm.

The uterus was small.

There was an equivocal appearance of a remaining hymen.

The symptoms in this case having induced a suspicion that the veins were inflamed, they were particularly examined in different parts of the body. No phlebitis was, however, discovered, yet in some of these vessels the blood was coagulated, and from its appearance had probably been in this state a short time before death.

CASE VII.

September 21st, 1828. Martha Newton, aged apparently about 25 years, a patient of Dr. Bright's, in Dorcas's ward, into which she was admitted on the 17th instant. She had come to town from Brighton, and described herself as labouring under intermittent fever, but her appearance did not altogether accord with the idea of ague. She stated that she had been taking bark prior to her coming to town, and a repetition of bark or sulphate of quinine was prescribed. Her pulse was not remarkable either for quickness or irregularity, and none of her complaints suggested a suspicion of disease of any of the viscera of the thorax. She had one paroxysm shortly after her admission, which was reported by the sister of the ward to differ from the ordinary paroxysm of ague. She was seen by Dr. Bright in another of these paroxysms on the 19th. The quinine or bark was continued, but some local visceral disease rather than ague was suspected. She died suddenly on the morning of the 20th, after eating a moderate breakfast.

The body was pale and not emaciated, and rather œdematous, the areola round the nipple was but faintly discoloured. The abdomen bore no marks of parturition.

The head was carefully examined, but no morbid appearance was detected in the brain or its membranes, except some thickening, and a whitish deposit in very minute opake particles in the plexus choroides.

There was a great deal of old pleuritic adhesion on the right side, less on the left, and a small quantity of clear but discoloured serous effusion on both sides, infiltrating the adventitious cellular structure. Both lungs had more than the natural firmness, but not the character of hepatization. They were of a darkish livid colour, very œdematous, contained very little air, and no tuberculous nor other deposit.

The pericardium contained two or three ounces of serum, which was very sanguinolent. This state of the serum, not only in the pericardium, but also, though in a less degree, in the pleura, was probably more the result of transudation after death than before it. There was a strong adhesion in the form of a ligamentous bridle between the close and the reflected pericardium on the left side. The pericardium on the auricle was roughened by minute elevations.

The heart appeared distended, and on being laid open by a transverse section it was found to be dilated, with thinning rather than hypertrophy of its parietes. The muscular structure was flabby and pale, and less evidently fibrous than in health. The right ventricle was nearly as much dilated as the left; no valvular disease was detected, but at the mouth of the pulmonary artery there was a singular original formation. There appeared to be four valves instead of three, a small part of one of them being cut off by a thin membranous partition.

The quantity of fluid in the abdomen was inconsiderable. There were no adhesions except in the neighbourhood of the spleen, where they were considerable, old and strong, especially between this organ and the diaphragm.

In the spleen there was a defined mass of about the size of a walnut of a light colour, which, as in some specimens before observed, appeared to depend on an infiltration into, or degeneration of the structure of the part.   This mass appeared to be commencing the process of softening.   The structure immediately adjoining it was, however, much more softened, so as nearly to have effected its separation, it was of a dark or almost black colour.   The remainder of the spleen, though not similarly affected, was soft, probably from cadaveric change.   There was, however, one part of its substance in which a change resembling the infiltration before mentioned was commencing.

The stomach contained scarcely any food, and with the intestines appeared to be tolerably healthy.

The liver and pancreas were likewise healthy.

The kidneys were pale, and in the right there was a yellowish white mass in which a degeneration similar to that noticed in the spleen appeared to have taken place, the traces of the original structure being still visible.

The ovaries presented several cicatrices, the tubes were free from adhesions.   The uterus rather large. A vascular peritoneal cyst was attached to one of the broad ligaments.

-209-

ON THE OBJECT OF POST MORTEM EXAMINATIONS,

Being an Address delivered to the Pupils of Guy's Hospital, on the Opening of the Theatre of Morbid Anatomy, Jan. 1828,

By Dr. Hodgkin.

———

* * * *

THOUGH it is needless for me to say any thing to enforce the importance of attention to morbid anatomy, since those whom I have now the honour of addressing, by their presence here, give proof that they are fully impressed with it, and are doubtless convinced that, while it affords the best, and in many instances the only test of our diagnosis, it is not less valuable in relation to the formation of therapeutical principles ; yet it may not be inexpedient for me, before I proceed to explain the plan by which I hope not altogether to fail in discharging the duty allotted me, to call your attention to the objects which it is our place to observe in making *post mortem* examinations.

These objects admit of various modes of classification. On the present occasion I shall divide them according to the order of time, and shall commence by the most recent, under which head I mean to include those changes which have been termed cadaveric. Phenomena of this kind may depend on gases exhaled, or developed in the tissues—on the permanent fluids, or on the solid parts of the body.

The first, or those of a gaseous nature, though they have hitherto been very much neglected, are by no means devoid of interest. On them depend not only the remarkable and often rapidly produced emphysimatous state of the subject, but the odour exhaled by the bodies of the dead. That this smell is peculiar when death has been occasioned by some kinds of poison, as by prussic acid, for instance, is well known; and, though less frequently mentioned, it can scarcely have failed to attract the observation of those who are in the habit of attending inspections, that the smell present on these occasions is by no means uniform. This variety, though in part dependent on causes operating either on the body when dead or on the individual in the act of dying, ought doubtless, in some instances, to be referred to changes effected in the animal matter during life; hence, though strictly cadaveric, they will be found on investigation to possess a greater degree of pathological importance than has hitherto been assigned to them. Such, at least, is the conjecture which repeated observations have induced me to entertain. I am not aware that this subject has ever been made a special object of investigation; and though it is one in which numerous difficulties would be met with, amongst which the want of a definite nomenclature for odours would not be the least, still I would recommend it to the attention of those who have time to devote to it.

In the Preface to Dr. St. John's work on Chemical Nomenclature, published in 1788, there are some remarks which point to an object of great practical importance to be gained by an accurate discrimination of the odours exhaled by the bodies of the dead. As the work is but little known, an extract from it will not be uninteresting.

" I have sometimes observed," says the doctor, " a phenomenon to take place during the putrefaction of human bodies, and which I cannot but think of very great importance to be inquired into and known. This is the exhalation of a particular gas, which is the most active and dreadful of all corrosive poi-

sons, and produces most sudden and terrible effects upon a living creature. This I more than once had an opportunity of remarking in the dissecting-room of M. Andravi, at Paris. I know that the carbonic acid gas produced by the combustion of charcoal, from liquors in fermentation, and by the respiration of animals, as well as all other elastic fluids, except vital air, is incapable of sustaining life; but the aeriform fluid which is exhaled at certain times from animal bodies in putrefaction, is infinitely more noxious than any elastic fluid as yet discovered; for it is not only incapable of sustaining life in the absence of vital air, but is dreadfully deleterious, and does not at all seem to abate in its corrosive property even in the presence of the atmospherical fluid: so that it is utterly dangerous to approach a body in this state of putrefaction. I have known a gentleman who, by slightly touching the intestines of a human body beginning to liberate this corrosive gas, was affected with a violent inflammation, which, in a very short space of time, extended up almost the entire of his arm, producing an extensive ulcer of the most foul and frightful appearance, which continued for several months, and reduced him to a miserable state of emaciation. He then went to the South of France, but whether he died, or escaped with the loss of his arm, I have not been able to learn. This is only one example of many which I have seen. I have known a celebrated professor who was attacked with a violent inflammation of the nares and fauces, from which he with difficulty recovered, by stooping for an instant over a body which was beginning to give forth this deleterious fluid. It is happy for mankind that this particular stage of putrefaction continues but for a few hours; and what may appear very remarkable, this destructive gas is not very disagreeable in smell, and has nothing of that abominable and loathsome fetor produced by dead bodies in a less dangerous state of corruption, but has a certain smell totally peculiar to itself, by which it may be instantly discovered by any one that has ever smelt it before."

Though the doctor has doubtless exaggerated the deadly properties of the gas of which he speaks, and in one instance, at least, appears to have attributed to it effects which ought rather to have been ascribed to contact with the viscera, I see no reason to dispute his accuracy in connecting a particular condition of the body, which renders it a source of danger to those engaged in the dissection of it, with the evolution of a gas of a peculiar and recognizable odour.

The cadaveric phenomenon dependent on the permanent fluids being more evident than those of the class of which I have just spoken, are consequently much better known. They are either dependent on the gravitation of the fluids, by which some parts are gorged, whilst others lose the portion which naturally belongs to them. As an example of the first, we may take the purple blotches so frequently to be seen on the backs of dead subjects; whilst the proverbial paleness of death is a familiar instance of the second. Or the fluids themselves undergo a change, of which an example may be found in the dark lines marking the course of subcutaneous veins, and which are produced by the transudation of the altered blood contained in these vessels.

The solids of the body are liable to no less remarkable phenomena, commencing long before putrefaction has had time to take place, nay even with the extinction of life, and undergoing a series of changes, modified by external circumstances, until entire decomposition, or the formation of a new and permanent substance, is effected. The source of vital heat being extinguished, the inert mass, more or less quickly, acquires the temperature of surrounding bodies; the muscles become rigid, though not always to the same degree, and continue in this state for a longer or shorter period, the duration of which appears to be in proportion to the rapidity with which it supervened: the longer the muscles have been acquiring their rigidity, and the later it commences, the longer they are likely to retain it.

The various tissues lose their power of resisting, if not of preventing, the transudation of the fluids. Hence the parts in the neighbourhood of the gall-bladder become tinged with bile, the coats of the blood-vessels stained by the blood which they contain, and sometimes, though more rarely, the mucous membrane of the intestines participates in the colour of the fæcal matter.

If no precautions are taken to suspend it, putrefaction advances, the soft parts of the body deliquesce, and generally acquire a dark colour, exhaling the odour peculiar to the decomposition of animal matter. This change, however, belongs to a much later period than that at which cadaveric inspections, except under very particular circumstances, are likely to be made.

My attention, however, has been repeatedly attracted by two very different states in which animal matter far advanced in putrefaction is to be met with. In the one the sulphuretted hydrogen, which probably proceeds from the decomposition of albumen, is insufferably offensive. The other is characterized by the copious evolution of ammonia, which at times seems to be totally unaccompanied by any adventitious smell. Nothing, to my knowledge, has been attempted, to ascertain the causes on which these two strikingly different states depend, and my own observations are scarcely sufficient to warrant my hazarding a conjecture. I have, however, repeatedly remarked that the production of the ammoniacal odour is accompanied by the presence of vast numbers of the larvæ of the musca putrex, or common meat-fly; and as albumen enters largely into the composition of these animals, I have thought it not improbable that their growth, at the expense of the decomposing substance, might be a wise provision of nature to obviate the production of a gas like sulphuretted hydrogen, at once deleterious and offensive.

When a sufficiency of moisture is supplied, and decomposition impeded by the exclusion of atmospheric air, the soft parts are converted into a substance having the characters of fatty matter, and known by the name of adipocere, in which state they may retain their original form to an almost indefinite period.

The bones exhibit few, if any, cadaveric changes, and, from their superior density, resist decomposition for a much longer time than any of the other tissues; but even these at length give way, not only in those cases in which bodies have been exposed, as is the custom in the present day, to causes which favour their decay, but even where much care and art have been spent in the attempt to prevent it. I saw a striking proof of this at the opening of a mummy presented to the Museum of Natural History in Edinburgh. The catacombs in which it had been found were those to which the highest antiquity is attributed. Hence it is by no means improbable that the individual of whose remains this mummy consisted had been dead full three thousand years. Although the atmospheric influence was to a great degree excluded by a very strong case, and by numerous layers of linen closely wound round the body—and notwithstanding that decomposition was still further opposed by abundance of antiseptic drugs—not merely the soft parts had crumbled to powder, but the bones, though still retaining their form, were passing into the same state, and several had already lost part of their extremities.

The phenomena of which I have next to speak constitute the class with which it is the most important that the morbid anatomist should be intimately and practically acquainted : in fact they form the principal object of research with those who undertake the inspection of the dead.

You will doubtless have anticipated me when I say that I now allude to the phenomena which are in immediate relation to the death and last illness of the subject. The greater number of these are the result of a pathological state, with the essence of which we are still by no means well acquainted. They are the product of inflammation. Whilst, however, a very large number of morbid appearances are justly to be attributed to this cause, too much care and attention cannot be paid to discriminate between these and a similar, but in their nature very distinct, order of appearances, which owe their origin to congestion. This discrimination is at no time more important than in the investigation of the pathological condition of the brain, and of the mucous membrane of the air passages and alimentary canal.

The want of a due attention to this distinction has doubtless led into numerous errors the ultra-partizans of a new medical sect, which, whilst it must be admitted to have done much for the cultivation of pathology, has become almost as exclusive as it is arrogant and conceited. The devoted disciples of the *sei-disant* physiological doctrine will see nothing but inflammation, and see inflammation everywhere.

Amongst the morbid appearances belonging to the class of which we are now speaking, serous effusions (of which very large collections are frequently met with) possess a character too distinct and remarkable not to have a separate order assigned to them. They must, however, be considered as constituting two very distinct divisions.

Many we must agree with Blackall and Geromini in considering as of an active character, and consequently allied to phenomena dependant on inflammation; whilst others are still regarded as possessing that passive and asthenic nature ascribed by the older authors to most of these effusions, and which allies them more nearly to the order of congestions.

Sanguineous effusions or hæmorrhages, which constitute another order of this class, are subject to a similar division with the preceding.

To the morbid appearances which I have now mentioned, must be added the preternatural softening and hardening of the different tissues, respecting the nature of which I shall not now attempt to offer an opinion. By many they are considered as the result of inflammation.

In the last order of this class I would place those causes of death which consist either of solutions, of continuity, or of displacement, and which depend on violence done to some organ or organs, either from internal or external causes. As examples of these I may mention rupture of the heart or large vessels, intussusceptions, fractures of the cranium and vertebræ, &c. &c.

In the next place we may consider the important class of adventitious structures ; since, though the fatal tendency of many of them very naturally connects them with the class of which we have just been speaking, the length of time which they may often exist with comparatively little derangement of the health, and which, consequently, allows of life being terminated by some other cause, will necessarily connect them with the succeeding class.

The adventitious tissues have been divided, by a very distinguished pathological anatomist, into the *analogue*, or those which resemble tissues naturally existing in the body; and the *heterologue*, in which the structure is altogether new. The latter is by far the more important, comprising scrofulous tubercle, scirrhus, cancer, fungus hæmatodes, the encephaloid tumor, melanosis, and cirrhosis.

In the fourth class we may place the result of chronic diseases not included in the preceding class, and not immediately connected with the cause of death, and also those appearances which owe their origin to diseases no longer existing, but which have left the permanent traces of their influence in the structure of the parts which they affected.

The detection of morbid appearances belonging to the first of these orders would throw light on the symptoms which may have accompanied the latter period of the individual's life, and illustrate the pathology of a troublesome and obstinate class of diseases.

A careful investigation of those of the second order will teach us the extent to which the human frame is capable of repairing the breaches which it may have sustained; and, in shewing us the mode in which these reparations are effected, may afford us important hints in our attempts to direct the progress of disease.

The fifth class, which in their origin carry us back to the earliest periods of life, comprise a set of morbid or anomalous appearances of which we cannot expect to meet with many examples in hospital inspections; they are, however, too important and interesting to allow me to pass them over without offering a few general remarks respecting them.

Of these appearances, which are designated by the terms malformation, *lusus naturæ*, or monstrosity, a very few not being incompatible with the life of the individual in a state of separate existence, and occasionally claiming the attention of the surgeon, possess an interest immediately connected with practice, besides that which belongs to them in common with other cases included in this class: such are the hare-lip and cleft palate. Others, and these are by no means numerous, though they allow the prolongation of life beyond the term of fœtal existence, materially disturb the functions, and occasion symptoms, which, although not within the reach of our remedies, it is, nevertheless, desirable to refer to their real causes. Examples of this kind are met with in the sanguiferous, and perhaps also in the nervous system. Others, again, productive of no notable

effect during life, remain unsuspected until accidentally brought to light in the course of cadaveric inspection: of this kind are intestinal appendices—the distinct termination of the pancreatic and common gall ducts—the persistence of supernumerary ribs, &c.

Far the greater number of malformations, and those which exhibit the most considerable deviation from the normal condition, are only met with in the fœtal state.

The investigation of these is too apt to be regarded as productive only of loss of time, and of vain and useless speculation.

It is to combat this erroneous opinion that I am induced to dwell the longer on this subject on the present occasion.

It has been remarked by Tiedmann— "Every man of reflection—every man who does not think that it is the only, or even the chief object of anatomy to describe organs, to expose their structure, and to draw conclusions applicable to medicine and surgery—will be convinced that it can only attain to the rank of a true science when it shall have made known the history of the formation of the animal body, and the laws which preside over this formation. Now a knowledge of this kind can be acquired in no other way than by the anatomy of inferior animals and of the fœtus, which alone unveils to us the curious fact of the gradual multiplication of organs, of their development, of their progressive complication, and of their degree of importance in relation to life."

For the elucidation of the subject to which Professor Tiedmann has alluded in the preceding passage, the anomalous formations which we are now considering appear to be quite as important as the phenomena presented by the perfectly normal development of the fœtus. Meckel, who has paid more attention to this subject than any other individual, makes the following strong, but perhaps not untrue, assertion:—" That original malformations are more interesting than most of the changes in structure and deviations in form which take place during life, will scarcely be denied, except by teachers without originality, or the students they mislead, who estimate the value of a study by the extent of pecuniary advantage they may expect to derive from it, rather than its scientific tendency, and the degree of influence it is calculated to exert over other studies."

It can scarcely escape the observation even of those who have had but little opportunity or inclination to acquire a knowledge of comparative anatomy, that a certain degree of similarity may be noticed in the structure of a great variety of animals; even amongst those which at first sight appear extremely different.

To illustrate this position I will call your attention to the upper extremities of man. The extensive motion of which they are susceptible, their antagonism, and, above all, their termination in the hands—instruments endowed with the most delicate sense of touch, and so wonderfully adapted for every variety of prehension that by some they have been regarded as the chief cause of man's superiority—might seem to place these limbs above all comparison with the superior or anterior extremities of inferior animals. A slight examination of their skeletons will, however, suffice to convince us that, in the mammalia at least, the formation of these organs may be referred to the same plan, and that, by a regular and almost uninterrupted series of degradations, the human hand and arm may be connected with the fore-legs of the horse, though these are possessed of motions so much less various, and terminate so much more simply; and with the short and fin-like paddles of the cetacea.

I will endeavour to make good this assertion by a hasty survey of the first example which I have mentioned, viz. that of the fore-legs of the horse.

In some of the quadrumana, or monkey tribe, we have nearly, if not quite, the same extent of motion, and the same power of prehension, as in man himself; but the sense of touch is far inferior. We find a perfect clavicle, a humerus and radius admitting of pronation and supination, and a thumb more or less capable of being brought into apposition to the other phalanges. From the quadrumana we may proceed to the rodentia: in one of these, the Aye aye, or Cheiromys, a little nocturnal animal of Madagascar, we find not only the clavicle and the fore-arm capable of pronation and supination, but also an extremity, whose slender phalanges bear no small resemblance to the hand, from which circumstance the name of the

animal is derived. In the squirrels this similarity is much diminished; and proceeding to the rabbit, we find the clavicle reduced to a mere rudiment; the motions of the fore-arm are much more limited, and though the division of the extremity is still preserved, the power of prehension is absent.

From this last division of the rodentia we may pass to the reuminantia. In these we find no trace of clavicle, and no rotatory motion of the fore-arm; this, however, consists of two bones. In the ulna, though anchylosed to the radius, it is impossible not to recognise the olecranon and the sygmoid cavity. To the radius succeeds a carpus, of which the bones, though numerous, are fewer than in man. The metacarpus is obviously composed originally of two bones, which are anchylosed together at an early period, and only two phalanges are developed to complete the extremity. Yet in the camel, even these retain some resemblance to the claws of the animals which we have left, and form a step which conducts us to the cloven hoof of the more completely digitigrade animals of this order—such as the deer and the antelope. From the fore-leg of these animals to that of the horse the transition is easy and obvious—we see rudimentary bones in the metacarpus, but the extremity terminates in single digital bones.

The analogy, however, is by no means limited to the mammalia. Quitting them by the order cheirophera, of which the bats compose the principal number, we have an easy transition to the wings of birds, some of which possess a horny appendage somewhat allied to the human nails. We find ourselves at length arrived at the extreme point of degradation observable in this class, in the wings of the cassowary and penguin.

In many of the reptilia the resemblance reappears in a manner too striking to require pointing out. The hand-like extremity of the fore-leg of the frog must be familiar to you all. An Italian cook, who once dressed for my supper some of these animals, which he called *pesce que cantano*, or fish that sing, said that sympathy prevented him from eating them himself, such was the resemblance which he thought they bore to man. It is, however, in the class reptilia that we first meet with animals in which these organs are wholly wanting. From serpents we are naturally conducted to fishes, in which it seems in vain that we should look for any analogy to the human arm and hand.

The degree of similarity which I have endeavoured to point out as existing in the anterior or superior extremities of all vertebrated animals possessed of such organs, and which warrants us in referring them to one general model or type, is equally remarkable in other organs, and is especially worthy of notice in the viscera. In some of these the chain may be carried many links further. Instead of limiting ourselves to the vertebrated animals we may even descend to those which exhibit the lowest forms of life.

It is on these resemblances, traced out with respect not merely to particular organs but to their combination in the composition of an individual, that some philosophical anatomists of modern times have founded the doctrine of analogies, and of an unity of plan pervading the whole animal kingdom.

This doctrine, in itself extremely beautiful, and even sublime, and which affords a happy explanation of many remarkable phenomena in the organization of animals, would be liable to no objection had its advocates been always content to ascend from well-observed facts to conclusions carefully and legitimately deduced. Thus far it is admitted, and supported by one whom the opportunities which he has enjoyed, and the extraordinary talents which have enabled him to turn them to the utmost profit, justly place at the head of all natural historians,—by Cuvier, with respect to whom, in this department, there is no one " major, similis, aut secundus." It has happened, however, very unfortunately for this doctrine, that several amongst those who have been the warmest in its support, and the most active in collecting facts relating to it, have attempted to pursue the subject in the descending line, and to proceed from supposed principles, which, in the present state of our knowledge, must unavoidably belong to the domain of the imagination, and which in some instances have been deduced from abstractions wholly foreign to the animal kingdom ; from such principles, I say, they have attempted to descend to particulars, in doing which they have fallen into absurdities with which the doctrine itself has been unjustly reproached. You will have some idea of the hallucinations of the transcendental anatomists, when I tell you, that in some way or other they have attempted to shew a similarity between an individual animal and the globe which we inhabit, if not the universe itself; that in certain parts of the body, as, for example, in the head, they see reproduced the type of the whole body, the arms reappearing in the zygomatic arches, and the legs in the lower jaw.

Some who have kept clear of absurdities of this kind, whose talents and acquirements command admiration, and who by the benefits which they have conferred on science are justly entitled to lasting praise, have, in the zeal with which they have sought analogies, pointed out resemblances which it is difficult not to consider as forced. One, in drawing the parallel between the two extremities of the body, has made the testes the counterpart of the brain, and the corpora cavernosa that of the tongue.

Another has compared the ear to a bulb of hair, and a third has taught that the small bones of the ear are analogous to the bones of the opercula, or gill-plates of fishes.

You will, I trust, pardon this long digression, which appeared necessary before I could make myself intelligible to those who may not have turned their attention to the doctrine of analogies.

We will now return to our subject, and endeavour to shew the importance of the investigation of monstrosities, in reference to the doctrine at which we have taken a glance.

In ascending from the lowest forms of animal life to the most perfect, we observe a gradual development and increase of parts, and this we also observe to be most marked and regular in the most important organs, such as those of sensation and circulation. We observe, too, that in different classes of animals the development of these organs has attained to a particular stage which becomes characteristic of that particular class. Thus in insects the organ corresponding to the heart is a mere elongated tube, known by the name of the dorsal vessel. In most of the molusca, and in fish, in which animals the blood is propelled by the same impulse in the greater or aortic, and in the less or pulmonary circulation, we find the heart to consist essentially of one auricle and one ventricle; the first to receive,---in which the centripetal motion terminates; the latter to distribute the circulating fluid, and consequently commencing the centrifugal motion. In the molusca we find variations in the application of this principle, but these are points which it is needless here to dwell upon.

The batrachian reptiles exhibit a tendency to the separation of the auricle into two cavities, and in the higher divisions of reptiles we find the organ still further perfected. In these, two distinct auricles and a ventricle, possessing a septum nearly complete, conduct us, by an easy transition, to the double hearts of birds and the mammalia, both of which, as you know, are possessed of a complete double circulation.

Now in the human embryo, as well as in those of the more perfect animals, the heart in the progress of its development exhibits those forms which are permanent with the inferior animals. It would seem, however, that in proportion to the high degree of development to be ultimately attained to, is the rapidity of those changes by which the inferior animals are represented; consequently the small size of the embryo, and the delicacy of its structure, render the examination extremely difficult.

It is in this difficulty that we are helped by the examination of cases of monstrosity, for it appears that many of these depend on the suspension of development at particular stages. The growth of the organ not being suspended with the suspension of its development, it at length comes under examination of a size and texture much more favourable to correct observation.

In the malformations of the human heart, the organ which I have adduced by way of example, we find, though very rarely, a rudimental form analogous to the dorsal vessel of insects. The instances are somewhat more frequent in which the structure of the fish and the batrachian reptile is preserved; but a degree of development extremely analogous to that of the Saurian reptiles, of which lizards and crocodiles are examples, is by no means uncommon.

Besides these monstrosities which illustrate the development of organs by

passing through stages characteristic of inferior classes of animals, another description of malformation carries us back to an extremely early period of existence, in which the embryos of man, and other symmetrical animals, consist of two lateral and perfectly correspondent halves, which are subsequently united. This union may be irregularly effected. It may take place imperfectly, as we see in hare-lip; in the division of the nose, which I have seen in the dog, though never in the human subject; in cleft palate and uvula; in bifid enseform cartilage; in bifid penis or double uterus; and in spina bifida; or it may be excessive. I have frequently seen the eyes coalesced into one, forming a true cyclops. Imperforate anus and vagina are perhaps instances referable to the same head; the most remarkable example of which is perhaps to be met with in the union of the legs, by which they form an extremity somewhat resembling the tail of a fish.

Other cases of monstrosity appear to depend on more mechanical causes, such as the preternatural shortness of the umbilical cord. Of these and some other forms I shall say nothing at present, having, I trust, already advanced enough to prove the interest which I have ascribed to the class of malformations, and to render it needless that I should urge such of you as a zealous attention to the practice of midwifery may furnish with the means of pursuing the subject, by no means to neglect the opportunities of doing so.

The class just described, viz. that of monstrosities, is the last in the arrangement which I have employed in the review which I have been taking. I wish it to be understood that I do not bring forward this arrangement with any idea of its being calculated either for a nosological system or for the classification of specimens in a museum, but merely as presenting the most natural order in which I could bring under your consideration the numerous objects which the examination of the bodies of the dead is capable of affording.

I have already trespassed so long on your time, that but few minutes remain for me again to advert to the means which I would fain hope may conduce to render the inspections to be made on this table really advantageous to those whose zeal prompts them to come to this theatre—the first, I believe, which has been constructed specially for the purpose to which it is devoted.

The objects which we shall have to attend to, will, of course, be chiefly those phenomena which I have mentioned as forming the second, third, and fourth classes. Much of their interest and practical utility will manifestly be lost if we have not the means of connecting the morbid changes with the symptoms which they may have occasioned during life. I shall use my best endeavours that, in those cases which more particularly require my attention, this defect may be as small as possible: I am, however, fully aware that, were it to depend on myself alone, it would be far beyond my power, could I spend more time in the wards than I can reasonably expect to do, to become so intimately acquainted with every case that, in the event of its terminating fatally, the loss of which I have been speaking would not be sensibly felt.

Let me, then, for your common and mutual advantage, once more recommend the measure which I have pointed out on a former occasion—namely, that the pupils, and more especially those who are attached to the physician's practice, should enter into a combination which should enable them, by a division of labour, to draw up histories, if not of all, at least of the most interesting cases. The adoption of such a plan may probably lead some of you to distinction, whilst it will certainly prove advantageous to all. Nor can I for one moment doubt that, at the close of the present clinical course, many will prove the happy effects of industry, under good tuition, by their competence ably to perform the task which I have described. Should you be induced, by what I have said, to act on this suggestion, I shall be most happy to co-operate with you in the undertaking.

Before I conclude I feel it necessary, in order to conciliate your lenity in passing judgment on the mode in which I may execute the task assigned me, to make one remark on the operation of inspection, and on the extent of verbal demonstration with which it may be accompanied. You must all of you have observed, and many of you experienced, that the operation, at times, requires the exertion of considerable physical strength—that the state of the parts occasionally requires much caution as to the mode of their exposure or removal; and, at times, no small nicety of dissection. Any of these causes would afford, to a speaker far more fluent than myself, good grounds for indulgence, or even excuse, for his remarks not assuming the form of a continued discourse.

To many of those who may be present, the minute notice of appearances almost daily presenting themselves would be only a tedious repetition; and, on the other hand, to pass them over in silence would be an act of injustice to those who come here for the purpose of imbibing their first practical notions of morbid anatomy. I see no better mode in which I can obviate this inconvenience, than by inviting those of the latter class to visit the museum on the days on which it will be open for the inspection of the pupils, when I shall feel a pleasure in meeting them, and, as far as I may be able, affording those explanations which they may have found necessary.

I shall probably, on another opportunity, solicit your attention to a few hints on the steps and precautions to be taken in the conducting of post mortem inspections: for the present I shall conclude by assuring you that it will be my constant aim, whether I may be fortunate enough to reach the mark or not, to co-operate with those who are strenuously endeavouring to render the school of Guy's Hospital the first medical school in the kingdom.

CASES

OF

ALBUMINOUS URINE

ILLUSTRATIVE OF THE

EFFICACY OF TARTAR EMETIC, IN COMBINATION WITH OTHER ANTIPHLOGISTIC REMEDIES,

IN THE ACUTE FORMS OF THAT DISEASE.

BY GEORGE H. BARLOW, M.A. & L.M.

ALTHOUGH the researches of Dr. Bright, and his followers, Rayer, Solon, Christison, Gregory, &c. have left little to be added to the pathology of that formidable disease now commonly designated by the terms "mottled kidney," "granular degeneration of the kidney," and "morbus Brightii," it is, I think, nevertheless admitted, by all who have bestowed upon the subject the attention which it deserves, that much remains to be done towards ascertaining the modes of treatment most efficacious, either towards its cure, or palliation, in its different stages.

But far as we may be from the attainment of this desirable object, I am induced to lay the following cases before the public; being convinced, that whether the plan of treatment which was pursued with success in the greater number of them, be or be not the best which can be devised, I am nevertheless contributing to the general stock of experience upon a question of no small moment, and thus acting in accordance with the intention with which this work was originally commenced, and the spirit with which, I trust, it has been hitherto continued.

Every practitioner must be familiar with that form of anasarca which is so commonly met with as a consequence of scarlatina, and which, as is generally known, is accompanied by the presence of albumen in the urine. This form of the disease is often successfully treated by purging, diuretics, occasional bleedings, and sometimes diaphoretics; after which, the milder tonics are frequently employed with benefit. Nevertheless, I have, upon many occasions, observed that the recovery of patients thus treated, is, for the most part, tedious, and sometimes incomplete; and that the depletions, which are commonly found necessary, are often not well borne, and produce a depressing effect upon the constitution which is not easily removed.

I was accordingly induced to seek for some other remedy: and regarding the affection to be essentially of an inflammatory character, as evinced by the increased frequency of the pulse, and the state of the blood when drawn—and considering, moreover, the probably injurious effects of medicines which act as direct stimulants to the kidneys in the recent stages of this form of the disease, and the importance, consequently, of promoting, if possible, the secretion from the skin—I was led to make trial of tartarized antimony, which I found fully to answer my expectations. My next object was, to inquire whether this form of renal disease was identical with the degeneration of the kidney described by Dr. Bright, occurring spontaneously, or from other causes than scarlatina: and being led, by the similarity of the symptoms, to a belief that it was so (a belief which has been since confirmed by two observations to be detailed presently), I was induced to make trial of the same remedy in the early and acute stages of the idiopathic form of the disease, and, in many cases, with the same success. I wish it, however, to be distinctly understood, that I make no claim to having effected perfect and permanent cures in any but acute cases in the early stage; whereas it but too frequently happens, that the disease, in this stage, is either disregarded by the patient, or not recognised by his medical attendant; and, further, it is probable that, in the majority of cases, there is no acute stage at all, but the disease is, throughout, of a chronic and insidious character.

I shall first adduce a few instances of that form of the disease which occurs as a sequela of scarlatina.

I find that, in the years 1835, 1836, I made short notes of

five cases of anasarca with albuminous urine, and no other
complication of importance: these were all treated with
small doses of acetate of ammonia and tartaric emetic, and
occasional purgatives of jalap and tartrate of potass, and
all recovered speedily.

The case which I am now about to relate was of a more
formidable character.

Case 1.

*Anasarca, and Ascites, consequent upon Scarlatina—Urine
highly albuminous—Cerebral Affection—Complete
Recovery.*

WILLIAM COWLEN, aged three and a half years (Sept. 29, 1835),
a fine boy, who has generally been healthy, was five weeks
ago the subject of scarlatina, from which he in a great
measure recovered, but did not regain his former liveliness
and activity. About a week ago he began to swell, first in
his face and hands, and afterwards in his whole body; which
swelling has continued to increase. About the same time
he complained of headache, and became more and more
drowsy; and for the last five days his mother has observed
his urine to be of a deep dingy-red colour. At present he is
much swelled over the whole surface of his body; his skin is
harsh and dry, but not hot; his eyes nearly closed; tongue
covered with a yellowish fur; pupils contracted: the child
evinces a great objection to the slightest motion or exertion,
and seems to take no notice of any one: pulse sharp, small,
and frequent: bowels not open during the last thirty-six
hours: urine scanty, of a dingy-red colour, and coagulating
upon boiling to such a consistence, that it remains in the
spoon when inverted.

> Pulv. Jalap. C. gr. x. st. sumend.
> Ant. Tart. gr. i. Sacchar. purificat. ʒi. m. fiant pulv. xvi. e
> quibus sumat i. quartâ quâque horâ.—Hirud. ij. pedibus.

Sept. 30. His bowels have been copiously acted upon.
The first dose of the tartarized antimony made him sick;
but the following ones did not produce that effect. He is
to-day much relieved, and the anasarca is less; but there is
a considerable quantity of fluid in the abdomen: tongue

still furred : pupils nearly natural : urine scanty, of a dingy-red colour, and very coagulable.

Pergat.—To be fed on bread and milk.

Oct. 1. He is to-day much worse : face exceedingly swollen : pulse sharp, small, and very rapid : tongue much furred, and it is necessary to force his mouth open, in order to see it. At present he appears in nearly a comatose state ; but I am told that during the night he screamed violently, and appeared delirious. Bowels not open for twenty-four hours.

Hirud. iij. temporibus.—Pulv. Jalap. C. gr. x. statim.
Rep. Pulv. tertiâ quâque horâ.

2. Is in all respects much better ; and answers, when spoken to. The anasarca is much diminished, but the quantity of fluid in the abdomen remains the same. Bowels freely acted on : urine increased in quantity, less dark, freely coagulable, but less so than at first ; sp. gr. 1009 : pulse less frequent, and rather softer : skin harsh and dry.

3. Continues to improve : pulse 100, softer : bowels not open for twenty-four hours.

Rep. Pulv. Jal. C. statim, et p. r. n.—Pergat.

5. Anasarca diminishing : appetite increasing : slight pain in loins, extending across the epigastrium : pulse 100 : skin dry : urine natural in quantity, and less coloured by red particles ; it is, however, still very coagulable ; sp. gr. 1009.

Fnt. Pulv. xvj. ex Ant. Tart. gr. ifs. Sumat i. tertiis horis.
Hirud. ij. lumbis.—Balneum callid. o. n.

6. The pain in the loins has nearly ceased. He perspired slightly, after being taken out of the bath ; and his skin is to-day softer and more perspirable than I have hitherto observed it.

Rep. Pulv. secundâ quâque horâ.

7. Urine natural in quantity, improved in colour ; less coagulable than when last examined, but still very much so ; sp. gr. 1010 : bowels rather confined.

Ol. Ricini ʒij. p. r. n.—Pergat.

9. He continues to improve. Perspired profusely during the night ; and his skin is now very moist. No fluid in the abdomen, and merely a vestige of the anasarca in the right hand and ancle : bowels regular : tongue cleaning.

Rep. Pulv. tertiâ quâque horâ.

From this time he went on steadily improving: his bowels, which were rather torpid, being regulated by castor oil. The tartarized antimony was gradually diminished in frequency, and the bath used at longer and longer intervals. Under this treatment, his urine gradually lost the dingy-red colour, and regained its natural appearance: its specific gravity also gradually increased, till it reached about 1023: his appetite became very hearty; but animal food was, throughout his convalescence, very sparingly allowed. By the end of November he was, to all appearance, in perfect health; full of flesh, with rosy cheeks, and a clear complexion. His urine, upon the most careful examination, did not afford the slightest evidence of the presence of albumen. I ascertained that this child was in perfect health in October last, or four years after the illness which I have just described.

I have adduced the above as an instance of a very severe case of this disease following scarlatina, successfully treated by occasional depletion, gentle purgatives, and tartar emetic. I ought to mention, that in a very severe case of the same kind, which occurred to me about a year ago, I used the tartar emetic in larger doses, in proportion to the age of the child; but did not, from the state of its general powers, think it advisable to have recourse to bleeding in any shape; and that the child went on very well, excepting that after the anasarca had disappeared the remedy was continued (the child having been removed into the country) and obstinate diarrhœa ensued, which was, however, at last allayed; and the child ultimately recovered, and was, to my knowledge, a short time ago, in perfect health.

I will now briefly relate two cases, shewing the identity of the anarsarca with albuminous urine, which follows scarlatina with the "morbus Brightii," arising from other causes; and then proceed to describe cases in which the same plan of treatment was applied in the latter form of the complaint.

CASE 2.
Scarlatina—Anasarca—Death—Kidneys diseased.

THOMAS WATERS, aged 16, (Jan. 16,1836,) had a febrile attack about nine weeks ago, which was attended with sore-throat and great heat and redness of the skin, followed by disquamation, from which he in a great measure recovered; but a month ago he began to swell, first in his hands and face, and then over his whole body: for this he was attended by Mr. Howitt, of Walworth, under whose care he greatly improved, and about ten days ago he was nearly free from swelling; but about five days ago, it again returned, and has continued to increase up to the present time. He is now generally anasarcous; and there is a considerable quantity of fluid in the peritoneum. He has much pain in the loins, extending across the abdomen towards the umbilicus; and there is some tenderness, upon pressure, about the situation of the kidneys, especially of the right. Urine of a dingy-red colour, much loaded with albumen.

He was ordered small doses of tartar emetic, in combination with hyoscyamus; which he continued to use, with slight benefit, till the 3d of February; when he was removed to Guy's Hospital, where he continued only five days: after which he was taken home at his own request, and died within two days. Through the kindness of Mr. Howitt, I obtained a view of the kidneys, which were very large; and the whole of the cortical structure of both was interspersed with a large proportion of pale-yellow granular matter.

There can, I think, be little doubt that, in this case, the primary disease was scarlatina: and I was informed that the lad's previous health had been remarkably good.

CASE 3.
Scarlatina—Anasarca—Partial Recovery—Relapse—Death— Kidneys large, and white.

ELIZABETH DAWKINS, aged 11, (March 23, 1839). Has generally enjoyed good health. A month ago, she suffered from severe and well-marked scarlatina; from which she was slowly convalescent, when it was observed, a few days ago, that her face was swollen. This swelling has continually increased to the present time; and she is now universally œdematous. She complains of headache, and pain across the chest, aggravated by inspiration. Tongue furred : bowels confined : pulse sharp : urine scanty, of a deep dingy-red, and very albuminous.

She was treated with purgatives ; tartar emetic, with acetate of ammonia ; and small doses of ipecacuanha. On the 26th, she was apparently so much better, that all the precautions which I gave, respecting exposure, clothing, diet, were disregarded ; and on the 2d of April I saw her in a state of insensibility, with well-marked symptoms of severe cerebral disease, and extensive anasarca. From this state she was recovered with some difficulty ; and appeared to be gaining ground rapidly for a few days, when symptoms of effusion in the chest suddenly came on, and in a few days ended her life.

The body was examined by Mr. Nettlefold and myself, forty hours after death ; when a large quantity of purulent fluid was found in the right pleural sac. About half-a-pint of serum was contained in the pericardium, with shreds or flocculi of fibrin, and the left ventricle of the heart was hypertrophied. The kidneys were large and lobulated ; and a greyish-white colour, with but little trace of the natural structure, pervaded all the cortical substance. The tubuli were dark, being of a deep chocolate colour.

I look uopn this case as very important, in shewing the identity of the anasarca, and albuminous urine following scarlatina, with that form of disease so generally known as the "morbus Brightii" : for not only does it agree with it, as regards the primary disease of the kidney, but also in the complications observed in other organs.

As it appears, then, that the renal disease consequent upon scarlatina is generally amenable to the method of treatment which I have detailed above, and as the two last-mentioned cases tend to establish the identity of this form of disease with that occurring independently of scarlatina, it seems reasonable to expect that the same plan of treatment should be successful also in the latter case ; and that it frequently is so, when adopted sufficiently early, is, I think, shewn by the following cases.

CASE 4.

Anasarca—Albuminous Urine—Complete Recovery,

GEORGE STANLEY, aged two years and a half, a well-grown child, who in the winter of 1834—35 suffered from a cerebral affection, from which he recovered under the use of small doses of calomel, was brought to me on the 4th of September 1835, having been for four days previously complaining of pain in the back of the head, and tightness across the epigastrium; and he was at the same time observed to be drowsy, and unwilling to move. Tongue furred: pulse sharp: bowels confined: general anasarca. I was informed that his urine was thick, and high-coloured.

Ant. Tart. gr. ¼. Liq. Ammon. Acet. ℥i. Aq. distillat. ℥ij. Sumat. cochl. i. amplium quater quotid.

Sept. 5. I had to-day an opportunity of examining some of his urine: it deposited a fawn-coloured sediment, and contained a considerable quantity of albumen. The first dose of his medicine made him sick yesterday, and he vomited a greenish fluid: he has, however, continued to take it without further inconvenience.

Pergat.

7. He is to-day more lively: tongue less furred: skin harsh: pulse less sharp: anasarca diminished.

Rep. Mist. tertiâ quâque horâ.

9. Better. Urine contains less albumen than on the fifth.

Sumat. Mist. cochl. ij. minim. quater quotid.

12. Continues free from pain: bowels rather confined: tongue clean: pulse 96, natural: skin softer: urine natural in appearance, slightly coagulable: sp. gr. 1013.

Sumat. Mist. cochl. iij. minim. quàrtis horis. Ol. Ricini ʒij. statim, et rep. p. r. n.

15. He is lively, and free from pain; and in every respect much improved. Pulse 83: skin soft: no anasarca: urine natural in appearance: sp. gr. 1015. There is a scarcely-perceptible turbidity, produced by the application of heat and nitric acid.

Sumat. Mist. ℥fs. quater quotid.

19. Continues much the same: urine scarcely at all affected by heat or nitric acid: sp. gr. 1017.

From this time he went on improving : in a few days more no albumen could be detected in the urine : and he appeared in perfect health, which he has continued to enjoy till Aug. 1839, when I ascertained that he was in good health, and that his urine was free from albumen.

Case 5.

A similar case has lately occurred to me, in a child, WILLIAM PERKINS, aged 5 years, who complained of headache and flushings of heat, followed by general pain. I saw him Sept. 19, 1839, five days after his first attack, when his limbs and face were much swollen, and his urine albuminous. He was treated in the same manner as the last case, except that the compound jalap powder was used, instead of castor-oil; and on the fifth of October his urine was free from albumen, and the child apparently well.

It will be observed, that the last two cases occurred in children; and it may be said that there is no proof that they might not have been the subjects of scarlatina a short time before I saw them, but in so mild a form as to have escaped the observation of the parents. However, I made strict inquiries upon this point, and was assured, in both instances, that they had been for months before in good health. And further, my own experience inclines me to believe that the idiopathic form of this disease is by no means rare amongst the children of the lower and middling classes in London.

The following cases may perhaps be regarded as more satisfactory, from their having occurred in adults.

Case 6.

Anasarca, and Ascites—Albuminous Urine—Complete Recovery.

PATRICK QUEENLAND, aged 49, Aug. 22, 1839, a stout powerful man, of temperate habits, employed as a porter in a hop-warehouse. A year ago he was under my care for acute rheumatism; since which he had good health, till ten days ago, when he was attacked with headache, and pains in his loins, extending across the epigastrium : ten days afterwards he observed that his feet and scrotum were much swollen, and that his face was puffy in the morning.   At present, there is general anasarca, especially of the scrotum, with some ascites.

> Pot. Acet. Ði.   Sp. Æth. Nit. m. xx.   Vini Ipecac. m. x. ex
>> Mist. Mucilag. t. d.
> Pil. Scillæ C.   Extr. Hyosc. āā gr. v.   b. d.

Aug. 24. Little alteration, excepting that he complains of increased thirst.   A specimen of urine which I saw to-day gave a copious precipitate with nitric acid: skin dry: pulse hard and sharp: bowels rather torpid.

> C.C. lumbis ad x.
> Ant. Pot. Tart. gr. $\frac{1}{8}$.   Mag. Sulph. ʒfs   Liq. Ammon. Acet. ʒfs.
>> ex Mist. Camphor. t. d.
> Pulv. Ipecac. Comp. gr. v.   o. n.

27. Skin still dry: pulse softer: tongue cleaner: pain in the loins much relieved.

> Aug. dos. Ant. Pot. Tart. ad gr. $\frac{1}{4}$.—Pergat.

29. Œdema much reduced: pulse soft: urine less albuminous: slight perspiration at times.

> Pulv. Jal. C. ʒfs. alt. auroris.
> Cont. Mist. sine M. S. et Pulv. ut antea.

Sept. 7. The œdema has entirely disappeared, excepting a little about the ancles: the powders have acted very slightly: no albumen in the urine.

> Pulv. Elaterii, gr. $\frac{1}{4}$.   Pulv. Jalap. C. Ðij. alt. auroris.—Pergat.

12. The last powders have produced rather watery dejections: pulse soft: tongue clean: perspires freely: a little albumen in the urine.

> Pulv. Elaterii gr. $\frac{1}{3}$.   Pulv. Jalap. C. Ðij. bis in hebdomadâ.
> Adde M. S. ʒfs. sing. dos. Mist. cont. Pil.

17. No albumen: no anarsarca.

21. Continues well: no albumen.

I have ascertained that this man is now [seven months since his illness] in good health.

CASE 7.

Anasarca of two weeks' standing—Albuminous Urine—
Recovery apparently complete.

ELIZA ROSE. aged 32, a married woman, who had borne children, and generally enjoyed good health, was admitted under my care at the Surrey Dispensary, Feb. 27, 1839. She stated, that fourteen days before, after having been exposed to cold, she felt weight and pain in her loins, extending across the epigastrium; and that a few days afterwards she perceived that her eyelids were swollen when she arose in the morning. At present, her face and legs are œdematous; tongue white; pulse sharp; bowels regular. She was ordered to take five grains of Dover's powder, night and morning; and one-eighth of a grain of potassio-tartrate of antimony, with acetate of ammonia in camphor mixture, three times a day. On the 1st of March she brought me a specimen of her urine, which yielded a copious deposit of albumen, upon the addition of nitric acid. On the 4th, the quantity of the antimony was doubled; and she continued to take it without inconvenience till the 11th, when it caused frequent vomiting. She was then much improved, her skin was moist, and her pulse softer; and the œdema had disappeared. Urine slightly albuminous. The dose of the tartar emetic was reduced to one-eighth of a grain; which she continued to take, as well as the Dover's powder, till the 26th; when she was discharged, apparently in good health; her urine being free from albumen.

It may perhaps be thought that the treatment pursued in this case can hardly be supposed adequate to the removal of so formidable a disease; but, upon the other hand, it should be remembered, that it was sufficient to excite nausea and vomiting, and that this occurred contemporaneously with the mitigation of the symptoms. But whatever may be thought of the treatment, it is evident that in this instance the disease was not dependent upon structural change, and the organ affected was in a state susceptible of recovery.

CASE 8.

Scarlatina at the age of Eight.—Anasarca, with Albuminous Urine, at the age of Twenty.—Recovery complete.

ELIZABETH RAINSCROFF, aged 20, a stout young woman, with dark hair and eyes, was under my care at the Surrey Dispensary, early in the summer of 1837. When I first saw her, I was told that twelve days previously she had felt slight rigors, headache, and a dull pain across the loins; that two days afterwards her face and legs became puffy, and that the swelling gradually extended to the loins and abdomen. When first seen by me, her skin was harsh and dry. She complained of thirst, headache, and slight pain in the loins extending across the epigastrium. Face, hands, feet, loins, and surface of abdomen, œdematous. There was also, perhaps, some little ascites; but of this I was not satisfied, owing to the œdema of the integuments: pulse sharp: tongue white: bowels torpid: urine of less than natural quantity, clear, and coagulating freely upon the application of heat, or addition of nitric acid. This patient was put upon the use of purgatives of jalap and supertartrate of potass; a draught, containing one-eighth of a grain of tartar emetic, with acetate of ammonia and camphor mixture, three times daily, and one-fourth of a grain of tartar emetic, with four grains of ext. of hyoscyamus, every night. The dose of the tartar emetic in the mixture was, after two days, increased to one-fourth of a grain, which she continued to take for a fortnight, when the anasarca had disappeared, and her skin was perspirable; but there still remained some albumen in the urine. The dose of the tartar emetic was then reduced to one-eighth of a grain, and the other medicines repeated. She continued to improve, perspired freely at night, and at the end of a month was discharged, free from complaint.

This patient was again under my care in November 1839, with slight dyspnœa, apparently of an hysterical character, which soon yielded to purgatives, and small doses of sp. æth. sulph. c., with tincture of hyoscyamus. I availed myself of the opportunity of twice examining her urine; when, on both occasions, it was found to be perfectly free from albumen.

This patient, I was informed, had been the subject of scarlatina when eight years old, but had since then enjoyed very good health. I think, therefore, that this must be regarded as a case of idiopathic renal disease, rather than as any way dependent upon the exanthem from which she suffered so long before.

The three last cases, I think, afford a proof that the disease under consideration does sometimes make its attack, in the adult, in the form of an acute affection, the time of the invasion of which is well marked; and they further shew, that when thus occurring, and when met sufficiently early with decided treatment, it is susceptible of cure. Of this treatment I believe that the use of tartar emetic forms an essential part:—and I take this opportunity of expressing my opinion of its utility, partly with a view of explaining a statement made by Dr. Bright in the Second Volume of this work, that I had believed it to exert almost a specific influence in this disease. This is, perhaps, more than I ever intended deliberately to affirm, as I much doubt the existence of a specific in any disease whatever. But I believe that, in this instance, the tartar emetic is more;—it is a remedy suggested by the nature of the affection, and calculated to fulfil the most obvious and important indications, namely, equalizing the circulation, subduing the inflammatory action, and restoring the functions of the skin. At the same time, I am far from recommending its use to the exclusion of other means calculated to aid in fulfilling the same indications: and among the most valuable of these adjuncts, I would reckon moderate local depletion, hydragogue cathartics, the warm bath, or, what is perhaps of equal value when this cannot be employed, the investing the loins in a large linseed-meal poultice.

I am aware that a great difference of opinion exists with regard to the diaphoretic plan of treatment in this disease, of which plan the tartar emetic may be regarded as a part; though I am far from regarding it exclusively in this light;— Dr. Osborne having warmly advocated its use; whilst Dr. Christison says, that it disappointed the expectations which he formed from a perusal of the elegant little treatise of the former; and extols the advantages of diuretics, and seems inclined to regard the apprehensions entertained by many, respecting the ill effects which may be expected from their use, as utterly groundless. But, for my own part, I do not think that sufficient stress has been laid by either of these authors upon the different treatment which must be necessarily required by difference in the period and form (whether acute or chronic) of the disease: for I believe that opposite remedies may be useful in its different stages; just as we know that in bronchitis, a disease which bears no very remote analogy to that under consideration, a decidedly antiphlogistic plan of treatment is imperatively called for in the acute and early stage; but that when the inflammatory action has been subdued, or the disease has passed into the chronic form, stimulating expectorants are frequently of essential service, although their inappropriate or too hasty exhibition is attended with the worst results.

Again, it should not be forgotten that copious diaphoresis may occur, either spontaneously or from the effect of remedies, without any concomitant amendment taking place; which happened in the case of Dawkins (Case 3 of present communication), and in Case 7 of Dr. Bright's communication upon this subject, in the First Volume of this work*.

But it is not merely as a diaphoretic that I would recommend the tartar emetic in the acute form of this disease: it is on account of its power of lowering the heart's action, as well as "its local effects upon the capillaries, when it reaches them through the circulation†;" whereby it diminishes the inflammation in the superficial capillaries of the lining membrane of tubuli uriniferi: for that such a state of the tubuli exists in the early stage of the disease is, I think, made apparent by the condition of the kidneys, in all the recent cases which have been examined.

It may be objected, that there is, not unfrequently, so great an irritability of stomach as to preclude the exhibition of the tartar emetic. This state of stomach has, within my observation, been confined mostly to the more-advanced stages of the disease; for I have only met with it in one recent case, which was complicated with extensive peritonitis, involving the peritoneal coat of the stomach.

With regard to the dose of the remedy, I would observe, that where the pulse is hard and full it may be given in such doses as in the first instance to produce nausea; but where there is a low state of the system, the antimony may be given in smaller doses, frequently repeated, so as to reach

* Guy's Hospital Reports, Vol. I. p. 361.
† Dr. Billing's Principles of Medicine, p. 65.

the capillaries without producing depression*. I have never found it necessary to give more than half-a-grain at a dose to an adult; neither have I attempted to push it to the greatest extent possible;—the object not being to give heroic doses of the remedy, but, if possible, to cure the patient.

CASE 9.

Anasarca, with Albuminous Urine—Partial Cure—Relapse, after two years—Complete Recovery.

EDWARD CARTER, a plasterer, addicted to the use of ardent spirits, was admitted under my care at the Surrey Dispensary, in February 1840. This man, I was informed, had before been a patient at the same institution, under the care of my friend and colleague, Dr. Hughes, to whose kindness I am indebted for the following particulars:—

He was first admitted Nov. 8, 1836, suffering from catarrh, and recent but exceedingly well-marked renal dropsy; pain and tenderness upon the loins; face pale and puffy; legs, and abdominal parietes, œdematous; urine scanty, pale, and very coagulable.—He was bled to ten ounces; ordered occasional purgatives of jalap and supertartrate of potass, and put upon the use of a draught containing one-fourth of a grain of tartar emetic and half-a-drachm of sulphate of magnesia in solution with acetate of ammonia in camphor mixture, and was shortly afterwards cupped in the loins. He was soon relieved of all his symptoms, except the dropsy; but there had hitherto been no perspiration. He was then kept in bed, a large linseed-meal poultice applied over the loins, and the same medicines continued. He perspired freely, and the dropsy disappeared. He felt himself well, but his urine remained coagulable; and he was discharged at the end of nine weeks.

He was a second time admitted under Dr. Hughes's care, Feb. 1, 1839, with the same symptoms as before, though less severe: his urine, however, was very coagulable. He said that he had continued well since he was before under Dr. Hughes's care; but that he got wet, and the disease returned. He was cupped twice on the loins, and put upon the same treatment as before. He was discharged well, with his urine free from albumen, at the end of six weeks.

---

* Billing, op. citat.

He afterwards enjoyed good health, till he was again admitted under my care, as above stated, with a slight attack of rheumatism, which he ascribed to getting wet; from which he quickly recovered. I availed myself of the opportunity of examining his urine, which I found perfectly free from albumen.

The above case is worthy of notice, from the circumstance that the recovery was complete in the second attack, though there is no proof that it was so in the first: still, I think it much more probable, that although the albuminous state of the urine had not ceased at the time he first left Dr. Hughes's care, it did so soon afterwards, than that it continued until he again became his patient; and I am inclined to regard the second attack merely as a recurrence of a disease from which he had before suffered, but had completely recovered: for it is by no means improbable that the function of the skin having been restored, and a return to a healthy action of the kidneys commenced, by the judicious treatment adopted by Dr. Hughes, the cure was afterwards spontaneously completed. The circumstance, that rheumatism, and not his former disease, was induced by the exposure to which he was subjected a short time before he became my patient, is, I think, an evidence that the kidneys had perfectly recovered their healthy state.

The plan of treatment recommended above will not be found useless in acute attacks supervening upon the chronic form of the disease, provided a change of measures be adopted as soon as the acute symptoms have subsided; when, as has been already suggested, tonics and moderately stimulating diuretics will be found serviceable, as is shewn in the following case.

CASE 10.

Albuminous Urine, probably of Two Years' standing.—Recent Aggravation.—Partial Recovery.

GEORGE SHEPPARD, aged 49, was admitted, under my care, at the Surrey Dispensary, July 18, 1839. He informed me that he had been for two years gradually losing his strength; and during that time he frequently observed his face to be swollen, especially about the eyelids, when he arose in the morning; and that his legs and ancles often swelled: that a year before he had suffered from general dropsy, attended with pain in the loins and across the epigastrium; for which he was admitted as an out-patient at Guy's Hospital, and obtained considerable relief, though the weakness never ceased entirely: and that about three weeks before he became my patient he was again similarly attacked, which he ascribed to having got wet through.

At the time I first saw him, his legs, hands, and face, were œdematous, as were the integuments of the loins and abdomen; though I could not ascertain the existence of any fluid in the peritoneal cavity. He complained of aching in the loins, and pain across the epigastrium. His appearance was leucophlegmatic, pulse sharp and frequent, tongue furred, bowels regular. I had not then an opportunity of examining his urine; but having little doubt of the nature of the disease, I ordered him to take one-eighth of a grain of potassio-tartrate of antimony in solution with acetate of ammonia, in camphor mixture, three times daily: five grains of Dover's powders every night: and half-a-drachm of compound jalap powder twice a week: to live chiefly on bread and milk.

On the 20th, I had an opportunity of examining his urine, which was much loaded with albumen. He was then much relieved, and said he had perspired a little on the preceding night.

On the 5th of August, the anasarca had nearly disappeared; as it merely shewed itself in his face in the morning, and in his legs. His pulse was then soft, and skin perspirable: the pain in his loins was only felt after walking, and he made no complaint of uneasiness across the epigastrium: urine less albuminous. He was now ordered,

Sp. Æth. Nit. m. xx. Tinct. Ferri Sesquichlorid. m. xv. ex Infus. Gentian. Comp. t. d.

Pulv. Ipecac. C. gr. v. o. n.

Pulv. Jalap. C. ʒfs. bis in hebdomadà.

On the 16th of October he said he felt much stronger, and

free from pain. The anasarca had ceased, but the urine still contained albumen. He was directed to feed sparingly on meat, to continue the bread and milk, and to take a pint of porter daily; the medicines being continued as before.

On the 16th of November he left the Dispensary, saying he was quite well; though there was still some albumen in his urine.

I saw him in January last, when he was able to follow his employment, as a carter.

There can be little doubt that the recovery in the last case was only partial and temporary: at the same time, I consider it worthy of attention, as illustrating the applicability of even opposite remedies in different stages of the complaint; for I am disposed to think that much of the difference of opinion which exists respecting the treatment of this most formidable malady is to be ascribed to a neglect of this distinction. At the same time, I cannot conclude without hazarding the expression of the belief, that the chance of recovery may in some measure depend upon the particular tissue of the organ affected; for it is by no means improbable that there may be varieties of the disease, as different in that respect as pneumonia and bronchitis. But were I to dilate upon this department of the subject, I should exceed the limits which I assigned to myself at the commencement of this essay, and enter upon an investigation which is fortunately in far abler hands, namely, of the physician with whom it originated.

ON

DIABETIC BLOOD.

BY G. O. REES, M.D. F.G.S. &c.

THE experiments of some of the most careful and experienced chemists have failed to detect sugar in the blood of
diabetic patients; and up to a very recent date, it was
supposed that the serum was free from contamination, even
in the most virulent and lengthened cases of diabetes. Some
late experiments, made by Mr. M'Grigor of Glasgow, seem to
shew that sugar is present, not only in the blood and urine,
but likewise in several secretions and excretions. The re-
actions obtained by that gentleman certainly rendered it very
probable that sugar was present; but I am not aware that it has
ever yet been separated, in its characteristic form, from the
serum of diabetic blood; except by Ambrosiani, who relates a
method by which he succeeded in extracting it in a crystallizable state. His process is as follows. The blood is to be
diluted with water; and boiled, in order to separate as much
as possible of the albumen and hæmatosine: the clear liquor
is then filtered away, and precipitated by di-acetate of lead.
The excess of lead is to be removed by a stream of sulphuretted
hydrogen gas; and the precipitate being allowed to settle, the
liquor is to be poured off, cleared by being boiled with white
of egg, filtered, and evaporated to the consistence of a syrup:
this, on being allowed to remain exposed to the air for some
weeks, deposits crystals of diabetic sugar. By this process,
Ambrosiani asserts that he has succeeded in extracting sugar:
and though I have not followed his process, yet I am inclined
to consider it calculated to afford a satisfactory result; for I
have observed that the presence of urea in the blood of

diabetic patients interferes with the demonstration of the sugar; and the performance of this process would tend greatly to destroy that principle.

The method I have adopted will yield sugar of considerable purity; though it will not enable us to determine, with precision, the weight of the principle. The process is as follows :—

The mass of blood * is to be evaporated to dryness, over a water-bath; the dried mass to be comminuted, and digested for several hours in boiling water : the aqueous solution is to be filtered off, evaporated to dryness, and the dried residuum digested in alcohol of sp. gr. 0.825 : the alcoholic solution so formed is to be filtered, or carefully poured off, evaporated to dryness, and the dry mass treated several times with rectified ether, which dissolves out urea, and also some fatty matter ; leaving behind the sugar, in admixture with osmazome and chloride of sodium : this mass, on being dissolved in alcohol, and the solution allowed to evaporate spontaneously in a flat glass dish, affords mixed crystals of alkaline chloride and diabetic sugar ; which are easily distinguishable from each other, and allow of being separated mechanically, by shaking them up in alcohol, when the chloride sinks; and the sugar, being principally collected above, may be removed, for examination, by careful use of the spatula : the alcohol must not, of course, be allowed to remain long in contact with the crystals, as it would re-dissolve them. It is a matter of surprise to me, that sugar has not been long ago detected in the blood of diabetic patients, though not separated from it; for the alcoholic extract of the serum, when mixed with water, will, after a few days, give off carbonic acid; which, in addition to the sweetish taste, and, I may add, syrupy smell of the evaporated alcoholic extract, is a sufficient evidence of the presence of sugar. I subjoin the analysis of 1000 grains of diabetic serum, obtained for me by the kindness of Dr. Bright. The sp. gr. of this patient's urine was 1048; and the contents of the serum as follows :—

* 12 ounces were used in these experiments.

Water	908.50
Albumen (yielding traces of phosphate of lime and oxide of iron, on incineration)	80.35
Fatty matters	0.95
Diabetic sugar	1.80
Animal extractive, soluble in alcohol, urea	2.20
Albuminate of soda	0.80
Alkaline chloride, with traces of phosphate . . . Alkaline carbonate, and trace of sulphate, the results of incineration	4.40
Loss	1.00
	1000.00

I should wish the proportion of diabetic sugar given here to be considered merely in the light of a close approximation; as it is impossible to separate it completely from impurity; and, moreover, the loss sustained by it during manipulation, which must be considerable, does not admit of estimation.

The alkaline salts contained a trace of an earthy phosphate in admixture; which is a curious fact, to which I have alluded in my paper on the analysis of the liquor amnii.

It will be observed, on comparing this analysis with that of the serum of healthy blood, that we have here a great excess of matters soluble in alcohol, while the albuminate of soda is rather less than in health. The alkaline salts are also in very small proportion, being only 4.40 gr. in 1000 grains of serum, while in health they amount to from 7 to 8 grains per 1000.

I attribute my success in obtaining sugar, in its characteristic form, from diabetic blood, principally to the use of ether, which extracts from it the urea and fatty matter. I find that the ether of the shops of sp. gr. 0.754, which of course contains some alcohol in its composition, is an active solvent of urea, while it exerts no action on the diabetic sugar.

ON THE PROPORTION

OF

UREA

IN CERTAIN DISEASED FLUIDS.

BY G. O. REES, M.D., F.G.S.

PHYSICIAN TO THE NORTHERN DISPENSARY.

———

THE existence of urea in the blood, in several forms of disease, has long ceased to be a matter of doubt in the minds of chemists. I am not aware, however, that the *proportion* in which that substance exists in morbid blood or secretions, has yet been very accurately determined. In attempting to throw some light on this subject, I have at different times examined fluids obtained from patients at Guy's Hospital; and now have the advantage of being able to refer to Dr. Bright's report of two of those cases, from the subjects of which I obtained, through his kindness, the specimens for analysis. Before relating the results of my examinations, I wish to describe the method which I have adopted in order to separate the urea perfectly free from contamination, and at the same time to avoid that loss which is inevitable when obtaining that substance for estimation in the form of nitrate.

Those who are accustomed to the manipulations of animal chemistry will at once recollect the uncertainty they have felt, as to whether the whole of the urea were separated by nitric acid from the mother liquor; and how tedious and unsatisfactory have been the subsequent processes of evaporation, to crystallize the remaining nitrate.

The relation of urea to ozmazome, as regards solubility in various menstrua, has rendered its separation from that substance a matter of great difficulty; and there is every reason to believe, that when nitrate of urea crystallizes from the extractive matter, its weight is much increased, by an unavoidable adherence of the latter principle. I am quite satisfied in my own mind that this cause of increased weight in our results greatly outbalances any loss which occurs by the imperfect crystallization of the nitrate before alluded to; for by the more perfect method which I now employ, I have always obtained a far less proportion of urea than formerly, although the risk of losing any of the principle present is not nearly so great as that incurred by the usual process.

The delicacy of the plan I now adopt is very great; so much so, that urea can be obtained perfectly pure from an animal fluid, which contains it in the proportion only of 0.15 per mille. The analysis is performed as follows:—The serum, or effused fluid, is evaporated to dryness, at a heat sustained somewhat below 212° Fahrenheit; the dry mass is broken up; boiling water thrown upon it, and allowed to digest several hours. This liquor being carefully poured off, a second portion of water is added, and allowed to digest; after which, the whole is thrown on a filter, and the solid matters washed with distilled water till the percolating fluid ceases to effect a solution of nitrate of silver. The digested and filtered liquors are next evaporated to dryness, by a gentle heat; and the extract, so obtained, digested in a stopper-bottle, with common ether of the shops, of sp. grav. 0.754. This menstruum extracts the urea only; and by digesting successive portions of it until the last added yields no deposit of that principle on evaporation, we obtain the whole of the urea present, and thus directly estimate its weight. As obtained by this process, urea is quite pure and colourless. It once happened to me to observe some slight contamination of the urea, obtained as above, by fatty matter which had escaped separation with the albumen: this, however, was easily got rid of, by dissolving the urea in distilled water, and throwing the solution on a filter previously moistened, when the fatty matter remained behind, and allowed the urea to pass through, perfectly pure.

The first fluid which I shall mention, as examined by this process, was obtained from John Gillmore, Dec. 18, 1839, a case of albuminuria. It was an effusion on the brain, and 210.4 grs. were obtained for examination. From this quantity 0.05 gr. of urea was obtained, equal to about 0.415 per mille. This fluid yielded but slight traces of albumen.

The second case, from which I obtained the serum of the blood, and likewise a portion of fluid which was procured from the cellular tissue by making punctures in the scrotum, was that of John Wiseman, a boy in Job's Ward, under the care of Dr. Bright *. The serum of this patient was of sp. gr. 1015, and contained only 23.49 gr. of albumen in 500 grs.; whereas the same quantity of healthy serum affords about 39.75 grs. It contained 0.2096 per mille of urea. The fluid obtained from the scrotum was of sp. gr. 1007.9 : the analysis of 500 parts gave,

Water	492.400
Albumen	0.800
Extractives and Salts. . . .	6.725
Urea	0.075
	500.000

the proportion of urea being equal to 0.150 per mille.

The third case, from which I obtained the serum of the blood at two different times, and also the fluid effused into the pericardium, was that of Susan Smalling, a patient of Dr. Bright †.

The first specimen of blood was received on March 4th. The specific gravity of its serum was 1025, being somewhat lower than natural : the analysis of 500 grs. yielded,

Water	452.10
Albumen	32.50
Extractives and Salts	15.15
Urea	0.25
	500.00

We here observe a deficiency of albumen, an increase of extractives and salts, and the presence of an ingredient foreign to the serum. The second specimen of blood which I received from this patient was obtained by cupping; and

* Vide No. 8 of Dr. Bright's Cases.
† Vide No. 21 of the same Cases.

not from the arm, as was the case with all the previously-mentioned specimens. It was sent to me on the 30th of April. The specific gravity of its serum was then 1029, or natural: the analysis of 500 parts was as follows:—

$$
\begin{array}{lr}
\text{Water} & 448.3 \\
\text{Albumen} & 40.8 \\
\text{Extractives and Salts} & 10.65 \\
\text{Urea} & 0.25 \\
\hline
& 500.00
\end{array}
$$

The effusion into the pericardium of this patient was of sp. grav. 1028. It yielded urea, but only a trace in 500 grs. of the effusion.

It will be observed, from the analysis quoted above, that the largest proportion of urea which I have detected in the blood is 0.5 per mille, and the least 0.2096. The effusion on the brain gave 0.415; the fluid effused into the cellular tissue of the scrotum, 0.150 per mille; and the pericardial fluid merely a trace in 500 grains.

The condition of the blood in the patient Susan Smalling is worthy of consideration, inasmuch as the serum of the blood underwent a great change between the dates of March 4th and April 30th: it being sp. grav. 1025 on the former, and 1029 sp. grav. on the latter date: the proportion of urea, however, remaining the same. The serum of the 30th April, if we except the existence of urea, may be considered as normal; the albumen being present quite to the natural extent; indeed, if any thing, somewhat beyond the amount generally found in the serum of healthy blood.

The case from which the scrotal fluid was obtained, affords an instance of great decrease in the specific gravity of the serum of the blood. The lowest specific gravity mentioned by Dr. Christison, in his lately-published valuable work, is 1019: this specimen was, however, only 1015 sp. gr.

Feeling great confidence as to the delicacy of the process which I have described as applicable to the detection of urea, I was anxious to apply it to the examination of the serum of healthy blood, which, by some authorities, has been stated to contain urea. Before the present method of analysis occurred to me, I had examined the serum of healthy venous blood without being able to detect urea in it. I determined, however, to examine the serum of healthy arterial blood by this new method, in order more completely to satisfy my mind on the subject. For this purpose, serum was obtained from blood drawn from the temporal artery, and submitted to the new process, but no evidence of the presence of urea could be obtained; though I know, from previous experiments, that I could not have failed to detect it, had it existed even in so small a proportion as 0.2096 per mille.

OBSERVATIONS ON THE BLOOD,

WITH REFERENCE TO ITS PECULIAR CONDITION IN THE

MORBUS BRIGHTII.

BY GEORGE OWEN REES, M.D. F.R.S.

PHYSICIAN TO THE PENTONVILLE NEW MODEL PRISON.

THE examinations of diseased blood which I had an opportunity of making at Guy's Hospital during the past summer, and the results of which will be found appended to each Case as given in the present Number of the Reports, have shewn much matter of interest in their general bearings; and as it is my intention to compare these diseased conditions with the healthy standard, and moreover to enter upon observations connected with the intimate structure of the blood, I may perhaps be excused for premising my remarks by detailing a few experiments, made with a view of proving the anatomy and true mechanical relations of the blood-corpuscle. The diseased condition, to which I have above referred, interferes with many of the physical attributes of the blood; and I am therefore anxious that medical readers should be satisfied on several points relating to the physical condition of the blood in health, before venturing to draw conclusions from what has been observed in disease.

It is hoped that the experiments about to be described may shew the necessity for a correct knowledge of physical structure on the part of those who are occupied in the chemical examination of the blood; and, also, that it may appear how we occasionally possess means of proving on large masses the views to which we have been led by microscopic examination—a method of inquiry which, valuable as it certainly is, must always be received with the distrust naturally felt towards a means of investigation so tempting to the imagination, and which, it is to be feared, has already been productive of much mischief in the hands of the ingenious and unscrupulous.

A careful perusal of the various anatomical and chemical works published on the blood will shew to the reader, that the writers on both branches of science begin to be at fault at one and the same point; that being, when they treat of the colouring matter of the blood, and its true relation to the corpuscle. They know well that the blood, while circulating, is composed of blood-corpuscles, suspended in a liquor; and they describe how this liquor, when the blood is drawn, deposits fibrin, and retains its albumen, extractives, and salts in solution, forming serum: they know, too, that the fibrin adheres to the blood-corpuscles; and the two together make up the mass called crassamentum: but from this point the subject becomes confused; and the anatomist who refers to chemical works for assistance will be equally at a loss with the chemist, who contents himself with a review of the present state of microscopic science, as applied to this branch of physiology. The most recent works on the chemistry of this subject shew a complete want of information concerning the physical conditions under which the red colouring matter is placed; and the processes recommended for its extraction are very unsatisfactory to the microscopic anatomist, who, if he refer to any recent work on the chemistry of the blood, (take for instance the quarto of Lecanu,) will, from the knowledge he possesses of physical structure, be not only dissatisfied, but thoroughly convinced that such a process as that recommended for the extraction of hæmatosine can scarcely be looked upon otherwise than as a means of obtaining a red matter changed by the action of powerful re-agents, and in admixture with the various products of the action of sulphuric acid on animal membrane. Let us imagine a physiologist referring to the work above mentioned;—and how will he be assisted? The process for the extraction of hæmatosine commences as follows:—The blood, fresh drawn, is to be deprived of its fibrin by beating it with twigs while coagulating, and then sulphuric acid is to be added to the remaining red liquor until it becomes brown and nearly solid. There is no occasion to enter further on this process. I shall, I trust, be able to shew how this first step is grossly inconsistent with what we know of the physical structure of the blood. Now, if it can be proved that the red colouring matter is contained in a vesicle, that vesicle with its inclosed coloured matter making up the blood corpuscle, we at once perceive the extreme awkwardness of this process, which, instead of first exposing the colouring matter mechanically, and then proceeding to extract it, subjects it, or rather its containing sac, to the action of a powerful re-agent; thus attacking it only after the formation of inconvenient products consequent on the destruction of an albuminous membrane by sulphuric acid; making it a difficult matter to believe that we at last obtain it in a form to exhibit the properties it possessed while circulating. Had the chemist been aware of that which I shall now notice, he would have been enabled, first to separate the blood corpuscles, then to burst them, and so obtain their coloured contents in solution for chemical examination.

In proceeding to treat of the red colouring matter as a constituent of the blood-corpuscle, I must premise that great confusion has arisen from the terms, red particle, red globule, and red corpuscle, being regarded as synonymous with hæmatosine or colouring matter; the latter expression meaning, in its correct signification, nothing more than one of the constituent parts of the red corpuscles; there being a white matter also present in those bodies, which chemists have only noticed within the last few years, and have never yet ventured to define more particularly than as the white matter of the corpuscles.

Assisted with the evidence afforded by some recent microscopic observations, I have been led to determine on a larger scale what I believe to be the true relation between the red colouring principle or hæmatosine and the white matter of the corpuscles. The microscopic experiments to which I allude[*] demonstrated that the red corpuscles were closed sacs, containing a fluid within them; and made it a matter of interest further to ascertain whether the fluid were red; or, on the contrary, that the corpuscle owed its colour to the redness of the enveloping membrane, the fluid within being without colour. The former of these views is certainly the

[*] Rees and Lane on the Structure &c. Vide Guy's Hospital Reports, No. 13.

most generally entertained by micrographers, though we find Schultzé regarding the latter as the more correct:—and it is not easy to devise means for testing the truth of either position by microscopic examination.

In considering this question, it occurred to me, that if the blood corpuscle were a closed sac, and capable of being burst by the addition of water (a point proved by the microscopic experiments above alluded to), we might, by thus treating a large quantity of collected corpuscles and bursting them, be enabled to collect the burst cases in mass at the bottom of the water, which would hold their contents in solution;—that we could thus examine their colour, and by this simple experiment set the question at rest. With this view, the serum was decanted from a specimen of coagulated blood: the clot was next carefully washed in the serum, in order to get as many red corpuscles as possible into the liquor: it was then removed, and the serum set aside to allow the red corpuscles to subside. Subsidence being complete, which occupied several hours, the supernatant serum was decanted, as nearly as possible without disturbing the deposit, and the deep-red thick mixture at bottom poured into distilled water, in order to burst the membranes of the corpuscles. This aqueous mixture was then well stirred, and set aside; when, after a few hours had elapsed, I observed a white deposit at the bottom of the containing vessel, while the supernatant liquor remained quite clear, and of a fine red colour. Now, with a previous knowledge that the blood corpuscles are burst by water, and likewise that they are sacs containing a fluid, this experiment makes it pretty certain that the containing sacs are white, and the contained liquor of a red colour.

I do not wish here to enter at length on the description of what I feel confident in my own mind should be regarded as the nucleus of the blood-corpuscle; but merely have to state, that the microscopic examination of the white precipitate to which I have above alluded has completely confirmed my former views of this question; satisfying me that the deposit is made up of burst membranes of corpuscles, and of nuclei; the latter being apparently the same structures which some writers have regarded as corpuscles deprived of their red colouring matter—a condition which, from what has already been demonstrated concerning the corpuscle, can never occur; inasmuch as destruction of the inclosing membrane of the corpuscle is necessary before its colouring matter can be extracted: after which violence, it is obvious that any soft solid maintaining a definite form, and which can be seen and measured under the microscope, must be some constituent of original organized structure, which has now become disintegrated.

The opinion, that the membranes of the blood-corpuscles, notwithstanding their extreme tenuity, possessed in common with other animal structures the property of admitting the passage of fluids in accordance with the law of endosmose, and which was first noticed and described by Mr. Lane and myself in the Guy's Hospital Reports, has been, up to the present time, entirely supported by microscopic evidence. I am anxious, on the present occasion, to prove the truth of this view, by relating some experiments conducted on large quantities of blood; not only more firmly to establish a necessary premise to my conclusions, but also to shew that the correctness of opinions, the results of microscopic examination, occasionally admits of being proved by experiments conducted on masses visible to the unassisted eye. Now, if it be true that liquors pass in and out of the blood-corpuscles in proportions bearing a ratio to their specific gravities, then, if a large quantity of corpuscles be collected, we ought, by treating them with solutions of different densities, to be able to produce conditions which will differently affect their contents; the higher specific gravities taking out large proportions of those contents; the lower specific gravities removing less from within the corpuscle: and our liquors obtained after deposition has occurred ought to be differently coloured accordingly: some should be deeply tinged with red; others almost white, having, from their less-specific gravity, entered the corpuscle in large proportion, and only drawn out a very small quantity of its coloured liquor.

The results obtained from experiments conducted as above described have been in exact accordance with those microscopic views, the correctness of which they were intended to test: thus, when a quantity of corpuscles obtained by subsidence from serum were mixed with a solution of common

salt, as nearly as possible of the specific gravity of the liquor
by which the corpuscle was surrounded, and consequently of
the same specific gravity as the liquor within, the mixture
deposited the corpuscles unaltered, and the supernatant
solution was colourless, owing to the difficulty of any admixture occurring between liquors of the same specific gravity
through the membrane containing the red colouring matter.
When, however, a liquor of higher specific gravity was mixed
with another portion of these subsided corpuscles, then the
conditions were completely altered; the subsided corpuscles
exhibiting a darker colour at the bottom of the vessel, owing
to their aggregating more closely from being to a certain
extent collapsed; and the supernatant liquor, instead of
being colourless, was tinged of a deep red; the liquor of
higher specific gravity having extracted a large quantity of
the contents of the corpuscles. When the reverse of this
experiment was performed by making the mixture with a
solution of less-specific gravity than the liquor within the
corpuscle, then the subsided mass was less compact, and
somewhat lighter in colour, but still red; and the supernatant liquor exhibited but a feeble and scarcely perceptible
tinge of pink, owing to the small quantity of colouring matter
which could escape from within the corpuscles; while the
liquor of less-specific gravity would enter in large proportion from without, swelling them, and thus making them
occupy more room as a precipitate. It may be stated here,
that a solution of any salt which does not act as a precipitant of serum, or even sugar, will serve to shew these effects;
the conditions produced being then entirely governed by the
specific gravity of the solutions, and in no way resulting
from the chemical qualities of the salt. The next point to
which I must allude, in connection with the subject of healthy
blood, is the condition of the iron, and its true position in the
organization of the corpuscle. It has already been proved
that the red colouring matter is a fluid contained within a
vesicle; which vesicle allows of the passage of fluids from
without to within, and *vice versâ*, according to certain fixed
laws: and I shall now endeavour to shew that the iron of
the blood is contained in this red liquor, and not in any
other of the constituent parts of the corpuscle. If we repeat

the first experiment which I detailed, and which consisted in bursting the vesicles of a mass of corpuscles, and so destroying them by the addition of distilled-water, we can obtain a solution of their coloured contents, either by allowing the subsidence of the cases and nuclei and pouring off the clear liquor, or by performing a careful filtration through doubled blotting-paper. If the clear solution so obtained be now evaporated to dryness, I find, by incineration of the dried mass, that it contains the whole of the iron of the corpuscles; while the white matter which subsides (composed of burst cases and nuclei), if well washed from adhering colouring matter, does not yield the slightest indication of the presence of the metal. We may therefore conclude that the red liquor of the corpuscles contains the whole of the iron, and in a very soluble form.

Those who have studied the appearances put on by the blood-corpuscles, as seen under the microscope, whatever may be their opinion concerning the method of re-production, will, I am sure, allow that corpuscles of a smaller size are constantly to be detected mixed up with those of mature growth; and I have myself, on several occasions, been satisfied, by experiment, that these smaller corpuscles possess precisely the same physical attributes as the larger ones, in relation to endosmodic phænomena. Now, it must be a necessary part of the process by which these small corpuscles arrive at maturity, that iron enter within the envelope, to supply one of the constituents of the red colouring matter; and to ensure this effect, two conditions are required:—
1. A liquor containing iron in solution must be applied to the membrane of the corpuscle; and, 2. This liquor must be of a specific gravity less than that contained within the corpuscle, or it will not enter it in quantity. Both these required conditions are to be found as physico-chemical characteristics of the mixture of chyle and lymph, which enters the blood by the thoracic-duct, to which fluid all experimenters have given a lower specific gravity than the liquor sanguinis. Thus the specific gravity of the contents of the thoracic-duct in the human subject, which I lately analysed[*], was 1024, while that of the liquor sanguinis may be given at about 1052, at the least.

[*] Vide Philosophical Transactions for 1842. Part I.

From other experiments, on the cat, the dog, and the ass, I am satisfied of the general truth of this statement. The iron which exists in the chyle is not contained in the crassamentum, which forms by coagulation; but we find it, on the contrary, as a constituent of the serum in a perfect state of solution, so that it may enter with facility through the membranes of the corpuscles: so perfect, indeed, is this solution, that, even after evaporating the chyle to dryness, we are enabled to extract the iron from the albuminous matters by digestion in water. It exists, in fact, dissolved in that constituent of the chyle which is called the aqueous extractive, and most probably in the form of lactate. Nature has, then, in this admirable manner provided for the introduction of iron into the corpuscle, by presenting it in a perfectly soluble form to the enveloping membrane, and dissolved in a liquor of a specific gravity suited to effect the necessary endosmodic actions.

Having thus shewn the reason why iron exists in the serum, and not in the crassamentum of the chyle—and also, why the contents of the thoracic duct are of less specific gravity than the liquor sanguinis—I wish to direct attention to the series of pathological phænomena which may be expected to arise when this due balance and arrangement of the physical properties of the fluids becomes destroyed, and when, by a diseased condition of longer or shorter duration, the blood so far varies from its normal standard as to present obstacles to the performance of those actions on the part of the chyle which must be considered as necessary for the preservation of animal life.

From what has been demonstrated at the commencement of this Paper, it is evident, that as the important changes of respiration occur in the colouring matter of the corpuscle, and since that colouring matter is contained within a membrane, a healthy condition of this envelope, such as admits of the transmission of liquors and gases according to certain fixed laws, is as necessary for the maintenance of life and health as is the perviousness of the larynx, trachæa, or bronchi; and any general cause acting upon the corpuscle, so as to interfere with those properties, may be expected to destroy life as rapidly as would the closure of any of the openings communicating between the atmosphere and the internal pulmonary surface.

Again, let the blood become deranged so that its specific gravity is lessened, and we may feel assured, that if the physical qualities, more especially the specific gravity of the chyle, be not simultaneously affected, and that, too, in a due proportion, the result must be, that the red colouring matter, the great oxygenator of the blood, is no longer produced in its ordinary quantity ; the ferruginous serum of the chyle not being able to enter the blood-corpuscle as in health. Again, if the degeneration above alluded to take place, we must recollect that all the solids of the body through which the blood courses are formed with pores and of material admitting of endosmodic action ; and that it is impossible for the solid constituents to preserve their health if constantly acted upon by the blood at a specific gravity of 1030 to 36, instead of 1052 to 57 ; the equilibrium of health being no longer preserved, and the watery blood inducing a like condition in the other solids. In throwing out these suggestions, I am prompted by a desire to draw the attention of the Profession to the great importance of the study of endosmodic action, as applied to pathology ; many of the phænomena of the Morbus Brightii being apparently attributable to a condition of blood such as I have above noticed.

On examining the Table (which will be found at the end of this communication, and consulting the Cases with chemical notices appended, the following will appear the prominent features to which attention should be more especially directed :—1. The excessive quantity of water in the blood. 2. The existence in the blood of one of the ingredients of the urine. 3. The existence of the same ingredient of the urine in the milk, and also in the fluids effused into various serous cavities. 4. The absence or deficiency in the urine of one or more of the natural ingredients of the excretion. 5. The general watery condition of the urine. 6. The existence of albumen in the urine.

When considering the part taken by the blood in producing the Morbus Brightii, it must not be too rapidly concluded that those changes which are observed in more advanced stages of the disease are identical in kind, and differing only in degree from those occurring at the commencement of a severe and fatal case ; or that they are the cause of the symptoms, terminating in perfect recovery, which we so often observe in mild cases of anasarca with coagulable urine following scarlet-fever. The diseased conditions of the blood noticed in the Table may, however, I think, well be considered the cause of the train of secondary symptoms attendant on the Morbus Brightii ; and the first morbid condition induced may be (as has been rendered more than probable by the late ingenious researches of Mr. Robinson) simply a congested state of the kidney—a mechanical derangement of circulation—giving rise to a filtration of the albuminous matters of the blood into the urine ; a drain on the system which, by impoverishing the vital fluid, may, in its turn, make the blood a cause of further symptoms, such as would never have developed themselves had not the primary disease been manifest. All, indeed, that we know of the history of this degeneration of the kidney, the mild character of some of the cases, and the facility with which the disease, as following scarlatina, admits of cure—tends to shew, that in the commencement the blood may be perfectly healthy, and the albumen in the urine the result of congestion by blood in its normal state.

There is, however, a fact in the history of this affection which does not render it altogether improbable that the presence of an excess of water in the blood may, in some cases at least, assist in bringing about the effusion of serum into the urine. I allude to the frequency of a dry skin, observed in some early cases. The probability that such a state of the cutaneous surface acts as a cause is considerably increased by the tendency to this kind of dropsy after the cutaneous surface has been involved by an attack of scarlatina, which produces a form of Morbus Brightii, for the most part easily admitting of cure. The difficulties which must necessarily occur in freeing the blood of water when the action of the skin is lessened or entirely stopped must be considered as very great, when we remember the large quantities of fluid daily given off from the cutaneous surface, and the small excess only in the quantity of urine characterizing any form of Morbus Brightii ;— the greater number of cases, indeed, passing less than the natural quantity. In making the above suggestion, I in no way wish it to be inferred as my belief that congestion alone is incapable of producing coagulable urine; indeed, as stated before, direct experiment has shewn to the contrary: but it is certain that the tendency to the entrance of albumen into the urine will be increased by dilution of the blood; and we frequently observe a condition occurring, at the very outset of the disease, favourable to the production of this form of deterioration in the circulating fluid.

The secondary symptoms of the Morbus Brightii—such as effusion into the large serous cavities or the ventricles of the brain, general cellular effusion, and the peculiar anæmic appearance which, even when no swelling of the face exists, is frequently so characteristic as to attract the practised eye— are easily explicable as results, when once we are acquainted with the watery state of the blood, and the physiological conditions necessary to preserve the integrity of the blood-corpuscle. The obvious mechanical assistance which an excess of water must afford for the production of general effusion needs no comment; but it may be a matter of difficulty to some, to explain how it is that the blood loses its red colouring matter; and which, to be clearly understood, requires an insight into the more minute changes occurring in the fluid, as a result of its aqueous condition. I have before shewn, that if the chyle does not accommodate itself in relative specific gravity to the blood, the necessary endosmodic actions cannot take place between the two fluids; and we may consequently expect difficulty in the production and growth of the red corpuscles, inasmuch as the iron cannot be supplied for the formation of colouring matter, the ferruginous serum of the chyle no longer entering through the membrane of the blood corpuscle in virtue of its less specific gravity: and I think it may be maintained as the correct view, that this is really the cause of that great diminution in the proportion of colouring matter observed in the blood of patients affected with the advanced stage of the Morbus Brightii. This diminution in the proportion of red corpuscles does not occur in early cases of the disease, however confirmed in character: an example of which may be seen by referring to the history of George Moore, 14 Job Ward, a mild case, probably admitting of permanent cure, in which the blood contained more than the normal proportion of fibrin and corpuscles; the albumen being very deficient, the serum light, and the water of the blood in about its natural quantity. We here see the first effects of the disease—the blood becoming deprived of its albuminous ingredients; a condition which, if it continue, will produce the next change; viz. a deterioration in the specific gravity of the contents of the corpuscle, owing to the liquor sanguinis becoming lighter, and endosmosing that structure: this state again soon succeeded by a lessening of the number of red corpuscles, attributable to the requisite actions no longer taking place on the part of the chyle, in the manner described in a former part of this Paper. The occurrence of inflammation in this disease, as will be seen by the analysis of the blood in the case of Holywell, produces the usual increase in the quantity of fibrin in the blood: this, however, did not happen to any considerable degree in the case of Charles Scott.

The existence of urea in the blood, and effusions obtained from the patients in the male and female wards, and also in the milk of a patient in Lydia Ward, has been satisfactorily proved: indeed, I have never yet failed to obtain it in sufficient quantity to shew its physical and chemical characters. The process employed for the blood and effusions is described in the Tenth Number of the Guy's Hospital Reports; and I find it to be, with slight variation, the best calculated for extracting urea from the milk. For this latter purpose the milk must be evaporated to dryness; and then several times digested with æther, which will extract the whole of the fatty matters, together with the urea; the latter being easily separable by heating the dry ethereal extract with water, and stirring it well during the digestion. After this process the urea exists dissolved in the water, which may be poured off from under the fatty matter, the latter having caked above the liquor on cooling.

As regards the urine in the Morbus Brightii, the deficiency of urea, and occasional deficiency or absence of lithic acid, its watery condition, and the presence of albumen, the two former states may in all probability be attributed to the derangement of the kidney alone; and the two latter, in some measure, to the condition of the blood. I am not aware that the total absence of lithic acid from the urine has been before observed. That such was the case, however, was proved by rigorous chemical and microscopical examination; the former consisting in evaporating the urine to a small quantity, adding muriatic acid, and carefully analysing any precipitate so obtained.

Albuminous urine, when viewed under the microscope, exhibits granules and corpuscles of varying form and size; the larger of which might be mistaken for the pus-globule by careless or inexperienced observers. The true source, however, of these bodies is, in all probability, the serum of the blood, which I find deposits analogous granules and corpuscles when diluted by a liquor of light specific gravity; which may easily be proved by pouring distilled water on serum, and submitting to the microscope the precipitate which collects after a few hours have elapsed. In other respects, coagulable urine presents the ordinary appearances under the microscope; the solid ingredients or crystallizable products exhibiting, when present, their usual characteristics. Some specimens shew very well the large form of granulated mucous globule known as the secretion of the prostate.

In concluding this communication, I cannot help expressing a hope that the many points of interest which the study of the Morbus Brightii affords may receive the early attention of physiologists; believing, as I do, that careful observation of the phænomena occurring in this disease must eventually throw much light both on the true nature of the blood-corpuscle and the all-important offices of the function of respiration.

TABLE *of* RESULTS *of* EXAMINATIONS *of* BLOOD *and* URINE *in* MORBUS BRIGHTII.

Whence obtained.	Blood: Composition in 1000 parts.	Urine.	REMARKS.
WILLIAM CURTAIN, 22 *Job Ward.*	Water . . 853·11 Solid matters } of serum } 81·28 Fibrin and } corpuscles } 65·61 Serum in 1000 parts: Albumen . . 69·5 Urea . . . . 0·5 Alkaline salts, 6·0	18 fluid oz. were passed in 24 hours, each oz. yielding 5·2 gr. of albumen (dry): sp. gr. of urine 1015: urea 8·1 per 1000. No lithic acid could be detected in this urine, in any form, either combined or free.	Specific gravity of serum was 1023: it not milky. The blood very slightly buffed
CHARLES SCOTT, 3 *Job Ward.*	Water . . 835·85 Solid matters } of serum } 82·54 Fibrin and } corpuscles } 81·61	32 fluid oz. passed in 24 hours: sp. gr. of urine 1011, each ounce containing 2·05 gr. of albumen. Lithic acid present, in small proportion.	Blood buffed and cup
JAMES BACK, 2 *Job Ward.* Disease complicated with Phthisis.	Water . . 828·92 Solid matters } of serum } 76·98 Fibrin and } corpuscles } 94·10	Containing 7·75 gr. of albumen in each oz.: urea 8·73 per 1000.	Serum contained 6 parts of albumen in 1
GEORGE HOLYWELL, 4 *Job Ward.* Disease accompanied with effusion into the Pleura.	Water . . 777·06 Solid matters } of serum } 71·14 Fibrin and } corpuscles } 151·80	For particulars, see the Cases in present Number.	Blood buffed and cup sp. gr. of the serum 1 containing in 1000 p albumen 64 and salts parts. Urea detec but not estimated
GEORGE MOORE, 14 *Job Ward.*	Water . . 782·86 Solid matters } of serum } 73·14 Fibrin and } corpuscles } 144·00	. . . .	Serum of sp. gr. 1 containing in 1000 p albumen 72, and urea parts.
ELIZABETH MⁱINNES, 5 *Lydia Ward.*	Water . . 805·71 Solid matters } of serum } 85·56 Fibrin and } corpuscles } 108·73	Sp. gr. 1012, containing 1·5 gr. of albumen in each oz., and no trace of lithic acid in any form.	Serum of sp. gr. 1 alkaline salts 7· per parts of serum.
From a healthy individual, for comparison.	Water . . 792·20 Solid matters } of serum } 87·85 Fibrin and } corpuscles } 119·95	Sp. gr. 1022: urea 30·1, and lithic acid 1·0 parts per 1000. No trace of albumen.	Serum of sp. gr. 102 30, containing albumen . . . 79 alkaline salts 7 in 1000 parts.

TRIAL FOR MURDER

BY

POISONING WITH ARSENIC,

BERKSHIRE LENT ASSIZES, 1845.

POST-MORTEM APPEARANCES; CHEMICAL ANALYSIS;
DETECTION OF THE POISON AS SULPHURET, TWENTY-EIGHT
DAYS AFTER INTERMENT.*

BY ALFRED S. TAYLOR.

Thomas Jennings was charged with the murder of his infant
son, Eleazar Jennings, a child aged three years and eight
months, by administering to him arsenic on the 23d of
December 1844.

From the statement of the case for the prosecution, it appeared that the prisoner resided in a small cottage with his
family, consisting of a wife and four young children, including Eleazar, the deceased. The only direct evidence
against the prisoner was in a statement made by his niece,
Maria Carter, a young girl, who had lived with him about a
year, and took care of his children. She stated, that on the
Monday before Christmas Day (December 23d), the prisoner,
his children, and herself (the mother being absent) dined
together on bacon and potatoes; that there was a salt-cellar
on the table, from which all the party, except the deceased,
took salt; that as soon as they began to eat their dinner the
prisoner went to the pantry, and brought out, between his
finger and thumb, a pinch (as the witness described it) of
something white, like salt, and put it upon the edge of the
plate out of which the deceased was eating his dinner.† The

---

* This case is drawn up partly from the brief for the prosecution, and
partly from notes taken at the trial.

† A question arose at the trial respecting the weight of a pinch of arsenic.
It was stated that it might be about twelve or fifteen grains. Actual
weighing afterwards proved that a good pinch of the powder was equal to
seventeen grains. Medical men are often asked to state the weights of particular measures of the poison in powder, as of a teaspoonful, a tablespoonful,
&c.

deceased dipped his potatoe into it, and swallowed the whole of it. In the afternoon of the same day, about half-an-hour after dinner, the deceased complained of pain in his belly; on the next day he was sick, and brought up something like water; and on Wednesday (Christmas Day) he died. It appeared further, from the examination of this witness at the inquest and trial, that the deceased said his belly was bad all the afternoon on Monday; he went once or twice to the necessary, but did not go often on Tuesday: that he was very thirsty on Tuesday, and mint-tea was given to him: that he was very sick on the Wednesday, and died about the middle of the day. As far as could be ascertained, the whole duration of the illness was about forty-eight hours. At the last moment, the prisoner went for a medical man, at the request of his wife; but before assistance arrived, the child was dead.

An inquest was held on the 27th December; and there being at that time no suspicion of poison, no inspection of the body was made, a verdict of natural death was returned, and the child was buried. About a fortnight after this oc-currence, another of the prisoner's children was taken ill, and died somewhat suddenly. An inquest was held on the body of this child on the 11th of January 1845. This body was inspected, and there were marks of inflammation in the stomach and intestines. A rough analysis of the contents of the stomach was made, but no poison could be found. A verdict of natural death was returned, and the second child was buried.

Mr. Lamb, surgeon, of Newbury, who had assisted in this investigation, had a strong suspicion that arsenic was pre-sent in the case of the second child; and he forwarded to me, for examination, an ounce phial filled with a portion of the liquid contents of the stomach. On subjecting them to analysis, arsenic was clearly found to be present, although in small proportion.

Suspicion being thus once excited, it was supposed that Eleazar Jennings, the first child, had also died from poison;

&c. I have found a teaspoonful of powdered arsenic to weigh 150 grains, and a tablespoonful to weigh 530 grains. These weights are liable to vary; but the results may be taken as sufficiently correct for all medico-legal purposes.

and after the result of the analysis in the second case, the Coroner issued his order for the disinterment of the body of Eleazar. This accordingly took place on the 24th January 1845, i.e. *twenty-eight* days after interment. The prisoner was present in the churchyard, and identified the body ; and on some remark being made that there was a suspicion that the children had been poisoned, he said there was no more poison in them (*i.e.* the two children), than there was in him. The stomach and intestines of the child, unopened, were placed in a clean bottle by Mr. Lamb, and brought to London. They were examined by himself and me, at Guy's Hospital, on the 25th January, and the result of the examination will be found in our evidence. This evidence is so fully given in the brief for the prosecution, that it is unnecessary to make any addition or alteration in it.

Arthur Lamb, is a surgeon, and resides at Newbury, Berks. On Monday, the 6th day of January, he was at the prisoner's house. The prisoner stated to him, in the presence of another witness, that he had had no arsenic in his house for two years, but that he had some in a cottage in the wood, and he had not used any since March last. That he (witness) received an order to make a post-mortem examination of the body of Eleazar Jennings, and an analysis of the contents of the stomach, and attended at the parish church at Thatcham, on the 24th January last, for that purpose. The body of Eleazar Jennings was disinterred that morning, in the presence of the constable of Thatcham. It was stated on the coffin that the child was three years and eight months old.

Witness found that decomposition had but slightly taken place in the body ; that the stomach and intestines were distended with gas, and externally exhibited marks of inflammation. He removed the stomach and intestines entire, having placed a ligature on the cardiac orifice of the stomach and on the rectum, in order to prevent the contents from escaping. He took them to London the next morning, the 25th January, and proceeded, with Mr. Taylor of Guy's Hospital, to make a further examination of them, as well as an analysis of their contents. On making an examination of the stomach of the deceased, Eleazar Jennings, witness found that the internal surface was inflamed and ulcerated. He was present when Mr. Taylor tested the contents of the stomach by various processes, and the result was, that arsenic was found by every one of the tests used.

The estimated quantity of arsenic discovered in the stomach was from five to six grains. He is of opinion that Eleazar Jennings died from the effects of arsenic. Raisins, currants, and suet, were also found in the stomach.

Alfred S. Taylor, is Lecturer on Medical Jurisprudence at Guy's Hospital. The last witness brought to him, on the 25th day of January last, the stomach and intestines of a child, and, assisted by this gentleman, he made an examination of them, and an analysis of their contents. The results of the examination were reduced to writing. The following is a copy of the notes made at the time :—

POST-MORTEM APPEARANCES.—Decomposition had but slightly advanced. The viscera were distended with air, and presented patches of a deep red colour externally: this was especially noticed in the duodenum.

The stomach. The central portion externally was of a deep green colour, an appearance which, according to the statement of Mr. Lamb, had come on since the exhumation. On opening the stomach a quantity of gas escaped, and about two drachms (two teaspoonfuls) of a reddish-coloured thick liquid was drained from it. The central portion of the mucous membrane was of a greenish-brown colour, but at the cardiac and pyloric ends it was of a deep cinnabar-red hue, especially at the cardiac extremity and along the greater curvature : at the pylorus, the mucous membrane was rather pale, so as to form a distinct boundary between that organ and the duodenum. Hard masses of a solid white substance were found scattered over the surface of the stomach, which, on examination, turned out to be lumps of suet. Besides this, there were a few currants undigested, and the skins of raisins. About an inch above the greater curvature, and near the cardiac extremity, was a long irregularly oval patch on the mucous membrane, of a deep mustard-yellow colour, about an inch in length, and less than half an inch in width. This yellow matter was closely intermixed with the husks of raisins, and in and about the spot the mucous membrane was ulcerated. By slight friction it was readily detached in layers of a yellow colour. Streaks and small patches of the same yellow-coloured matter, were also found towards the centre of the mucous membrane on the posterior wall of the stomach.

Duodenum. The mucous membrane was of a deep red colour, and the mucous glands were considerably enlarged: there were no yellow stains to be seen. The small intestines presented patches of redness through part of their course. The *rectum* was unusually pale, and contained a lumbricus about seven inches in length.

CHEMICAL ANALYSIS.—The hard white solid matter diffused over the mucous membrane of the stomach was found to be fat, by placing it on white blotting paper, and then passing beneath the paper a heated spatula, when it was entirely melted and absorbed by the paper, forming a greasy transparent stain, and leaving no solid residue.

Liquid contents of the Stomach.—The liquid obtained from this organ amounted to two drachms: it was of a deep red colour, turbid, and contained particles of fatty matter and mucus floating in it. It was neither acid nor alkaline. 1. When a small portion was boiled with copper and muriatic acid, the copper was only tarnished after some hours. 2. The liquid was diluted with its bulk of distilled water, acidulated with acetic acid, boiled three quarters of an hour, and filtered. The filtered liquid was nearly colourless, and sufficiently clear to allow of the direct application of the chemical tests for arsenic. (*a.*) It acquired a yellow colour when exposed to a current of sulphuretted hydrogen gas. (*b.*) It gave a light yellow precipitate with ammonio-nitrate of silver. (*c.*) It gave a light grass-green with ammonio-sulphate of copper. These re-actions clearly indicated the presence of arsenic. The effects, however, were, on the whole, so slight, as only to justify the inference that the small quantity of the liquid (ʒii) found in the stomach contained faint traces of that poison.

Solid contents of the stomach.—The yellow-coloured matter was carefully removed by an ivory spatula from the mucous membrane of the stomach, and allowed to dry spontaneously by imbibition on several folds of white blotting paper.

When the deposit was examined with a glass there were observed white-looking crystalline particles, like sand, intermixed with the yellow substance.

1. A small portion of this was boiled with copper and pure muriatic acid, when an iron-grey deposit, indicative of arsenic, immediately appeared on the metal. Several slips of fine copper gauze were then successively placed in the liquid, and a considerable quantity of the iron-grey deposit was thus obtained. On drying the copper, and gently heating it in a small reduction tube, a white crystalline sublimate was produced, bearing all the physical characters of arsenious acid.

2. Another portion of the yellow substance was now mixed with incinerated acetate of soda, well dried; and, on heating the mixture in a reduction tube, a distinct and well-formed crystalline ring of metallic arsenic was immediately procured. The part of the glass containing the ring was filed off and broken, and the fragments were then heated gently in a wide tube, when a white crystalline crust, apparently of arsenious acid, was immediately obtained. On dissolving this in a few drops of water, and adding the ammonio-nitrate of silver and the ammonio-sulphate of copper, a rich lemon-yellow precipitate was obtained in the former case, and a bright grass-green in the latter. Sulphuretted hydrogen also gave, with another portion, a golden-yellow precipitate.

These results, thus corroborating and confirming each other, proved beyond all doubt that the deposit in the mucous membrane of the stomach was a compound of arsenic. The poison had been obtained in the metallic state by Reinsch's process, and by reduction with soda flux. The metal had been reconverted to arsenious acid, and this, dissolved in water, had given the usual re-actions with the two liquid and the gaseous tests.*

---

* The reader will perceive that Marsh's process was not employed. This was considered unnecessary, because the existence of the poison was so clearly established by the other processes and tests. By avoiding the unnecessary multiplication of proofs, the objections taken to chemical evidence in cross-exami-

Opinion.—From all the above-mentioned results, the following conclusions were drawn:—

1. That arsenic was present in the stomach of this child, and the total quantity might be estimated at from five to six grains.

2. That it had been introduced into the stomach as white arsenic, but had become partially changed to sulphuret or orpiment, by the decomposition of the body.

3. From the deeply-reddened state of the mucous membrane of the stomach and duodenum, and from the fact of the poison being incorporated with the ulcerated membrane of the stomach, there is no doubt that the arsenic so found was taken during life, and was really the cause of death.

4. From the fact that the husks of raisins, currants, and suet were closely intermixed with the poison, it is not improbable that the arsenic was taken with plum-pudding.

In conclusion, I may remark that the quantity of arsenic which would probably suffice to kill a child of this age would be about two or three grains, and, under favourable circumstances, perhaps even less.

———

Notwithstanding that the deceased was not seen during life, the post-mortem appearances in the stomach, which were unusually well marked, and the result of the chemical analysis, left no doubt in the minds of Mr. Lamb and myself that arsenic was the cause of death: hence there was but little room for cross-examination on this head.

It may, however, be as well to mention, that the points on

examination are of course considerably reduced. It should be remembered, that, in evidence founded on chemical analysis, "*whatever does not strengthen, weakens.*" It cannot be said of such evidence, "*superflua non nocent,*" because the cross-examination is sure to be directed to the fallacies of superfluous tests, just as it is always directed to the irrelevant details of a post-mortem examination.

I may also observe that arsenic was subsequently detected in the tissue of the liver of the deceased, into which it had been obviously absorbed. The liver was cut up in slices, dried and boiled with one part of pure muriatic acid and eight parts of water (Reinsch's process). After two hours the solution was filtered, and arsenical deposits were obtained on copper gauze. These yielded octohedral crystals of arsenious acid by sublimation, and on dissolving the crystals in water the liquid tests gave the characteristic re-actions for arsenic.

which the counsel for the defence dwelt were—1. The power of judging from post-mortem appearances so long after death; but it was stated that arsenic had, in this respect, remarkably antiseptic properties. That evidence of this kind, however, might not rest solely on description, an accurate drawing of the stomach, as it appeared at the time of the analysis, was made by Mr. Hurst, of Guy's Hospital, and some precipitated sesquisulphuret of arsenic mixed with gum was employed to give the correct appearance of the yellow patch found near the greater curvature.   2. It was a question why this child should not have died sooner, had its death been caused by arsenic: to which it was replied, that the period at which death took place from arsenic was subject to great variation according to circumstances: that some persons died within a few hours, while others lingered for several days: that, in short, no definite rule could be laid down on this point.   3. Whether arsenic was not a natural or *normal* constituent of the human body, and whether this was not the opinion of the celebrated toxicologist, Orfila?   It was stated in answer, that such an opinion was not held by chemists who had experimented on the subject, and that Orfila had himself been obliged to abandon it, as his experiments performed before the Institute, in 1841, had entirely failed in demonstrating its existence in the healthy human body.   The fact that a question of this kind was put, shews how long an error in medical jurisprudence may continue to find circulation among lawyers after it has been rejected by the medical profession.   The question, however, was here entirely misplaced, because the arsenic was found in a *solid layer*, lying on the surface of the mucous membrane of the stomach, and was not extracted by solution, incineration, or carbonization.   The fallacy involved in the question was immediately displayed to the jury, by the learned Judge asking, whether it was medically possible that any person could spontaneously generate within his stomach *five grains* of solid arsenic!   4. The last question turned upon the validity of the tests for the poison—Whether there was not some kind of objection to every known test for arsenic, although the same objection might not apply to all the tests?   This was an ingenious question.   The reply given was, that no single substance, nor any mixture of substances, was known in chemistry which would give all the re-actions for arsenic that had been obtained in this case.

The evidence chiefly bearing against the prisoner, as the person who administered the poison rested, as it has already been stated, with his niece. Before poison was discovered in the body of the deceased, the prisoner denied that he had had any arsenic in his possession for two years. After the discovery, he confessed that he had had some arsenic for destroying vermin, but had given it away. It was proved in evidence that a short time before Christmas he had given away a quantity of a white powder (some of the arsenic) to a neighbour, in the presence of his niece. She saw him poke it out of a bottle with a stick, and he then threw the stick in the fire. She did not see whence he took the bottle, or what he did with it. The prisoner admitted, in his voluntary statement, that he kept the bottle on the top shelf of the dresser in the pantry adjoining the room in which they had their meals; and it was from this room that he was seen to come by the niece with a pinch of white powder between his finger and thumb, which he placed on the plate of the deceased as if it were salt. He said he cautioned the witness Carter not to touch the bottle, which she denied. The fact that arsenic was there at the time the deceased was taken ill was made evident by the testimony of several witnesses. The prisoner made several contradictory statements with the view to save himself by incriminating Maria Carter — alleging that she had poisoned the children.

Two bottles of white powder were produced by witnesses at the trial, to whom the prisoner had given them after the death of his children. One of these bottles was pronounced by the witness Carter to be similar to the one out of which she had seen the prisoner take the white powder to give to a neighbour.

It was then necessary to determine the nature of the contents of each bottle, and for this purpose an analysis was required to be made during the trial. Each was found to contain white arsenic in fine powder, unmixed with any other ingredient, and the quantity in the two bottles, could not have been less than five ounces. Another bottle of a brown powder was also traced to the possession of the prisoner: this was proved to be nux vomica, which he had been in the habit of using for poisoning crows.

In the defence it was urged that the symptoms observed might have depended on the worm found in the rectum; that the prisoner could have had no motive for poisoning his children; and that it was more likely, if the deceased had been poisoned, that the arsenic was administered by Carter the niece. The Jury, however, were satisfied with the evidence, and the prisoner was convicted, and subsequently executed.

OBSERVATIONS

ON

URINARY CONCRETIONS AND DEPOSITS;

WITH AN ACCOUNT OF THE

CALCULI IN THE MUSEUM OF GUY'S HOSPITAL,

BY GOLDING BIRD, A.M. M.D. F.L.S.

A QUARTER of a century has elasped since an account of the urinary calculi in the Museum of Guy's Hospital emanated from the pen of the late Dr. Marcet, in an Essay on the Chemical History and Medical Treatment of Calculus Disorders; a work in which the resources of medicine and chemistry were brought to bear on this, at that time, nearly unexplored portion of pathological science. From the labours of his contemporary and friend, the late Dr. Wollaston, of Drs. Prout, Yellowly, and many others, who have directed their time and talents to the investigation of the composition and characters of urinary calculi, and concretions generally, so much light has been shed over the whole subject, that the task devolving on any one who now attempts to give an account of even a large collection of calculi becomes comparatively easy. To Dr. Prout, for his successful and original researches into the composition of calculi generally, as well as of the ultimate constitution of their organic elements, a great debt of gratitude is due; whilst the account of the urinary concretions in the splendid collection at Norwich, by Dr. Yellowly*, will ever remain a model of patient and careful research.

* Since the above was written, Science has had to mourn the loss of this very excellent physician and philosopher. The same spirit of industry which characterized Dr. Yellowly in his early career, continued to inspire him in age. In a letter I received from him a few weeks before his death, he expressed his intention of completing the examination of calculi added to the Norwich Museum since the publication of his essay : these amounted to 95, of which he had just finished the analysis of 75.

In the year 1817, when Dr. Marcet published his Essay, the Museum of Guy's Hospital contained but 228* calculi. During the last twenty-five years, this number has been augmented to 363; all of which have been divided so as to exhibit their internal structure, with the exception of 21. The great majority of the calculi added since Dr. Marcet's publication have been analysed at different periods, as they were placed in the Museum, by Dr. Babington, Dr. Rees, and myself; and in every instance, the examination has not been limited to the composition of the external crust, but has been particularly directed to the chemical constituents of the ingredients composing each layer. Attention has in every instance been particularly directed to the composition of the nucleus, in contradistinction to that of the body of the concretion. This is of very great importance; for when once a few solid particles of any substance aggregate and form a mass in the bladder, they very readily induce a crystallization of oxalate of lime, uric acid, or triple phosphate; or a deposition of urate of ammonia, phosphate of lime, or other amorphous ingredient, according to the lesion of function and state of irritability or innervation present. Hence, if ever, by medical treatment, we shall be enabled to prevent the formation of a calculous concretion, or remove one already formed, it will, in all probability, be by means directed by the character of the matter which there is a tendency to deposit as a nucleus. On this account I have adopted a classification of the calculi in Guy's Hospital Museum, founded not upon the number of alternating layers, but upon the character and composition of the nucleus. In the following Table, it must be borne in mind, that all the distinct constituents present in each concretion have not been mentioned; those only being inserted which were present in such quantity as to constitute a considerable portion of either body, nucleus, or crust of the concretion. Those ingredients, which existed in mere traces, or in very minute quantities, have been omitted; as they are rather to be regarded as accidental contaminations, and not as essential elements of the calculus. No urinary concretion, indeed, ever exists perfectly pure and unmixed; for there are very few in which some traces of

* Including 142 removed from one patient.

uric acid, or phosphates, are not observable: and even if these be absent, the colouring matter of urine or blood prevents the calculus being regarded as perfectly pure.

CALCULI IN GUY'S HOSPITAL MUSEUM,

OF WHICH SECTIONS HAVE BEEN MADE,

ARRANGED ACCORDING TO THE CHEMICAL COMPOSITION OF THE NUCLEI.

GENUS I.—NUCLEUS, URIC ACID. 245.

Species 1. *Calculi nearly entirely composed of Uric Acid or Urates.*

A. Nearly all uric acid		31
Uric acid, nearly pure	18	
Stained with purpurine	2	
Contained urate of lime	2	
. . . . and ammonia	2	
. . . . urate of soda and lime	1	
. . . . oxalate of lime	3	
. . . . phosphate of lime	1	
. . . . triple phosphate	2	
	31	

B. Body consisting chiefly of urates		169
Contained traces of urate of soda	142	
. . . . and lime	22	
. . . . urate of lime	4	
. . . . uric acid in the body	1	
	169	

Species 2. *Bodies differing in composition from Nuclei.*

A. Bodies consisting of oxalate of lime		10
Oxalate of lime and uric acid alternating	2	
Uric acid in the body, with an outer layer of carbonate of lime	1	
Oxalate, chiefly confined to external layers	1	
Oxalate of lime in the bodies nearly pure	6	
	10	

B. Bodies consisting chiefly of earthy phosphates		22
Bodies composed of fusible calculus	14	
. . . . phosphate of lime	3	
. . . . triple phosphate	5	
	22	

C. Body consisting of carbonate of lime . . . . 1 . 1

D. Alternating calculi 12

Body:	Crust:	
Urate of ammonia . .	Fusible	1
Oxalate of lime . . .	Uric acid	3
. . . .	Fusible	3
. . . .	Triple	1
. . . .	Phosphate of lime . .	3
Fusible	Uric acid	1
		12

GENUS II.—NUCLEUS, URATES OF AMMONIA OR LIME. 17

Species 1. *Calculi nearly all composed of Urate of Ammonia* . . . 7

Urate of ammonia, nearly pure	5
Uric acid, in tubercular patches on crust . . .	1
Traces of urate of soda and phosphate of lime . .	1
	7

Species 2. *Bodies differing from Nuclei* 9

Body:	Crust:	
Uric acid and fusible .	As body	1
Urate of ammonia . .	Uric acid	1
. . . .	Oxalate of lime . . .	1
. . . .	Posphate of lime . . .	1
. . . . and oxalate of lime . .	Uric acid, with oxalate and phosphate of lime	1
Urate of ammonia and fusible	As body	1
Urate and phosphate of lime	Ditto	1
Oxalate of lime . . .	Fusible	1
Fusible	As body	1
		9

Species 3. *Nucleus, Urate of Lime.*

A. Body fusible . . . . 1 . 1

GENUS III.—NUCLEUS, URIC OXIDE.—*None.*

GENUS IV.—NUCLEUS, OXALATE OF LIME. 45.

Species 1. *Calculus, nearly all Oxalate* 18

Uric acid in nucleus	1
Crust, covered with opaque octohedral crystals .	1
. . . . transparent	2
. . . not covered with crystals	14
	18

Species 2. *Bodies differing from Nuclei.*

A. Bodies consisting of uric acid or urates 8

    Uric acid, nearly pure 7

    . . . . covered with urate of ammonia . . . 1

                             8

B. Bodies consisting of phosphates 13

    Phosphate of lime 6

    Triple phosphate 4

    Fusible mixture 3

                            13

C. Body compound 6

     Body :   Crust :

    Uric acid . . . . Fusible 2

    . . . . Oxalate of lime . . . 1

    Urate of ammonia . . Phosphate of lime . . 1

    1. Uric acid . . . . ⎫

    2. Oxalate of lime . . ⎬ Oxalate of lime . . . 1

    3. Uric acid . . . . ⎭

    Cystic oxide 1

                            6

Genus V.—Nucleus, Cystic Oxide.

Species 1. *All Cystic Oxide* 11

    Colour, greenish blue 1

    . . . dirty greenish grey 9

    . . . fawn brown 1

                          11

Genus VI.—Nucleus, Earthy Phosphates. 21.

Species 1. *All Phosphates of Lime* . . . . 2 . 2

Species 2. *All Triple Phosphates* . . . . 1 . 1

Species 3. *All Fusible Mixed Phosphates* . . . . . 18 . 18

Genus VII.—Ingredients of Calculus mixed, with no evidence of arrangement in concentric layers . . 3

A. Uric acid and triple 1

B. . . . . . phosphate of lime 1

C. . . . urates of soda and ammonia, with oxalate

    and phosphate of lime 1

                            3

ABSTRACT VIEW OF NUCLEI.

Nuclei, consisting of uric acid or urates 262
. . . .   cystic oxide 11
. . . .   oxalate of lime 45
. . . .   phosphates 21

                                                   339
Mixed calculi 3

                                                   342

    I have not included in the above Tables the fibrinous calculus of Dr. Marcet, in consequence of its differing so totally from other concretions; as it must be regarded as a portion of dried inspissated albuminous matter exuded from an irritated kidney, rather than as a calculus produced under circumstances at all analogous to those of other concretions. Several specimens exist in the Museum, of the pelves of kidneys and ureters being obstructed by clots of fibrin; but none of these present the hard, concrete condition of the calculus described by Dr. Marcet. I am not aware of this variety having been mentioned by any other author except Brugnatelli, who, in his Litologia Umana, describes some calculi as consisting of *crystallized* albumen (di materia albuminosa cristallizata di colore d'ambra): they were passed by one individual, and each was about the size of a nut. These pseudo-calculi appeared to consist of dried coagulated albumen, which not unfrequently presents considerable lustre and a vitreous fracture, although scarcely sufficient to justify its being regarded as crystallized.

    Among the other ingredients existing in calculi, in very minute quantities, and not enumerated in the Table, are, hydrochlorate of ammonia, oxide of iron, and carbonate of lime. The former has been described by Dr. Yellowly as a frequent ingredient, generally, however, existing in mere traces in calculi; the second has been described by Professor Wurtzer, Mr. Brande, and Dr. Brett, and is often present in uric-acid calculi; and the third is frequently present in phosphatic and oxalic concretions. None of these ingredients are so generally present, as to merit their being regarded as presenting much interest, in a pathological sense.

Calculi present the greatest possible variety in appearance; generally, however, having more or less of an ovoid figure. Of those in Guy's Museum, the urate of ammonia and uric-acid concretions are the most regular, nearly all being ovoid or circular[1], a few only reniform[2]; this species never presenting any very prominent processes or projections, unless fresh centres of deposition occur on their surfaces, as when crystals of uric acid are deposited on an ovoid urate of ammonia concretion[3]. The cystic-oxide concretions vary considerably in outline; when large, being generally oval and smooth, as in Fig. 6. Plate II.[4]; and when smaller, often presenting projections from their surfaces, as if they were made up of crystals radiating from a common centre[5]; sometimes being moulded to the figure of the organ which secreted it, as shewn in the curious ear-drop-like concretion, Fig. 7. Plate II.[6] The oxalate of lime is generally most irregular, as far as the surface is concerned; although its outline is generally tolerably defined, either bearing a close approximation to an elliptic, or even a rectangular figure: Plate I. Fig. 1. The most contorted and irregularly-figured calculus is the triple or fusible, it being often a complete cast of the pelvis and calyces of the kidney[7]; occasionally, however, it is almost regularly oval, and sometimes circular[8]; this variation, in all probability, depending upon the position occupied by the calculus, and upon whether it had been retained in the kidney, or passed down the ureter before it had become of any considerable size. The mixed calculi, or those not presenting any regular concentric arrangement or a distinct nucleus, are often moulded to the kidney[9]. The phosphate of lime calculus is generally smooth externally, and conchoïdal in fracture, sometimes appearing as if made up of several cohering portions[10]. The triple phosphate[11] and fusible mixture[12] are not unfrequently found deposited on one side of a previously-formed calculus, as if one surface only had been exposed to the urine containing the earthy

[1] No. 2118.   [2] No. 2119.   [3] No. 2125.   [4] No. 2143.
[5] No. 2145.   [6] No. 2145.   [7] No. 2163.   [8] No. 2161.
[9] No. 2136.   [10] No. 2148.   [11] No. 2198.   [12] No. 2154

salt in solution, which is then generally found under the form of elegant white vegetations [13].

The nucleus is usually found in the geometric centre of the calculus, or nearly so; sometimes, however, being remarkably excentric, as in some reniform concretions [14]; and in a few, several distinct nuclei or centres of deposition are met with [15]. In some rare instances, the concretion which forms the nucleus is found loose within the body of the entire calculus [16]; a circumstance in all probability arising from a layer of blood or mucus having concreted around the nucleus, and on which the matter forming the body of calculus became deposited. In this case, on the whole becoming dry, the mucus or blood would be diminished to a very thin layer, and the calculus would appear to contain loose matter in it. In a few instances, calculi appear to possess no nucleus, the centre being occupied by a cavity full of stalactitic or mammillated projections, giving the idea of the external layer having been first formed, and the mammillated portions subsequently formed in the interior. This state occurs only, so far as I have seen, in uric-acid calculi, one of which is figured in Plate I. Fig. 2.[17] In one specimen in the collection, the central cavity is lined with fine crystals of triple phosphate, resembling the crystals of quartz so often found lining cavities in flints.[18] Brugnatelli describes one of a similar kind [19].

Sometimes calculi present very remarkable appearances, as if they had been divided into segments: this, in some cases, can be explained by the attrition of calculi [20] against each other, where several exist at once. In some, they actually appear as if they had been divided by a fine-cutting instrument; and in one, in the Museum, the apparently divided portions seem as if they had again become cemented and framed in by a subsequent deposit: Fig. 4. Plate I.[21] I confess

---

[13] Two of them are figured in Vol. II. of these Reports, in the 5th and 6th Figures of the Plate accompanying Dr. Hodgkin's Paper.

[14] No. 2119.   [15] No. 2158.   [16] No. 2133.   [17] No. 2113.   [18] No. 2154.

[19] "Litologia Umana ossia recherche chemische et mediche sulle sostanze petrose che si formano in diverso parti del corpo umano." *Pavia*, 1819. p. 43.

[20] No. 2218.   [21] No. 2136.

myself quite at a loss to explain many of these very remarkable appearances.

In the following account of urinary concretions, I have
merely described those which I have met with in the Museum
of Guy's Hospital; and as regards the deposits, I have preferred describing those which I have myself met with,
without reference to the accounts given by other writers.
The only exception to this rule is the case of uric oxide, to
the re-discovery of which I am anxious to direct the attention of my professional brethren.

In the account of the deposits and the figures I have given
of them, many circumstances hitherto unknown, or at least
unpublished, are mentioned; and of which, without the aid
of the microscope, I should have still remained in ignorance.
The value of this instrument in investigations of this kind
can hardly be overrated; and if it only aids in the detection
of a previously-overlooked deposit of oxalate of lime, it can
scarcely be said to have been used in vain. A low power
is sufficient for the examination of urine: a good half-inch
achromatic object-glass, with a low eye-piece, is sufficient for
the examination of every case of crystalline sediments*.

URIC ACID.

This very important product of vital chemistry exists
naturally in the urine in solution; and appears as a deposit
only, when the normal proportion of fluid is decreased, the
quantity of the uric acid increased, or when a sufficient
excess of some other acid is present, which by its affinity for
the substance with which the uric acid is combined, determines its precipitation. The particular manner in which
uric acid really exists in the urine has been a subject of
considerable dispute, as the quantity of water present in
the secretion is insufficient to hold dissolved the proportion
naturally present. Some have supposed that it is retained
in solution in so small a proportion of water in consequence

---

* These deposits, after being washed and allowed to dry on a slip of glass,
can be beautifully preserved by means of Canada-balsam. In this way, I have
every variety of deposit which has occurred to me, rendered permanent; and
from these, the microscopic drawings in Plate III. have been made, either by the
aid of the camera lucida of Amici, or, what I find far preferable, the mirror of
Sömmering screwed upon the eye-piece.

of combining with it in a nascent state. Berzelius* seems inclined to regard the saline ingredients of the urine as the solvent, just in the same manner as a weak solution of common salt, or hydrochlorate of ammonia, is capable of dissolving more iodine than a similar bulk of mere water could. Duvernoy† has suggested, that the colouring matter of the urine aided the solubility of the acid ; and this view appears to be adopted by MM. Vigla and Quevenne‡ ; although these observers appear inclined to regard the acid as existing in a free state, whilst Duvernoy assumes it to be positively combined with the colouring matter. On the other hand, Dr. Prout‖ regards ammonia as the true solvent of uric acid, and that it exists in the urine in the state of saline combination. For my own part, I confess, that although it is not impossible that a certain proportion of uric acid may really be held dissolved by the agency of the saline, or colouring constituents of the secretion, still the great majority of chemical evidence is decidedly in favour of Dr. Prout's view ; which, moreover, very happily explains the nature of many of the deposits met with in urine, under the influence of a suppressed or impeded condition of the cutaneous functions.

Characters of Urine containing Excess of Uric Acid.—It very rarely happens that uric acid exists in diffusion in the urine at the moment of emission; it generally appears in proportion as the fluid cools. Urine containing an excess of uric acid, whether free or combined with ammonia, is almost always of a deeper amber colour than natural, sometimes even approaching a reddish-brown tint: it is always acid ; its action on litmus-paper being nearly in the ratio of the amount of deposit which appears by cooling. The behaviour of urine containing an excess of uric acid free and combined is shewn in the Table. When urine is of a specific character of about 1.020, it generally contains such a quantity of uric

* Traité de Chimie, Tome VII. p. 354. *Paris*, 1833.   In his Lehrbuch der Chimie, published the same year at Stuttgard, no opinion is offered, "*auf welche Weise diese Auflosung bewirkt wird, ist unbekannt.*"   Band. III. § 128.

† Chemisch-medicinisch Untersuchen des Menschlichen Harns, p. 16.

‡ L'Expérience, Tome I. p. 194.

‖ Stomach and Urinary Diseases. Pl. lxxiv.   1840.

acid in combination with ammonia, as to let fall a copious deposit of this salt in the state of an amorphous powder, on reducing the temperature of the fluid: this phenomenon may in winter be readily observed, by merely setting the urine aside for a short time in a cool room; and in summer, by immersing the vessel containing it in a freezing mixture. This fact, indeed, affords very considerable support to Dr. Prout's opinion of the state of combination in which uric acid exists in urine; for, excepting under diseased action, I never saw uric acid deposited in this manner in a free state, but invariably in an amorphous form, combined with ammonia. On warming urine thus treated, the deposit disappears; whereas, had it consisted of uric acid, it would have been unaffected; as when once this acid is separated by the action of any precipitant from urine, it does not disappear on heating the fluid.

An excess of urea is not very unfrequently met with in urine containing an unusually large proportion of uric acid; and hence crystals of nitrate of urea are frequently observed in the course of an hour or two after the addition of concentrated nitric acid to some of the urine in a watch-glass. This circumstance is, however, by no means constant; and I have never observed any definite ratio existing between the urea and uric acid, when an excess of the latter is present.

Recognition of Uric Acid free and combined.—The presence of urate of ammonia in urine is very readily demonstrable, either by exposing it to a low temperature, or by evaporating the fluid in an air-pump vacuum. In either case, the sides of the containing vessel become covered with a deposit of urate of ammonia, which under the microscope appears amorphous. I have never met with this salt in the form of needles, as described by M. Vigla, although during the past winter I have examined with the microscope some hundreds of urinary deposits; and hence, although I do not feel warranted in stating with M. Donné that it never exists in the acicular form, I am confident that the pulverulent amorphous state is the condition in which it exists in the vast majority of cases, at least in this country.

The deposit of urate of ammonia which every day falls

under the observation of the physician varies extremely in
its colour, from snow-white to fawn-colour or reddish-brown;
not unfrequently, especially where portal derangement exists,
assuming a series of beautiful tints, varying from the most
delicate pink to the brightest carmine, or very nearly to the
deepest crimson. These two states constitute two well-
marked series more or less connected with very different
pathological conditions. In the white, fawn, or brick-red
deposit, a deficient state of the cutaneous functions is constant, at least so far as I have seen: in many cases, however,
the erythismal condition of the gastro-intestinal mucous
membrane constitutes the most prominent coincident disturbance; whilst, when the deposits presenting the various
streaks of pink or crimson occur, there is always more or
less evidence of functional or organic derangement of the
liver, spleen, or other organs influenced by the portal circulation. The most splendid purple deposits of this kind
I ever saw occurred in a case of ascites, depending on an
enormously enlarged spleen, produced by antecedent, neglected ague. When a deposit of urate of ammonia is examined under the microscope, it is found to be made up of a
series of amorphous granules, presenting no approach to a
crystalline arrangement; unless, as very frequently occurs,
free uric acid be present. On gently warming the drop of
urine submitted to examination, the deposit vanishes, and
then any crystals of uric acid that may be present become
perfectly distinct: the addition of a minute quantity of any
dilute acid to the still warm urine determines the production
of beautiful, well-defined crystals of uric acid, under one or
other of the forms described below.

Two, at least, very distinct forms of fawn-coloured deposits
of urate of ammonia are met with; one, in which the precipitate mixes readily with the supernatant fluid by slight
agitation and appears to form a very homogeneous mixture,
and subsides exceedingly slowly by repose. On attempting
to filter urine of this kind, it passes through the paper in a
turbid condition; or, if the paper be too fine to allow this to
occur, it permeates it with extreme slowness. This variety
is generally free from any admixture of free uric acid, at
least in a crystalline state. The other form is not quite so

frequently met with: in this, the urine is often very pale, and the deposit sometimes quite white, occasionally forming dense clouds in the fluid, like puriform mucus; readily, however, distinguished from it, by its solubility, on the addition of hot water, or the application of heat to the turbid urine itself. The deposit, instead of forming a nearly uniform mixture by agitation, is diffused through the fluid in detached bran-like particles, which readily subside, and are easily separable by the filter. In this variety, crystals of free uric acid are very frequent; and if not distinguishable at first sight with the microscope, become perfectly distinct, in causing the amorphous urate to disappear by warming the drop of fluid, or, what is sometimes preferable, by the addition of a drop of a solution of ammonia.

It frequently occurs, that deposits of urate of ammonia are not uniform, but are made up of two or more distinct layers, presenting each a distinct tint: thus we frequently meet with a pinkish layer reposing on a whitish one, or a pale fawn on a brick-red deposit. When urine, in which a deposit of urate of ammonia has already formed, is set aside, a semi-opaque layer, resembling mucilage or jelly in its character, is very frequently found: this consists of urate of ammonia, probably combined with water, as an hydrate. This gelatinous layer in a short time appears to concrete, and present the usual pulverulent character of deposits consisting of urate of ammonia.

Urine containing deposits of urate of ammonia occasionally presents a very remarkable phenomenon, by heating it to the boiling point, and keeping it at that temperature for a few minutes. The urate of ammonia, of course, soon disappears, and is replaced, as the ebullition continues, by a deposit which resembles albumen, in being totally insoluble in nitric acid: it differs from albumen however, in the urine containing it not being precipitable by nitric acid, and in the high temperature required for its precipitation. The nature of this substance is, like that of many others of the organic elements of the secretions generally, but ill understood: if, however, we may, in the present state of our knowledge, venture to give it a name, I feel inclined to refer it to the same category as the incipient albumen of Dr. Prout.

Uric acid is found in a free state, or at least only containing colouring matter, much less frequently than in the form of urate of ammonia : wherever it exists, the urine is always acid, often considerably more so than is met with in any other conditions of the urine. The quantity of uric acid which separates from healthy urine by repose is exceedingly small, and forms minute microscopic grains, which attach themselves to the sides of the containing vessel; this change being probably produced by the slow action of the minute quantity of free lactic or phosphoric acid present, on the urate of ammonia in solution. An addition of any acid to healthy urine considerably increases the quantity of uric acid separated, as well as the rapidity of its deposition. The minute crystals of uric acid thus obtained, contain considerable traces of colouring matter; and vary in hue, from pale yellow to brown or red, and in some few cases to positive black; appearing, when dry, like so many polished grains of gunpowder, powerfully reflecting light. When, from any cause, an excess of urate of ammonia is present in the urine, it is deposited, as above stated, in an amorphous state; unless, as frequently occurs under the influence of local irritation in the kidney, calculous diathesis, suppressed perspiration, &c., a considerable excess of some free acid is also secreted; in which case this acid unites with the ammonia, and consequently the uric acid is deposited in a crystalline form, having a varying proportion of colouring matter mixed up with it. Some obscurity hangs over the nature of the precipitating acid, and it is by no means certain that in every case it is identical. The lactic, phosphoric, and hydrochloric acids have each been suspected, and even proved to have existed. I have seen one case, at least, in which I feel tolerably satisfied that the precipitating acid was the sulphuric.

When uric acid is artificially separated by the addition of another acid, the crystals vary in colour with the amount of chemical action exerted on the colouring matter of the urine by the acid employed: hence the lightest-coloured crystals are obtained when acetic and phosphoric acids are used; whilst nitric and hydrochloric acids generally cause the deposition of deeply-tinted crystals, which present, under the microscope, evidence of a somewhat complex structure.

It frequently happens that crystals of uric acid are present in urine, so thin and diaphanous as to escape observation, until, by a careful adjustment of light, they become visible under a moderate magnifying power. It is rare to meet with nearly perfectly colourless crystals of this substance : we may, however, generally succeed in detecting them, mixed with urate of ammonia, in the very pale bran-like deposits above described. Uric acid is found most generally of a yellow, orange-red, or brick-dust colour; never, however, presenting the beautiful carmine tints occasionally possessed by urate of ammonia. It is sometimes met with, isolated and unmixed with any amorphous deposits ; but more generally is found in company with the urate of ammonia : and, by repose, two distinct layers are formed; the lowest consisting of uric acid, often in crystals sufficiently large to be distinguishable by the unassisted eye* ; and above this is a dense stratum of amorphous urate.

Some difficulty exists in the recognition of urate of ammonia in calculi, from the frequent presence of traces of the ammoniacal phosphate of magnesia; which, in consequence of its evolving ammonia when the calculus containing it is digested in a solution of potass, has led to erroneous conclusions. This difficulty, and I believe all others, may be readily avoided, by boiling a portion of the powdered calculus in pure water, filtering whilst hot, and adding to the filtered liquid a drop or two of pure hydrochloric acid. In this manner the urate of ammonia is dissolved and decomposed by the acid; and on cooling, a deposit of uric acid, in tables, occurs, readily recognisable under the microscope : it then only remains to determine the base with which it was combined : for this purpose, evaporate a few drops of the fluid, decanted from the crystals, on a slip of glass ; and the minute cubes of chloride of sodium, which the microscope enables us to detect, will at once inform us that soda existed, combined

---

* I was much surprised at the statement of M. Vigla, that uric acid, when visible in a deposit by the unaided eye, is always amorphous (L'Expérience, Vol. I. p. 195). Most certainly, in this country, the results of observation are totally opposed to the statement of this very talented and ingenious observer.

with the uric acid; whilst the appearance of tufts and fea-
thers of hydrochlorate of ammonia will shew, with equal
certainty, that ammonia was the base which rendered the
uric acid soluble in boiling water.

The following are the varieties, presented by the crystals
of uric acid, I have met with in the examination of urinary
deposit. The most interesting are figured in Plate III.

A. Rhomboïds, of a tolerably distinct lozenge-shape; being,
in fact, the natural crystalline form of the acid; and are
found either constituting the great mass of a deposit, or
much more generally mixed with amorphous urate of ammonia. It very rarely happens that all the angles possess their
proper sharpness; the acute angles are generally well preserved, whilst the opposite obtuse corners of the lozenge are
rounded off, so that the whole crystal represents a long elliptical figure with sharp extremities, as shewn in Fig. 1, *a.*
Very perfect and nearly colourless crystals of this kind are
frequently met with in the bran-like variety of urate-of-
ammonia deposit. If we attentively examine one of these
crystals, especially if it happen to be deep-coloured, as is
generally the case, a very curious angular marking is observed in its centre, resembling a nucleus. This is constantly
visible; and may be observed, even in very transparent
colourless crystals, by moving the mirror, so as to obtain an
oblique pencil of light. This structure is shewn in the two
highly-magnified crystals, in Fig. 1, *b.*

B. The elliptic lozenge crystal is occasionally found curi-
ously modified, the acute angles being preserved, the obtuse
ones rounded, and a portion of the crystal removed near each
acute angle; so that the whole resembles a kind of spindle,
sometimes approaching a fleur-de-lys figure. Some of these
are represented in Fig. 2.

These very curious crystals are often of a beautiful amber
colour; and are generally found in very acid urine, mixed
with the lozenges above described. They sometimes constitute the great mass of a deposit; but I never met with
one entirely made up of them.

C. Not unfrequently, the outline of the crystal of uric acid
loses its acute angles: most generally they then represent
flat, rectangular tables, about twice as long as broad: more

rarely they resemble cubes, the surface of the crystal being completely square, as in Fig. 3; and then they generally constitute the whole of the deposit, whilst the tables are almost invariably found mixed with urate of ammonia.

In the cubes, evidence of the existence of some internal structure is distinctly visible by aid of the microscope; lines, arranged in parallelograms, as in Fig. 3, *b*, being readily distinguished, by means of an achromatic object-glass of half-inch focus. If these crystals be allowed to dry, and then be examined after immersion in a fluid, the edges of the crystal frequently become translucent, so that it resembles an opaque cube furnished with a transparent frame. This variety is figured in Fig. 3, *c*. Sometimes the tabular crystals are rounded, elongated, and excavated at their sides and extremities. This modification is of rare occurrence, and I never saw a deposit entirely composed of it.

D. In very acid urine, the long tabular crystals are sometimes seen serrated at their extremities, or so deeply shaded as to give the idea of their being edged with a series of dark compact lines. This state is never visible at the sides of the crystals, whilst it is constant at the extremities. This is very beautifully seen in the crystals obtained by warming urine containing a deposit of urate of ammonia, so as to dissolve it, and adding a small quantity of hydrochloric acid, or by acidulating healthy urine with this acid, especially after warming it. The uric acid is deposited in crystals on the sides of the glass; and after the urine is decanted, water should be poured in; and by slight agitation, the crystals become detached, and will quickly subside, so that they can readily be obtained for examination. They are rarely found rhomboïdal, still less frequently perfect tables, and never, so far as I have seen, cubical. In general, they present, in an exaggerated degree, the peculiar form above described : they are quadrilateral flat crystals, twice as long as broad, the sides being well and sharply defined ; the extremities being serrated, and marked with dark close lines, not all of equal length: a finer, and less distinct series of lines traverse the whole crystal, in the direction of its length : these are shewn in Fig. 4, *a*. Occasionally, these crystals are found broader than long : then the sides are often concave, and

strongly lined by minute serratures; these, indeed, sometimes extend quite across the table, from one side to the
other: this variety is figured in Fig. 4, *b.* The body of the
crystal is always strongly tinted, from its containing a
quantity of the colouring matter of the urine modified by the
acid used as the precipitant; being, in fact, sometimes black
and lustrous, so as to resemble, when dry, grains of gunpowder.
The microscope, however, renders these crystals of interest,
on account of the peculiar structure it developes; for in the
tabular portion of each, two transparent crescents are visible:
these are placed with their convexities towards each other,
the sharp ends of each pointing towards either angle of the
crystal. The convexities of these curious crescents sometimes actually touch: frequently, however, they are more
distant from each other. This structure is beautifully distinct, under proper illumination, in the nearly-black crystals
before referred to; as the crescents appear white and transparent, on a semi-opaque blackish-brown ground. Some of
these crystals are shewn in Fig. 5. more highly magnified
than the others.

E. Occasionally, the tabular, or more rarely the rhomboïdal crystals are found placed transversely in the form of a
cross, or united in rosettes or stars of various degrees of regularity: some of these, presenting a rich golden hue, form most
interesting objects under the microscope. These are more
frequent in the bright orange-red sand; and frequently are
found in abundance in the pink deposits of urate of ammonia.
This variety is figured in Fig. 6. Sometimes, as shewn in
Fig. 7. the long thin tables of uric acid cohere in fasciculi;
which, diverging from each other, cause the whole to present
the appearance of St. Andrew's cross.

F. I have sometimes met with a remarkably elegant
form of uric acid, mixed often in considerable quantity with
amorphous urate deposits. These crystals resemble quadrilateral tables, with sharp, well-defined angles, generally of
a straw colour, and presenting no evidence of complex internal structure. On carefully, however, adjusting the focus,
and using a proper play of light, these crystals resolve themselves into a series of short cylinders, lying on their sides, as
shewn in Fig. 8. The only writer who has described these,

so far as I am aware, is M. Vigla, who has figured them
in the Plate given with his Paper in the First Volume of
L'Expérience.

G. Irregular crystalline flake-like masses of uric acid,
always deeply tinted of an orange-red hue, are occasionally
met with in deposits of urate of ammonia; and often when
the latter is nearly white, so as to be readily visible by the
contrast in colour. These are often of considerable size,
being frequently a quarter of an inch broad. They very
closely resemble filings of the acid deposited on a vessel, and
scraped off: I am confident that such, however, is not their
origin, at least necessarily. Examined by the microscope,
these masses possess more or less of a distinct crystalline
lined structure, but still are, undoubtedly, the most amorphous form under which uric acid occurs.

H. Minute transparent modified crystals, consisting of
uric acid, are frequently met with in urine, either in the
meshes of the mucous net, deposited during cooling, or
mixed with deposits. These almost always possess more or
less of a lined structure, and often resemble obtuse lozenges
cut in half; or are like a series of these superposed upon
each other, as in Fig. 9. Other forms are frequently seen
still more irregular in their outline, resembling irregular
little crystalline masses, sometimes with well-defined edges,
like fragments of cubes or tables; and occasionally, they
resemble truncated cylinders lying on their sides.

The obstinacy with which uric acid attracts the colouring
matter of the urine is exceedingly remarkable; and that the
latter material modifies its crystalline form, is undoubted;
especially as the only form capable of being obtained artificially by precipitation from the alkaline urates is the table
and rhomboïd. Indeed, it has been remarked by Duvernoy,
in the work before quoted, that if an acid be added to urine,
the uric acid is precipitated, distinctly crystalline only, when
a less proportional quantity of colouring matter than natural
exists in the urine; whereas, if it be in excess, the precipitate
is always pulverulent.

In addition to the above microscopic characters, a deposit
may be recognised as consisting of uric acid, when it does
not disappear by heat, dissolves in hot solution of potass

without the evolution of more than mere traces of ammonia, and is precipitated in nearly white minute crystals when the solution is poured into any dilute acid. If any doubt remains regarding the actual presence of uric acid, the deposit should be dissolved, by aid of a gentle heat, in nitric acid, diluted with three or four times its bulk of water. On evaporating the mixture to dryness in a watch-glass, a pink residue is left, which becomes of a magnificent purple when held over a bottle containing ammonia, or when a few drops of its solution are added.

In the above remarks, I have altogether avoided referring to the presence of the alkaline and earthy urates in deposits, as I never met with them composing more than mere traces in amorphous sediments. They all dissolve on heating the urine, and preserve no trace of crystalline structure ; so that without a special examination, with the view of obtaining the nature of their bases, they would necessarily be confounded with urate of ammonia. It is stated, that urate of soda constitutes a white deposit in the urine of gouty people : I certainly have never yet met with it.

Presence of Uric Acid and Urates in Calculi.—No elementary constituent of healthy urine is met with so generally diffused in calculous concretions as uric acid and its compounds : indeed, very few calculi exist in which traces of this substance are not to be met with. The nucleus or central portions of a concretion around which the subsequent layers become deposited, consists, in the great majority of instances, of uric acid or its salts : thus, in the collection at Guy's Hospital, consisting of 342 calculi, exclusive of 21 which have not been divided, no less than 255 possessed nuclei in which uric acid predominated. Of these, in 231 the central portions consisted of the acid nearly pure ; in 16, it consisted of urate of ammonia ; in one, of urate of lime ; and in seven, of uric acid mixed with urates and earthy salts in varying proportions.

Calculi consisting entirely of uric acid are always smooth externally, at most covered with smooth tubercles, never presenting those rugged and acuminated processes so generally characteristic of the oxalate of lime calculus. Even in cases in which the concretion has been formed and retained in the kidney, and when we find the calculus moulded to the pelvis and infundibula of the organ, the projecting processes of the calculus are always rounded and smooth. The only exception, if exception it be, to this law, is found in a calculus, No. 2125, in the collection at Guy's: this presents numerous acuminated irregular projections from its surface, possessing the nearest resemblance, in external appearance, to the oxalate of lime calculus I ever saw. The body of this concretion consists, however, of urate of ammonia of a clay colour: on the surface of this, irregular masses of uric acid have been deposited, and these constitute the rough projections alluded to. The external surface of this calculus presents the rich brown so frequently met with in the oxalate of lime concretion; for one of which species this interesting specimen must, without chemical analysis, have been mistaken.

The colour of the external surfaces of uric-acid calculi varies from a pale-fawn to a rich brown; never being white, except from the presence of a crust of amorphous urate of ammonia, as in the specimen numbered 2218[80]; or of phosphate of lime, of which numerous examples exist in the Museum. The appearances presented by sections of uric-acid calculi vary extremely: generally, even when the concretion consists entirely of uric acid, a very distinct development of concentric layers is met with: each of these individually, and the whole in mass, also generally present more or less of a radiated or striated appearance. Sometimes, however, the section appears massive, or as if the portions of which it was made up were deposited in a more amorphous form than in the former, in which a tendency to a crystalline arrangement is often strongly and distinctly marked. In colour, great variety is met with in sections of these calculi: as a general rule, however, the fawn or brown prevails throughout the whole collection. Some present a fine reddish-brown, as in that marked 2194[25]: others resemble the colour of polished oak, as in 2192. The sections of some calculi in which uric acid prevails are often exceedingly beautiful, especially when this deposit alternates with some other. This is elegantly shewn in the calculus No. 2171, accurately delineated in Plate I. Fig. 3; in which a rich nut-brown deposit of uric

acid is deposited on an irregular fawn-coloured one of oxalate
of lime: the interstices between the various projections and
processes of the latter are so uniformly and equally filled up
with the uric deposit, that the surface of the calculus is
smooth, and its figure oval, so that from its external appearance no one would suppose it to contain so large a nucleus
of oxalate of lime.   The sections of this calculus, which bears
a fine polish, closely resemble some varieties of fortification
agate.   The external layer of uric acid in this concretion is
remarkable for the appearance it presents of possessing a
series of secondary nuclei arranged on one side of the peri-
phery, accurately shewn in the figure.

In some rare cases, we meet with the uric acid arranged in
an anomalous manner, the section presenting no trace of
even an approach to a nucleus: on the contrary, a central
well-defined cavity, studded with stalactitic nodules of the
acid, occupies the centre.   A fine example of this is numbered 2113 in the collection, and is figured in Plate I. Fig. 2.

Urate of ammonia in all probability is much more frequent in calculi than the labels affixed to them in collections
would lead us to infer.   All my own observations tend to
support the correctness of the opinion long ago given by Dr.
Prout, of the frequent existence of this salt in calculi.   It is
true, that in the collection at Guy's only seven consist
almost entirely of this substance; yet it is present, as an important ingredient, in upwards of 180 other calculi.   The
colour of calculi consisting of urate of ammonia, or chiefly
composed of this substance, is very generally characteristic;
being of a pale greyish-fawn or clay colour, often nearly
approaching to that presented by sections of oxalate of lime
concretions: not unfrequently, they more nearly resemble
pipe-clay in tint: indeed, this peculiarity in colour will often
enable us to suspect its existence in calculi supposed to be made
up of uric acid only.   Of this there is an excellent illustration
in the very remarkable calculi numbered 2213.   These are
112 in number, all of the same figure, being cubes rounded at
the edges and angles: they were all removed from the
bladder of one patient, by the late Sir Astley Cooper.   These
calculi have the colour of pipe-clay, and their bodies are
chiefly composed of urate of ammonia: although described

by Dr. Marcet as consisting of uric acid, as that excellent chemist and physician was not aware of the existence of this substance in calculi, when he examined them. The decrepitating property possessed by calculi when heated, and regarded by Dr. Marcet as characteristic of the presence of oxalate of lime, is very generally presented by those in which urate of ammonia enters as a constituent.

Urate-of-ammonia calculi seldom, if ever, present the concentric arrangement so generally presented by uric-acid concretions; a circumstance admitting of ready explanation, in the generally amorphous condition in which the urate is deposited in sediments, never presenting the crystalline appearance so frequent in uric-acid deposits.

With regard to the other salts of uric acid, the urates of soda and lime alone exist in the calculi I have examined: in no instance in the collection do they constitute the entire mass of a calculus; and frequently only exist in layers mingled with the urate of ammonia or uric acid. In one instance, however, I found the nucleus of a calculus to be composed chiefly of urate of lime.

CYSTIC OXIDE, OR CYSTINE.

This substance does not exist as an ingredient in healthy urine, and occurs but rarely as an element in the diseased secretion. It was first discovered by Dr. Wollaston*, forming the chief ingredient in a calculus given to him by Dr. Reeve of Norwich; and he soon after found one other specimen among the calculi in the Museum at Guy's Hospital. Subsequently, calculi composed of cystic oxide were met with by Dr. Marcet, Dr. Prout, and several other physicians, in the human subject; and by M. Lassaigne, in a calculus removed from a dog, and belonging to the collection in the Veterinary College of Alfort, near Paris.† Cystic oxide differs from all the other known elementary ingredients of calculi, in containing a considerable proportion of sulphur, no less than two atoms being present in each equivalent of the oxide.

Characters of Urine containing Cystic Oxide.—It is to be regretted that the urine has not been carefully examined in

* Philosophical Transact. 1810.   † Annales de Chimie, Tom. XXIII. p. 328.

the cases of cystic-oxide concretions. Indeed, the only recorded accounts of its existence in the form of an urinary deposit, that I am acquainted with, are those given by Stromeyer on the continent; Drs. Prout, Venables, and myself, in this country. The urine examined by both Dr. Prout and myself came from the same patient; and since the publication of my examination of this in a former Volume of these Reports, I have met with but one other instance in which cystic oxide existed in urine; at least, in an unequivocal manner.

Urine containing cystic oxide varies in colour, from a pale amber to greenish yellow and even apple-green. The first was the colour possessed by the urine passed by the patient from whom the calculus No. 2115⁵⁰ (Museum Catalogue) was removed; whilst Drs. Prout and Willis have met with specimens of the second variety of colour: and one instance of the third, or apple-green, occurred to myself, in the urine passed by an old lady, a patient of my friend Mr. Blenkarne of Dowgate Hill. In specific gravity, the specimens of cystic-oxide urine I have examined, varied from 1.012 to 1.0118: they were always acid, with one exception in which it was neutral. A smaller quantity of uric acid and urea than natural existed in these specimens; and Stromeyer observed the same circumstance in the case in which he met with cystic oxide as a deposit.

Recognition of Cystic Oxide.—This substance, when present in the urine, is always in a white crystalline state, never being found amorphous; and its microscopic characters afford the readiest mode of recognising it. When urine which contains a deposit of this kind is mixed with hydrochloric acid, it is not rendered clear, as it would be if turbidity were produced by earthy salts: on the application of heat, however, the cystine slowly dissolves.

When a deposit suspected to contain cystine is examined, it should be washed with boiling water, to remove the urates and any crystals of common salt which might be present, and then placed, in a drop of water on a slip of glass, under the microscope. Crystals of cystic oxide will then be readily distinguished, by their presenting one or other of two forms under which it occurs. In the first of these, it appears under the form of tolerably regular six-sided tables, sometimes transparent throughout, but more generally opaque in the centre: in the second, it occurs as roundish tables, opaque in the centre, and often quite so, somewhat crenate at the edges. The former state, which is the shape of the normal crystal, is shewn in Fig. 14. Plate III.; and the latter, which has been hitherto undescribed, is shewn in Fig. 15. The behaviour of urine containing cystic oxide towards reagents is shewn in the Table.

When cystic oxide is suspected to exist in a calculus, the readiest mode of detecting it is to digest some of the powder in a warm solution of ammonia, and to allow a drop of the clear fluid to evaporate spontaneously on a slip of glass. The crystals of cystic oxide, if present, will then be readily recognised, by microscopic examination.

A source of fallacy in the detection of cystic oxide in urine may exist in the curious modifications presented by common salt during its crystallization. Every one is aware that chloride of sodium, when allowed to evaporate from its aqueous solution on a plate of glass, leaves perfectly defined cubes, which are beautifully distinct under the microscope; and it has been long known, that when crystallized from fluids containing urea, the normal cubical crystal becomes replaced by octahedrons. Mr. Busk, surgeon to the Dreadnought Hospital-ship, first noticed the fact, that when common salt was dissolved in urine, or in a fluid containing urea, and the solution rapidly evaporated, the octahedrons were, in their turn, replaced by a series of elegant crystals, in the form of croslets and daggers; and this gentleman has proposed this peculiar change in the crystals of common salt, as a test of the presence of urea. When, however, this salt is allowed to evaporate slowly from its solution in urine, a very different state of things occurs—crystals are left in the form of tables which are sometimes eight-sided, and frequently six or three-sided, occasionally even forming acute rhomboïds. In the form of six-sided plates, common salt closely resembles cystic oxide, and might be easily mistaken for it; but these crystals are never opaque in the centre, as those of cystine generally are: next, they do not exhibit colours with polarised light, as the last-mentioned substance does; and lastly, they are soluble in water. These three characters will remove any difficulty that may arise in distinguishing between the modified crystals of common salt and those of cystine. The crystals obtained by the rapid evaporation of a solution of salt in urine are figured in Plate III. Fig. 17; and those by slow evaporation, in Fig. 16.

Presence of Cystic Oxide in Calculi.—Cystic oxide has, as yet, been met with in but few calculi: in the splendid collection at Norwich, consisting of more than 600 specimens, no concretion composed of this substance exists; and Dr. Yellowly has informed me, that none has been added since the publication of his Paper in the Philosophical Transactions. Ten calculi, composed almost entirely of cystic oxide, existed in the Museum of Guy's Hospital when Dr. Marcet published his work; and since that period, although five and twenty years have elapsed, the only additions made consist of the specimen described by myself in a former Volume of these Reports, and of a compound calculus which I found in the collection without any history connected with it, in which two concentric zones of cystic oxide existed, deposited on a nucleus of oxalate of lime: Plate II. Fig. 5. With a single exception, all the calculi of cystic oxide hitherto found have been nearly pure, containing but a small quantity of earthy phosphates: (No. 2168.)

Calculi of cystic oxide have generally a wax-like lustre, and are covered either with smooth tubercles or sharp projections externally: the latter are only met with in small concretions, as in those numbered 2145 in the Museum at Guy's. When recent, their colour nearly approaches that of the uric acid calculus, being of a pale brown: they undergo, however, a remarkable change in colour by long keeping, turning slowly from brown to grey or green. Thus the calculus figured by Dr. Marcet*, being the identical specimen in which Dr. Wollaston discovered the second case of the occurrence of cystic oxide, and which was brown in 1817, now possesses a rich blueish-green colour, accurately shewn in Plate II. Fig. 6. This colour it has possessed for twelve years,

---

* Essay on Calculous Disorders: supra citat.   Plate III. Figs. 1 and 2.

to my knowledge; but for how much longer, I am unable to state. The smaller calculi passed by Mr. Birkett in 1814, and referred to by Dr. Marcet in his work, have also undergone a similar change; but not quite so completely, being now greyish-green, and two or three are merely grey. One calculus, which in figure resembles an ear-drop, presents only a dirty grey colour: (Fig. 7.)

This change in colour, which cystic-oxide calculi undergo, has not been, so far as I am aware, mentioned by authors on this subject; and its cause remains very obscure. The specimen I examined three years ago [*], (No. 2145^{70},) has, as yet, undergone no change. It has been suggested to me, by both Dr. Prout and Dr. Willis, that this alteration in tint may in some way depend upon changes produced by the sulphur which is present as an elementary ingredient in cystic oxide. This opinion is at least extremely probable; and derives some support from a circumstance I noticed in Mr. Blenkarne's patient: here the urine either was green when first passed, or rapidly became so by keeping; and in a few days it developed enough sulphuretted hydrogen to blacken the glass vessel containing it.

Internally, the calculi composed of cystic oxide present a very imperfectly radiated structure, and exhibit no tendency to a development of concentric layers. When scraped, they yield easily to the knife, and form a perfectly white powder, whether the calculus be brown or green.

The curious instance of cystic oxide occurring in a compound calculus on a nucleus of oxalate of lime, I have described in a former Number of these Reports. It has been accurately figured by Mr. Hurst, in Plate II. Fig. 5; in which the two concentric layers of greenish cystic oxide are exceedingly well shewn.

URIC (XANTHIC) OXIDE.

WHETHER this curious substance be an element of healthy urine or not, it is extremely difficult to determine: it has indeed been suspected that a certain relation exists between it and one form of the colouring matter of urine. Considering, indeed, the very simple relation borne by this substance

---

[*] Guy's Hospital Reports, Vol. I. p. 492.

to uric acid, we should not be surprised if uric oxide be found, upon careful investigation, to exist in healthy urine.

Characters of Urine containing Uric Oxide.—These are totally unknown; as neither Dr. Marcet nor Professor Stromeyer, the only philosophers who have met with this substance, appear to have examined the urine passed by the patient from whom the concretions were obtained.

Recognition of Uric Oxide.—The account given by Dr. Marcet of the properties possessed by this substance is but meagre; and I trust this will serve as an apology for here transcribing, in an English dress, the peculiarities of uric oxide as observed by MM. Liebig and Wöhler, in the calculus in which Stromeyer discovered it. The calculus in which Dr. Marcet first detected this substance weighed but eight grains, and nothing is known regarding the portion not consumed in the analysis: it does not exist in the collection at Guy's Hospital; and neither Dr. Prout, Dr. Yellowly, nor Dr. Babington, can give any information on this point. This is a matter of great regret, as until the re-discovery of the uric oxide by Stromeyer, all trace of this curious substance had been lost for many years.

This calculus was removed by Langenbeck from a peasant's child, eight years of age, at Hanover. In shape, it resembled a flattened pullet's egg: it broke it into three pieces during the operation. The whole calculus weighed nearly 339 English grains: its section was partly of a lustrous bright brown colour, and partly earthy and pale. It was composed of concentric separable layers, without any appearance of a crystalline or fibrous texture: it possessed a distinct nucleus, which did not, however, differ in chemical characters from the body of the calculus. It was as hard as uric acid calculi generally are; and, on slight friction, it assumed a wax-like lustre. Its chemical characters were examined by Stromeyer shortly after its removal by Langenbeck: but very lately, MM. Wöhler and Liebig submitted it to a fresh examination, and determined its composition by ultimate analysis. In warm nitric acid, fragments of this calculus dissolved without effervescence; the solution, by evaporation, left a lemon-yellow residue; which dissolved readily in water, forming a yellow fluid; and in a solution of potass, with a similar but darker hue. In no way could the red colour, characteristic of the action of nitric on uric acid, be obtained. In a solution of potass, it dissolved : the solution was of a dark yellowish brown, with a tinge of green, like dilute bile : it was clear, but passed through the filter with extreme slowness. On passing a current of carbonic-acid gas through this fluid, a white precipitate of pure uric oxide fell down : this, by drying, formed hard fragments of a pale yellow colour, and, by friction, assumed the appearance of wax*.

The only mode of detecting this substance in calculi will be, to avail ourselves of the characters distinguishing it from uric acid, to which, in many respects, it has the close similitude which their resemblance in chemical composition would lead us to anticipate. I have therefore placed side by side the most important characteristic properties possessed by uric acid and oxide.

URIC OXIDE.	URIC ACID.
1. Dissolves slowly, and without any effervescence, in nitric acid.	1. Dissolves readily, with copious effervescence, in nitric acid.
2. The nitric solution leaves, by careful evaporation, a yellow stain.	2. The nitric solution leaves, by evaporation, a pink residue.
3. It dissolves in concentrated sulphuric acid ; and the addition of water does not render the solution turbid.	3. It dissolves in concentrated sulphuric acid ; and the addition of water produces a copious precipitate of uric acid.
4. Its solution in potass is not precipitated by hydrochlorate of ammonia.	4. Its solution in potass is precipitated by hydrochlorate of ammonia.
5. It is precipitated pure and free from alkaline combination, when a current of carbonic acid is passed through its solution in potass.	5. It is precipitated from its solution in potass, by a current of carbonic acid in the form of urate of potass.
6. When decomposed by heat, it does not yield any trace of urea.	6. Decomposed by heat, it becomes partly converted into urea.

From an examination of these characters, we learn, that readily as we may succeed in detecting uric oxide if it should again be met with constituting the great mass of a calculus,

* Annalen der Physik, Band 41. seite 393.

yet that extreme difficulty must attend its discovery when it only exists in mere traces, or mixed with uric acid. I certainly have occasionally suspected its presence in some calculi which present a remarkably wax-like lustre, but have never been able thoroughly to satisfy myself on the subject. In one calculus in particular, No. 2121, in which a large nucleus of urate of ammonia is surrounded by a mixture of uric acid and urate of lime, there exists a number of detached little masses near the circumference of the section, which, on scraping or rubbing, assume, with the utmost facility, a wax-like lustre; whilst the mass in which they are imbedded retains its primitive dulness. These little masses differ from any thing I have seen in mere uric acid; and although they certainly contain this substance, I have always suspected the probable existence of uric oxide in them.

PINK-COLOURING MATTER (PURPURINE).

THIS matter has been but imperfectly investigated; and, like some other products of vital chemistry, it is easier to shew what it is not, than what it is. It has been long known that urinary deposits often present more or less of a pink hue, sometimes, although more rarely, verging on a deep purple; and various hypotheses have been advanced, to explain this circumstance. On the continent, it has been generally asserted that a peculiar colouring matter is secreted by the kidney, as a product of diseased action; and in this country, Dr. Prout has stated his conviction that the colour of these deposits depends on the presence of purpurate of ammonia, the muroxide of Liebig. This opinion I ventured, some years ago, in conjunction with Dr. Hargrave Brett*, after a minute examination of some of these pink deposits, to oppose; and it is with great regret that I again am obliged to express my total dissent from the opinions of the excellent physician and chemist to whom this branch of science owes so much. The grounds on which I founded my objections have been long before the public: it is therefore unnecessary to refer to them, further than to state, that the experiments detailed in the Paper alluded to have been repeated many times, and have stood the test of many years'

* Medical Gazette, Book 14. pp. 600—751.

experience. In fact, although, when urate of ammonia is dissolved in a weak solution of purpurate of ammonia (muroxide), it is deposited of a pinkish tint, yet the pink deposits met with in disease bear no analogy whatever to those artificially tinted with the purpurate, except in colour; differing, *toto cœlo*, in every chemical character. On this account I have ventured, for the purpose of avoiding confusion and of steering clear of controversy, to propose the term "*purpurine*" for the colouring matter of pink deposits.

Presence of Purpurine in the Urine.—Urine is occasionally met with containing a colouring matter of a pink tint, generally verging on russet-brown. Such urine is acid, and on the addition of ammonia it assumes a fine crimson hue: on filtering it, to free it from the precipitated phosphates, and evaporating the fluid to a thick syrup, the addition of alcohol causes the deposition of the saline ingredients, and yields a purplish-red solution, the colour of which is unaffected by dilute acids or a solution of potass.

A pink colour, often of a very beautiful tint, is produced in most urine by the addition of nitric acid; but the most splendid hues are obtained by adding hydrochloric acid to previously heated urine. Generally, a fine rose-red, or lilac-pink, is thus obtained; but in some cases, in which the colouring matter was probably deficient, only the faintest inclination towards pink could thus be obtained. Whether the colouring matter thus developed by the action of acids bears any relation to the colouring ingredient of deposits, is yet a matter *sub judice*.

Recognition of Purpurine.—The colour, in the present state of our knowledge, is often the only guide we possess for the detection of this matter in deposits or calculi. Digestion in warm alcohol dissolves it, and, by this means, any pink concretion may be decolourised. The alcoholic solution is often faintly acid, and does not lose its colour by the addition either of acids or alkalies.

Presence of Purpurine in Calculi.—We occasionally meet with at least probable evidence of the presence of this body in calculi, by the pink colour they present. In Guy's Museum, a very interesting calculus, numbered 2170[50], exists:

this has an oval nucleus of uric acid, on which is deposited a body of oxalate of lime, a crust of uric acid surrounding the whole : delicate lines of bright pink define the edges of the several uric layers : these are shewn in Plate II. Fig. 9. In the calculus 2212[58], a line of purple surrounds the uric-acid nucleus ; and in a large uric-acid calculus, No. 2184, the exterior half inch, all round, is stained of a pale purple. There is a note in the Museum Catalogue referring to a friable calculus, No. 2159, to the effect, that the lad from whom this was removed, had some time before passed a pink deliquescent concretion, supposed to be purpurate of ammonia.

Mr. Taylor[*] has mentioned the existence of several calculi having pink layers, in the Museum of St. Bartholomew's Hospital ; but no one has recorded so many cases of this as Brugnatelli[†]. This philosopher has figured, in his very elaborate work, several calculi, not only containing pink layers, but some in which the nucleus was composed of pink deposit, or rosacic acid, as he termed it. This is shewn in his 34th Figure. He alludes to another case, in which several (*buon numero*) little pink calculi were passed by an individual : and in a large calculus, shewn in his 35th Figure, remarkable for the presence of a large central cavity, the urate of ammonia forming its walls was stained externally of a bright purple.

CARBONATE OF LIME.

As might be anticipated from the acid state of healthy urine, carbonate of lime is not a normal constituent of this secretion ; and, whenever it is present, it must probably, in every case, be regarded as a secondary production, from the re-action of carbonate of ammonia on the phosphatic salts present in the urine.

Characters of Urine containing Carbonate of Lime.—Urine containing this salt must necessarily be alkaline, and in all probability would contain free carbonate of ammonia. I have never examined a specimen of urine containing a deposit of carbonate of lime ; yet that it must occasionally be met

---

[*] Medical Gazette, Vol. XXII. p. 189.
[†] Litologia Umana, sup. citat., p. 43.

with, is evident, from the not unfrequent presence of this salt, in certainly small quantities, in calculi consisting of the earthy phosphates and oxalate of lime. There can be no doubt, when carbonate of ammonia is the precipitating agent, that it is derived from a re-arrangement of the elements of urea, probably under the influence of an extremely depressed state of the nervous supply of the secreting organs, as in the latter stages of adynamic typhus fever; of which cases have been recorded by Dr. Graves and others.

To obtain the elements of two atoms of carbonate of ammonia, all that is necessary, is, to add the constituents of two equivalents of water to one of urea. This may be readily seen in the following formula, in which the elements are represented by their initial letters.

	C. N. H. O.		C. N. H. O.
1 atom urea	$= 2 + 2 + 4 + 2$	2 atoms carbonic acid	2 4
2 atoms water	$=$ 2 + 2	. . . . ammonia	2 + 6
	$2 + 2 + 6 + 4$		$2 + 2 + 6 + 4$

Recognition of Carbonate of Lime.—If we meet with a deposit from an alkaline urine, which, after being washed with a little water, dissolves with effervescence in a dilute acid, we can have no hesitation in declaring it to consist of carbonate of lime. To detect it in a calculus, reduce a fragment to powder, cover it with a few drops of water, and add a little hydrochloric acid: a brisk effervescence will occur, if the calculus contained carbonate of lime. The addition of water, before adding the acid, is necessary, to prevent error occurring from the extrication of adherent air-bubbles.

Presence of Carbonate of Lime in Calculi.—No calculus consisting of this salt alone, exists in the collection; hence it may be regarded as a very rare occurrence: in one specimen only does it constitute the body of a calculus, in that instance being deposited, of a snow-white colour, on a nucleus of uric acid. Carbonate of lime exists in very small quantities in several of the calculi consisting of the earthy phosphates, as was first pointed out by Dr. Yellowly; and I have met with it in several calculi consisting of oxalate of lime.

OXALATE OF LIME.

THIS salt never exists in healthy urine, although its several constituents are present under one form or other; so that the generation of this very important ingredient of urinary concretions admits of a tolerably satisfactory explanation. Lime is always present, combined with phosphoric and perhaps other acids, in urine; and so great is the insolubility of oxalate of lime, and so intense the mutual affinity of its constituents, that the addition of oxalic acid as a soluble oxalate instantly determines the precipitation of the salt under consideration. The particular manner in which the evolution of the oxalic acid found in urine occurs, can scarcely be regarded as at all satisfactorily explained: most, however, seem to regard it as a secondary product of the oxidation of saccharine matter occasionally present in the secretions, and thus appear inclined to draw a close analogy between the diathesis in which sugar and that in which oxalic acid are generated. I confess that this has always appeared to me to be rather a forced analogy; and one at least, so far as I have examined the matter, by no means borne out by the chemical characters of the urine. To this subject I shall return, when speaking of the general causes of calculous deposits. The beautiful experiment of Liebig and Wöhler on the conversion of uric acid into oxalic acid and urea* is sufficient to shew how readily the latter acid may be generated under an oxidizing influence; and the moment that, from any lesion of the healthy function of the kidney, it is produced, it will instantly combine with the lime, which naturally exists combined with phosphoric or other acids, and produce the highly insoluble oxalate.

Characters of Urine containing Oxalate of Lime.—Urine depositing this salt has usually been described as possessing somewhat of a greenish tint. Such, however, has not been the case with the specimens I have examined; and within the last few weeks, several specimens, containing splendid oxalate of lime, have come under my notice, so that I am able to speak with some confidence on this subject. The

---

* Prof. Graham's Elements of Chemistry, 1842. p. 1004; or Dr. Kane's Elements, 1841. p. 1166.

urine, in each case, was acid; in tint, varying from a pale straw-colour to even deep amber, sometimes nearly limpid, much more generally containing a copious deposit of urate of ammonia of a very pale colour, rarely being tinged with pink; and frequently mixed with uric acid and numerous fragments of epithelium : the specific gravity generally exceeded the average density of healthy urine, but sometimes was below it, varying from 1.016 to 1.029. An excess of urea was frequently present; so that when the urine was above the density of 1.020, it crystallized very quickly after the addition of an equal bulk of nitric acid. When the urine contains no urate of ammonia, the deposit of oxalate, on account of its transparency, is generally nearly imperceptible; but on decanting the supernatant fluid, after a few hours' repose, and placing a few drops of the lowermost layers in a capsule, a white crystalline sediment is very readily distinguishable; and this, when examined under the microscope, presents a very beautiful appearance. The crystals are invariably sharply defined, and always entire, in figure perfectly octahedral, differing however materially in the acuteness of the terminal angles : if these are very acute, the crystals are seen lying on their sides with their angles and edges exceedingly distinct, as shewn in Plate III. Fig. 10, *b*.* When the octahedron is more obtuse, the outline of the crystal appears perfectly square, having another square outline in its centre, so arranged that the angles of the inner square are opposite the sides of the outer one. When these crystals are allowed to dry, and then examined either in a drop of water or Canada-balsam, the inner square remains transparent; whilst the outer becomes opaque, often absolutely black. Thus each crystal looks like two cubes, a transparent one enclosed in a black one. These appearances are shewn in Fig. 10, *a*. In no instance have I seen oxalate of lime in an

---

* The shape of these crystals is well shewn in the manner pointed out to me by my talented friend, Mr. J. W. Griffith, the resident Medical Officer of the Finsbury Dispensary, to whom I am under considerable obligations for the assistance he has afforded me in these interesting but tedious investigations. This gentleman added a few drops of alcohol to an oxalic deposit moistened with water : a series of vortiginous currents, perfectly distinguishable by the microscope, became excited by mixture of the two fluids; and in these, the crystals roll over each other, and their true figures become beautifully distinct.

amorphous form : wherever its presence was unequivocally demonstrable, it was always beautifully crystallized. When oxalate of ammonia is added to urine, and the deposit of oxalate of lime produced, examined under the microscope, it is found to consist of numerous little globules, transparent in the centre, having a marked tendency to become arranged in rouleaus, somewhat after the manner of blood-disks. This artificial oxalate has been figured by Rayer*, who does not appear to have ever seen the crystalline form now described; nor, indeed, does that very accurate observer, Dr. Prout, describe it, further than by alluding to the very rare occurrence of oxalic gravel : so that I believe I am justified in regarding the account now given of the form of oxalate-of-lime deposits as having some claim to novelty. The only writer who, to my knowledge, has described crystals of oxalate of lime in urine is Dr. Donné†; and he states that that they are capable of being readily produced, whenever a person is made to eat preparations of sorrel (Rumex acetosa, or Oxalis acetosella), or to take any preparation containing a soluble oxalate.

Urine containing the oxalic deposit occasionally gives a very copious precipitate with salts of lime, so as, at least, to render it probable that a soluble oxalate really existed in solution; and I have repeatedly observed fine needle-like crystals left by the evaporation of a few drops of urine on the plates of glass on which it had been placed, to submit it to microscopic examination, which were readily soluble in water, and certainly bore a very close resemblance to oxalate of ammonia. I only regret that want of time has prevented my examining this point more minutely; but I cannot help expressing my conviction that a soluble oxalate, probably the oxalate of ammonia, frequently exists in urine containing the oxalate-of-lime deposit.

Recognition of Oxalate of Lime in Deposits and Calculi.— In the majority of cases, oxalate of lime does not occur unmixed in a deposit : in the first case in which I recognised its existence, several years ago, it was mingled with a large

---

* Traité des Meladies des Reins, Tom. I. Tab. 3. Fig. 6.

† Journal de Chimie Médicale, Tom. V. p. 406.

quantity of red particles*, so frequently thrown out during
the high degree of irritation produced by an oxalate-of-lime
concretion. Since then, I have, in very few instances, found
the crystals subsiding in the form of a scanty white deposit,
not having the lustrous glistening aspect of the triple phosphate : this, however, was but an occasional occurrence. The
general rule, deduced from my own experience, is for the
oxalate to exist mixed with very white urate of ammonia,
sufficient in quantity to entirely mask the crystals of the
former, so that the whole appears like an amorphous deposit
of the urate : and as, when the latter was made to disappear
by warming the urine, the transparency of the crystals of
oxalate of lime rendered them nearly invisible, a tolerably
copious deposit of this salt might be very readily overlooked.
To avoid this, I adopt the following process; which I would
recommend to be used with all pale-coloured deposits, in which
the presence of oxalate of lime is suspected. Allow the urine
to repose for an hour or longer in a tall phial; pour off the
upper three-fourths of the fluid ; and, shaking the rest for a
few seconds, pour a few drops of the turbid fluid into a watch-
glass, and gently warm it, by holding it over the flame of a
taper or spirit-lamp, gently moving the capsule so as to
cause the fluid to assume a slow rotatory motion : by this
manipulation, a sort of vortex is excited in the urine, which
brings every trace of matter insoluble in the warm fluid to
the centre of the concavity of the watch-glass. Gently draw
off the clear fluid with a pipette, which can readily be
done without losing any of the deposit, and add a few drops
of distilled water. Then place the capsule under the microscope; and the minutest quantity of oxalate of lime may be
recognised by the form of the crystals; always in this state
resembling very small cubes; sometimes, from their minuteness, appearing like little globules; in every case, however,
being resolved into figures of a quadrilateral outline, on the
application of a higher magnifying power. On allowing a
drop of hydrochloric acid to glide down the sides of the

---

* This is the very case published in the Medical Gazette, Vol. XVII. p. 894.
and quoted by Rayer (op. cit. p. 207), as a type of the oxalic deposits. From
this circumstance, as well as from the perusal of his valuable remarks on the
whole subject, I cannot help concluding that this excellent physician has rarely,
if ever, seen a deposit of oxalate of lime.

capsule, the deposit is seen to vanish. Acetic acid and ammonia do not affect it. By these characters, no error can occur in the recognition of oxalate of lime; and I venture to suggest the probability of its being much more generally met with in deposits of urate of ammonia than has been suspected.

No difficulty can occur in the detection of oxalate of lime in calculi: all that is necessary, is, to break off a fragment, and ignite it before the blowpipe-flame: it readily burns into a white ash, which effervesces with acids, forming a solution from which lime can be precipitated by the addition of oxalate of ammonia. During the ignition, the calcareous salt is converted into carbonate of lime, by the evolution and combustion of carbonic oxide; and if the heat be too intense, the carbonic acid is driven off, and pure lime left.

I have very lately met with a very curious crystalline deposit, mixed with fawn-coloured urate of ammonia and the flake-like form of uric acid. It occurred in a case of aggravated dyspepsia, with great emaciation and dull heavy lumbar pains, in a woman of 40 years of age. On heating the urine, the urate dissolved, and left the uric-acid flakes, which had become paler by boiling, mixed with a white crystalline powder: this did not dissolve in acetic acid or ammonia, whilst in nitric and hydrochloric acid it readily disappeared. On being examined under the microscope, the powder was found to consist of crystals bearing some resemblance in figure to a dumb-bell; as shewn in the three drawn below, Plate III. Fig. 12. They were finely striated, their margins beautifully defined, and, among hundreds of them examined in different specimens of urine, not the slightest variation in figure was observed: in size, they about equalled the smaller lozenges of colourless uric acid so often found accompanying urate of ammonia. From their chemical character, I have felt inclined to regard these crystals as oxalate of lime; although, from the minute quantity at my disposal, I have by no means completely satisfied myself on this point*.

* Since the above was written, this opinion of the identity of these curious crystals with oxalate of lime has been remarkably corroborated by a change in the character of the deposit. Beautiful, large octahedrons of undoubted oxalate appeared first mixed with the curved crystals shewn on the figure, and at this time (Feb. 11) have completely replaced them: the deposit, which is very abundant, now consisting of octahedral crystals of oxalate of lime (Fig. 10, *b*), mixed with lozenges of uric acid and large fragments of epithelium.

PRESENCE OF OXALATE OF LIME IN CALCULI.

WHEN crystals of oxalate of lime cohere and constitute a calculus, the concretion presents certain physical characters, which will very generally enable us to recognise its composition, independently of chemical analysis.

Calculi of oxalate of lime, next to those of uric acid or urates, are the most frequently met with. They almost invariably present a tubercular, angular, or spinous surface; and, in tint, vary from gray to a rich brown; from which circumstance, conjoined with their rough exterior, they have gained the specific name of "*mulberry.*" I have never met with a calculus of this kind with a perfectly smooth exterior: sometimes the external surface is studded with spines so acute and slender as to resemble thorns*. Occasionally, their surfaces are studded over with acute octahedrons of transparent oxalate of lime, giving an extremely beautiful appearance to the concretion. A calculus of this kind, No. 2138, has been elaborately described by Dr. Rees, in a former Volume of these Reports. Sometimes these crystals are opaque, and the octahedron is remarkably flattened: the calculus then looks as if studded with pearl-spar: of this, the calculus marked 2139^{25} affords a good example. One-sixth of the calculi, consisting entirely of oxalate of lime, in the Guy's Hospital collection, are covered with crystals of this calcareous salt. On a superficial examination, some difficulty often exists in distinguishing between calculi containing layers of pale oxalate of lime and the clay-coloured urate of ammonia; so very nearly, in several instances in our Museum, do they approach in tint and physical appearance. The superior hardness, and irregularity of outline, will generally aid in distinguishing the oxalate from the soft and more regularly deposited urate: of course, their chemical character will at once readily distinguish between them.

It has been supposed that the spinous and irregular form of these calculi depends upon their being formed in the kidney, and that they were casts of the pelvis and calyces of the organ: this, however, is by no means sufficient to account

---

* An excellent example of this is seen in the calculi numbered 2077^{16}. One of these is figured in the Plate accompanying Dr. Barlow's Paper in this Volume.

for their figure, for no calculus so closely becomes a cast of
the interior of the kidney as the fusible variety, and yet this
ever presents a tolerably smooth surface, however contorted
in figure. It is therefore more likely that the constantly
crystalline state in which the deposit of oxalate occurs has
more to do with it; and, without calling to our aid any very
fertile imagination, a tendency to a cubic or octahedral outline can often be traced in the entire calculus. The specimen
numbered 2138, and shewn in Plate I. Fig. 1, affords a good
instance of the cubical figure occasionally presented by these
calculi.

Sometimes we meet with calculi whose section shews their
interior half to be composed of oxalate of lime, presenting
all the spinous and process-like appendages so characteristic
of these concretions; whilst upon this has been deposited
some substance which is usually amorphous in its character,
and has completely filled up the irregularities of the nucleus,
and given to the whole an ovoid figure. In the calculus
marked 2171, all the irregularities presented by a large gray
nucleus of oxalate of lime are concealed by a layer of brown
uric acid, so that the whole section presents the appearance
of fortification agate. This calculus is figured in Plate I.
Fig. 3. Sometimes the irregularities are concealed by a
layer of the phosphates. The converse of this is frequently
met with, oxalate of lime being deposited on an oval nucleus
of uric acid or urate of ammonia. Both these states are
often seen in calculi consisting of three distinct and equally
thick deposits, and several instances of this exist in the
Museum. Thus, in the calculus numbered 2199, a smooth
regular nucleus of uric acid is surrounded by an irregular
tubercular deposition of oxalate of lime; whilst all the spinous
projections and processes of the latter are completely concealed by a smooth amorphous layer of phosphate of lime.
In the section of another calculus (2195), the same thing is
observed; except that the mulberry deposit is covered up
by a crust of fusible calculus, instead of phosphate of lime.
In Fig. 8, the section of a calculus thus formed is shewn: the
nucleus is oval, and consists chiefly of uric acid; and on
this is deposited oxalate of lime; which, although forming a
by no means thick layer, is not deposited concentrically,
but arranged in rough projecting tubercular masses. This

calculus is numbered 2166[60] in the Museum Catalogue. Occasionally, the section of a calculus shews a layer of oxalate of lime arranged round the interior one with great regularity, and presenting a remarkably radiated appearance resembling a series of infinitely minute needles placed side by side, and presenting a perfectly porcellaneous lustre. This is well shewn in the specimen numbered 2196.

PHOSPHATE OF LIME.

This salt naturally exists in urine, notwithstanding its insolubility in water, being held in solution, through the agency of either lactic acid or phosphoric acid, either free, or in the state in which, according to Berzelius, it is present in urine, partly saturated with ammonia. On the addition of an alkali to urine containing a normal proportion of phosphate of lime, it is precipitated in an amorphous form; unless ammonia be used as the precipitant, in which case the deposit will appear crystalline, from the presence of a considerable quantity of the ammoniaco-magnesian phosphate.

Occasionally, an excess of phosphate of lime exists in the urine, and may be present in one of two distinct states: one, in which it is dissolved by the free fixed acid of the urine; and hence, on applying heat, it remains in solution: the other, in which it becomes deposited by the application of heat, or by exposure to the air. Some discrepancy of opinion has existed regarding the nature of the menstruum which, in these cases, holds the phosphate in solution; Dr. Rees[*] regarding the hydrochlorate of ammonia of the urine as the solvent, whilst Dr. Brett[†] is induced to consider, that, in cases where a deposit of phosphate of lime occurs on applying heat to urine, carbonic acid acts as the solvent, and the evolution of this in a gaseous form determines the precipitation of the calcareous salt. So far as my own observations have extended, I have certainly seen cases to which both these views will equally apply; and I feel inclined to regard both opinions as correct, within certain limits. Thus, among specimens of urine which deposit phosphate of lime on the application of heat, I have met with some which became

Guy's Hospital Reports, Vol. XVII. p. 847.
† Medical Gazette, Vol. I. p. 401.

turbid from the deposition of the phosphate, by mere exposure for a few hours to the air, or to an atmosphere of hydrogen gas—a circumstance admitting only of explanation by
supposing the evolution of some volatile solvent: and that
this really was carbonic acid, I conceive scarcely admits of a
doubt, since on placing a specimen of urine of this kind in
a flask furnished with a tube bent twice at right angles and
immersed in a solution of chloride of barium to which ammonia had been added, and applying heat to the urine, a
precipitation of carbonate of barytes appeared in the fluid in
which the tube was immersed, *pari passu* with the deposition
of phosphate of lime in the flask.   If, in addition to this fact,
it be borne in mind that a solution of phosphate of lime in
hydrochlorate of ammonia does not become opaque by exposure to the air unless heat be applied, it follows that we
are obliged to fall back upon the explanation given of these
cases by Dr. Brett.   On the other hand, I have repeatedly
seen specimens of urine which deposited phosphate of lime
only after the application of heat; and to these cases the
ingenious explanation given by Dr. Rees very satisfactorily
applies.   Hence we may fairly assume that phosphate of
lime may exist in urine dissolved in a fixed acid, in which
case it is not deposited on the application of heat; or held in
solution by carbonic acid or an ammoniacal salt: in either
instance being precipitated by heating the urine, and in the
former by mere exposure to the air, from the evolution and
escape of the gaseous solvent.

Characters of Urine containing Excess of Phosphates.—Specimens of urine containing an excess of phosphates are almost
always pale, often presenting scarcely more colour than mere
water: when the contrary occurs, and the urine presents a
near approach to the normal amber tint, it generally happens
that the presence of an excess of earthy salt is but temporary;
a by no means unfrequent circumstance in many chronic
ailments of a dyspeptic character, or in which a depressed
condition of nervous energy exists, as after fatigue, blows
over the spine, extreme senility, or excessive indulgence in
sexual intercourse.

Whenever a positive deposit of phosphate of lime exists,
the urine is generally alkaline, rarely neutral, although often
slightly acid at the moment of emission.   When urine con-

tains phosphate of lime in a state precipitable by heat, it is always more or less acid.—The chemical characters of urine containing an excess of phosphate of lime are shewn in the Table given at the end of this Paper.

No constituent of urinary deposits has led to more errors than the phosphate of lime: where it exists in solution in the urine, and precipitable by heat, it has been repeatedly mistaken for albumen; and where it has formed the great mass of a deposit, has as frequently been mistaken for pus or purulent mucus. Scarcely any thing can be conceived to resemble these morbid products more than many forms of phosphatic deposit; sometimes being found lying at the bottom of the containing vessel, in the form of a cream-like layer; and occasionally suspended in the fluid in thick ropy masses, which so closely resemble strings of puriform mucus as to deceive any one not aware of this very serious source of fallacy: of course, the solubility of the deposit in any dilute mineral acid will at once dispel the illusion and distinguish phosphate of lime, under any of its Protæan forms, from a puriform deposit. If, however, albumen be present in the urine, as in these cases not unfrequently happens, greater difficulty exists in identifying the true nature of the deposit; yet even here, if dilute hydrochloric acid be added to the urine before the application of heat, any opacity produced by the presence of phosphate of lime will disappear, and thus be readily distinguished from that produced by pus.

Recognition of Phosphate of Lime.—When we meet with a white urinary deposit readily soluble, after being heated to redness on a slip of platina, in hydrochloric acid without effervescence, precipitable from its solution by ammonia in an amorphous form, we may be certain it consists of phosphate of lime.

If a specimen of urine becomes opaque by heat, the opacity disappearing on the addition of a drop of hydrochloric or nitric acid, it contains phosphate of lime held in solution in one or other of the modes before described.

In calculi, phosphate of lime may be detected by igniting a fragment, dissolving it in hydrochloric acid, and placing a drop of the solution, on a slip of glass, under the microscope: the addition of a drop of a solution of ammonia will immediately cause the deposition of phosphate of lime in an

amorphous granular form, if it existed in the fragment submitted to examination.

Presence of Phosphate of Lime in Calculi.—Traces of this
calcareous salt are very generally met with in all calculi, and
it frequently forms a considerable portion of their mass:
very rarely, however, does it constitute the nucleus; and in
the collection at Guy's Hospital, it is only so found when
the rest of the calculus consists of the same substance, of
which there are but two specimens. It very frequently forms
a thin superficial crust over the surface of other calculi.

One of the calculi in the collection, consisting entirely
of phosphate of lime, presents a porcelaineous appearance
externally, admitting of a considerable polish by friction, is
conchoïdal in its fracture, and is of a greyish-white colour:
the other is more regular in figure, and is made up of a
series of concentric layers of the phosphate, readily distinguishable from each other by their tint, being alternately
white and fawn-coloured. In three specimens, the mass of
the calculus is made up of the phosphate deposited on a
nucleus of uric acid; in one instance, on a nucleus of urate
of ammonia; and in six, on oxalate of lime. In one calculus
in the collection, the mass is made up of nearly snow-white
phosphate of lime, deposited on several distinct nuclei of the
fusible calculus. Four distinct nuclei are visible in the section of the stone: these are semi-translucent, and radiated
like a zeolite; the phosphate of lime being deposited round
each in distinct angular masses; each separating from its
neighbour so readily, as to give the sides of the whole concretion an appearance of being made up of a series of calculi,
rather than of one. Each fragment presents a well-marked
conchoïdal surface, at its juncture with that next to it.

Calculi chiefly or entirely composed of phosphate of lime
are tolerably hard and smooth externally, not presenting the
angular asperities of the oxalate of lime, or the frequently
contorted and irregular figure of the fusible calculus: occasionally, we find them apparently composed of two or three
portions fitting into each other; one face of each piece presenting a concave, and the opposed one a convex surface.

Ammoniacal Phosphate of Magnesia (Triple Phosphate).—
It is doubtful whether this salt can, with justice, be regarded

as a constituent of healthy urine. The acid phosphate of magnesia exists in solution in that fluid; and on the addition of ammonia, is precipitated, in the form of the triple salt; the ammonia used as the precipitant forming part of the compound. In the same manner, when urine is kept for some time, crystals of the triple phosphate are formed; but even this affords no evidence of the salt having previously existed, as the ammonia coloured by the decomposition of the urine unites with the phosphate of magnesia in solution, and forms the triple combination.

Characters of Urine containing Triple Phosphate.—Where this salt exists in combination with phosphate of lime, forming the well-known fusible compound, the characters of the urine scarcely differ from those met with in simply phosphatic secretion; and the same remark applies to urine containing the triple salt, when a calculus concretion really exists in the bladder or kidney. It however frequently happens, that the triple phosphate is met with in the urine of patients labouring under an aggravated form of irritative dyspepsia. In this case, the urine is often of natural colour, and rather high specific gravity: on cooling, the salt is observed to form a crystalline pellicle on the surface of the fluid, after appearing tinted of the most gaudy colours from its marked iridescence. The triple phosphate can only be regarded as the product of diseased action; and differs from the phosphate of lime, which, in general, is the result of enervation, from the state of irritation generally present where this diathesis prevails. The urine is sometimes neutral, often acid, and never alkaline, unless the deposited phosphate is really a secondary result. On exposing to heat urine of this kind, the triple salt is deposited; the precipitation often being attended with an evident evolution of carbonic acid.

It frequently happens, especially in cases of disease attended with a marked degree of enervation, that urine depositing triple phosphate evolves a pungent, disagreeable, and even fœtid odour: this has been usually denominated ammoniacal: this, however, is an error; for if the urine be fresh, in all, or at least in the great majority of cases, it will be found to be acid, notwithstanding the pungently-fœtid odour it evolves.

Recognition of Triple Phosphate.—This salt exists in deposits in two distinct forms, each containing a different proportion of ammonia, and readily distinguishable by their crystalline form.

The first or neutral triple phosphate may be prepared artificially, by the addition of a solution of phosphate of ammonia to one of sulphate of magnesia, or by adding a very small quantity of ammonia to a considerable quantity of urine. This salt always forms a white glistening deposit; and is frequently met with constituting an iridescent pellicle or scum on the surface of urine : it is readily soluble in weak acids, even the acetic; and is unaffected by alkalis. By microscopic examination, this phosphate may be instantly recognised. If a drop of the urine containing it be examined under even a weak magnifying power, a series of beautifully-defined transparent crystals will be seen, all of them being either prisms or some modifications of them, often strongly shaded on one side, and illuminated at the edges and angles, unless they be immersed in water or some powerfully-refracting medium, when they appear perfectly transparent. In Plate III. Fig. 11. the various forms I have met with of this sort have been accurately delineated by Mr. Hurst.

The second or bibasic phosphate may be artificially formed, either by dropping an excess of ammonia into urine, or by adding a solution of phosphate of ammonia or soda, to which ammonia has been added, to one of phosphate of magnesia. This salt always occurs in alkaline urine, and in all probability is a secondary product. I never met with it constituting the entire mass of a deposit, but it frequently is found mixed with phosphate of lime. It not unfrequently occurs in small quantities in the pellicles or scum which form on the surface of urine by keeping. When artificially formed, by the addition of ammonia to urine, it always forms elegant stellar crystals, as shewn in Fig. 13 : when, however, it is formd naturally, it usually forms thin crystalline laminæ, resembling foliage, as shewn in Fig. 12; sometimes being traversed by a transparent cross; and in this state often, on account of its transparency, escapes detection, unless polarized light be employed.

Both these salts frequently exist in deposits mixed with phosphate of lime; and in this state it is most generally found in calculi. In this state it may be readily detected, by exposing a fragment to the heat of the blowpipe flame : it will very readily melt into a semi-translucent bead ; whilst the phosphate of lime *per se* can scarcely be made to fuse, even on the application of a very high temperature ; and the triple phosphate, when heated by itself very slowly, melts into an opaque enamel. Hence, when the two salts exist mingled, the combination is generally termed the fusible calculus. When a deposit, or fragment of calculus containing the phosphate, is dissolved in hydrochloric acid, and a drop placed under the microscope, its nature can be determined by the single addition of a drop of a solution of ammonia : this determines the precipitation either of an amorphous granular mass of a series of stellar crystals (Fig. 13), or of both these mingled together : in the first case, the calculus matter consisted of phosphate of lime ; in the second, of the triple phosphate ; and in the third, of the fusible compound.

Presence of Magnesian Phosphates in Calculi.—These salts rarely exist alone : there is, in Guy's Museum, out of twenty-one calculi entirely composed of phosphates, one only composed of triple phosphates, two of phosphate of lime, and nineteen of the fusible mixture. Crystals of the triple salt frequently occur disseminated through the bodies of calculi ; and are frequently met with forming distinct layers, easily recognised by their glistening appearance and fragile structure, sometimes being found filling up little cavities in the concretions. The fusible mixture usually forms a very white concretion, easily crumbling on pressure ; and is frequently met with in curiously-contorted figures, moulded either in the form of the pelvis of the kidney, as in No. 2163, or neck of the bladder, as pointed out long ago by Dr. Marcet. Both this and the triple salt are very frequently deposited only on one side of a calculus, forming remarkable cauliflower-like excrescences of a pearly aspect : of this, beautiful examples are met with in the calculi numbered 2198, 2154[84], 2154[26], 2200.

The magnesian triple phosphates, alone, or more frequently mixed with phosphate of lime, generally constitute the calculous masses deposited on foreign bodies accidentally or intentionally left in the bladder.

Relations of the various Constituents of Calculous Deposits to each other.—The examination of the natural relation of calculous ingredients is particularly important, especially in its practical bearings. For almost all of what little knowledge we possess of this subject we are indebted to Dr. Prout: and lately, both M. Rayer, and my talented friend Dr. Robert Willis, have devoted considerable attention to this point. It must be confessed, that much of the generally-received hypothesis connected with this question rests on speculative ground entirely; and ample room has been given to theories of this kind, by the discoveries of the conversion of proximate elements into each other—a series of metamorphoses, with which the science of modern organic chemistry abounds, and for which we are chiefly indebted to the master-spirit of the Professor at Giessen, the celebrated Leibig.

I dare not presume to occupy many pages with the consideration of this highly interesting subject, having already exceeded my assigned limits. I will therefore content myself by shewing how readily, by a slight re-arrangement of atoms, we can demonstrate the probable formation of the organic ingredient of calculous concretions from the constituents of healthy urine; reserving for a future opportunity a more minute examination of these interesting changes.

A. DERIVATION OF OXALIC ACID.

Liebig and Wöhler have shewn, that when uric acid is digested with the peroxide of lead, it is resolved into urea, oxalic acid, and allantoin, the characteristic ingredient of the fluid of the allantois of the cow. If we adopt the very probable view of Dumas, that urea is really an oxamide with two atoms of base (amidogene), the resolution of urea into oxalate of ammonia, on the addition of water, is shewn at least to be a very probable result of vital chemistry.

	C. N. H. O.		C. N. H. O.
1 atom of urea	$2+2+4+2$	2 atoms oxalic acid	$2+0+0+3$
2 atoms of water	$2+2$	. . . . . . ammonia	$2+6$
	$2+2+6+4$		$2+2+6+3$

From these formulæ, we see that the elements of two atoms of oxalate of ammonia are identical with those of one of urea and two of water, minus a single atom of oxygen.

If we admit the secretion of oxalate of ammonia to occur, the production of the calcareous salt admits of a ready explanation, in the manner before described.

B. DERIVATION OF CYSTINE (CYSTIC OXIDE).

The derivation of this substance is obscured by the copious elimination of sulphur attending its formation. That normal urine contains sulphur, not only in the state of acid, but in some way less firmly combined, is a fact demonstrable by boiling it in a silver basin, when a crust of sulphuret of silver is formed; a fact noticed long ago by Proust. Albumen has also lately been found to contain sulphur as a necessary ingredient; as, from the researches of Mulder *, this substance consists of ten atoms of Protein (Pr. $=$ C. 40, H. 31, N. 5, O. 12) *plus* two of sulphur and half an equivalent of phosphorus. Hence it is possible that the sulphur of cystine may be a derivative of albumen, if it be not merely the result of excessive elimination of a single element.

If we exclude sulphur, we cannot fail to observe the very simple relation which cystine bears to uric acid, urate of ammonia, and lactate of urea; so simple, indeed, as to shew the probability of the conversion of these substances into cystine, without calling in aid any marked development of a new diathesis or novel function. A glance at the following formulæ will be sufficient to illustrate the position here advanced :—

1. If from two atoms of cystine and four of nitrogen we suppose four equivalents of hydrogen and sulphur to be removed by oxidation or otherwise, we have the constituents of uric acid and urea.

	C.	N.	H.	O.			C.	N.	H.	O.	S.
1 atom of uric acid $=$	10	$+$ 4	$+$ 4	$+$ 6		2 atoms cystine $=$	12	$+$ 2	$+$ 12	$+$ 8	$+$ 4
. . . . . . urea $=$	2	$+$ 2	$+$ 4	$+$ 2		4 atoms nitrogen $=$		4			
	12	$+$ 6	$+$ 8	$+$ 8			12	$+$ 6	$+$ 12	$+$ 8	$+$ 4
							12	$+$ 6	$+$ 8	$+$ 8	$+$ 0
								4	$+$		4

2. The elements of one atom of cystine and two of urea are equal to those of urate of ammonia and water, *plus* five

* Vorläufige Resultate der Zerlegung verschiedener Thierischer Stoffe. In Pogg. Annalen, B. 44. s. 443.

equivalents of hydrogen and two of sulphur.

	C.	N.	H.	O.
1 atom urate of ammonia				
2 atoms of water				

1 atom urate of ammonia $= 10 + 5 + 7 + 6$

2 atoms of water $= 2 + 2$

$\overline{10 + 5 + 9 + 8}$

	C.	N.	H.	O.	S.
2 atoms of urea	4 + 4 +	8 + 4 + 0			
1 atom of cystine	6 + 1 +	6 + 4 + 2			

2 atoms of urea $\quad 4 + 4 + 8 + 4 + 0$

1 atom of cystine $\quad 6 + 1 + 6 + 4 + 2$

$\overline{10 + 5 + 14 + 8 + 2}$

$10 + 5 + 9 + 8 + 0$

$\overline{5 + 2}$

Again, if we oxidize three atoms of lactate of urea (a combination which, from the researches of M. Henry, appears to be always present in urine), by eight atoms of oxygen; we shall have the elements of three equivalents of water, two of nitric acid, and four of cystine, *minus* the sulphur.

———————

It must be admitted, that the above remarks are merely speculative; and I by no means venture to assert that the conversions alluded to necessarily occur: still, I would suggest the probability of the necessary existence of but two great classes of deposits, or diatheses in which they exist, instead of several different and distinct species of diseased action. I would venture to propose the division of deposits into two genera or classes; the first being organic, strictly the product of vital agency, not derived from without, and indebted for their origin to deranged function; the second, including those sediments which are wholly or in part derived from without, and often rather to be considered the result of wear and tear of the sane organs of the body than of active disease.

The first of these classes will include uric acid and urates, being the nearest approach to a healthy state of secretion. If, from any cause, less oxygen be eliminated, we have these replaced by the xanthic (uric) oxide; whilst, if the oxidating function of the kidney be exalted, oxalic acid is developed under the form of oxalate of lime. The tendency to an excessive elimination of sulphur will cause the replacement of uric acid, or urea, by cystine. To this category is also referrible the carbonate of lime, which I regard not as a secretion *de novo*, but a secondary product; the result of so great a state of enervation, that the bond of affinity, which in the healthy condition of the nervous system keeps firmly united the elements of urea, becomes loosened, a re-arrangement of atoms occurs, the urea becomes carbonate of ammonia, and, under the influence of ordinary chemical affinity, carbonate of lime is generated at the expense of the calcareous salts of the urine.

The second class contains the phosphates simple and mixed: the acid of these compounds may probably be really generated in the kidney by the oxidation of the, phosphorus present in the fatty matter and albumen of the blood; and, if so, the bases are alone derived from without. Under certain circumstances, it is pretty evident that the earthy phosphates are developed by a sort of vicarious function of the kidney; for in some few cases, in which the phosphate of lime has not been deposited in the osseous structure, as in mollities ossium and rachitis, the urine has been loaded with it. *Cæteris paribus*, of the two phosphates, the salt of lime appears more generally the result of enervation, and the magnesian combination the product of irritation.

If these views be substantiated—and I trust soon to bring evidence before the Profession of their probability—they would tend to simplify the generally-received doctrine of the existence of a series of distinct diatheses—a doctrine, of the correctness of which I confess myself by no means satisfied. To take a single instance:—If, from the mal-performance of any function, as that of the skin by the suppression of perspiration, the kidney be called upon to perform a supplementary or compensating duty, for the purpose of excreting that amount of carbon and nitrogen for which the skin is temporarily unfitted, we know that the presence of urate of ammonia in the urine is the immediate result. It is surely, then, not making too great a call upon one's imaginative powers, to conceive that, under slight predisposing causes or idiosyncrasies, this deposit may become replaced by the other organic ingredients, or even by carbonate of lime, according to the comparative amount of irritation or enervation present in the system in general or kidney in particular. I need hardly allude to the influence these views, if proved to be correct, would have on the treatment of calculous affections. I, however, merely thus briefly allude to them; trusting to the forbearance of the critic, until I have an opportunity of making known the data on which I have ventured to advance them.

Colour.	Nature of Deposit.	Action on Litmus.	Sp. Gr.	Ebullition before Filtering.	Ebullition after Filtering.

A.   Uric Acid.

Colour.	Nature of Deposit.	Action on Litmus.	Sp. Gr.	Ebullition before Filtering.	Ebullition after Filtering.
Pale Amber	Brick-red uric acid	very acid	1·027	—	—
Very Pale	Pale uric acid and mucus	acid	1·006	—	—
Dull Amber	Do. with white urate of amm.	acid	1·021	urate dissolves	—
Bright ditto	Ditto crystals more copious	acid	1·025	ditto	—
Dark ditto	Ditto, and mucus	acid	1·018	ditto	slight +
Pale ditto	Ditto	acid	1·015	ditto	

B.   Urate Ammonia.

Colour.	Nature of Deposit.	Action on Litmus.	Sp. Gr.	Ebullition before Filtering.	Ebullition after Filtering.
Pale	Chalk-like urate of ammonia	acid	1·026	ditto	—
Pale	Fawn-coloured ditto	acid	1·025	ditto	—
Pale	Pale pink	acid	1·026	ditto	—
Dull Amber	Brown urate	s. acid	1·011	ditto, but coagulates	dep. of albumen
Amber	Pale urate	acid	1·028	urate dissolves	
Carmine	Fine carmine urate	acid	1·025	ditto	urine deepens in colour
Amber	Pink urate	acid	1·020	ditto	

C.   Cystic Oxide.

Colour.	Nature of Deposit.	Action on Litmus.	Sp. Gr.	Ebullition before Filtering.	Ebullition after Filtering.
Pale Amber	Mucus and cystine	acid	1·0148	—	opacity
Pale Amber	Ditto	acid	1·0115	—	—
Apple-green	Ditto	acid	1·012	renders deposit denser	—

D.   Oxalate of Lime.

Colour.	Nature of Deposit.	Action on Litmus.	Sp. Gr.	Ebullition before Filtering.	Ebullition after Filtering.
Amber	Red muddy deposit	acid	1·026	dissolves the coloured deposit	—
Pale ditto	No visible deposit	acid	1·021	—	
Deep ditto	Pale urates	acid	1·020	ditto	
Amber	Ditto, and flaky uric acid	acid	1·016	dissolves part	—
Amber	Pink urates	acid	1·029	dissolves it	—
Amber	Fawn-coloured ditto	acid	1·016	ditto	—

E.   Earthy Phosphates.

Colour.	Nature of Deposit.	Action on Litmus.	Sp. Gr.	Ebullition before Filtering.	Ebullition after Filtering.
Very Pale	White powder	alkaline	1·020	—	—
Pale Amber	Crystalline powder	neutral	1·022	increases the deposit	+ soluble in acids
Amber	Mucous cloud	acid	1·020	copious + of triple phosph.	copious +
Pale Amber	Ditto, and few crystals	neutral	1·013	milkiness	ditto
Pale Amber	Copious white deposit	neutral	1·013	increases deposit	copious +
Pale Amber	White fusible powder	alkaline	1·011	s. increase	s. +

N.B. In the above Table, the following Abbreviati——

TAINING DIFFERENT DEPOSITS.

Hydrochloric Acid after heat.	Nitric Acid.	Acetic Acid.	Chlor. Calcium.	Ammonia.	Disease.	Microscopic Characters of Deposit.
A. Uric Acid.						
Rose-tint		—	—	+	Chorea	Rhomboids.
Ditto	—	—	—	—	2 Infants, æt. 3 mo.	Ditto.
Ditto	—	s. +	+	+	Dyspepsia	Fine rhombs and rosettes.
Ditto	—	—	—	+	Morbus Cordis	Ditto, very large.
Bronze-colour	s. +	—	—	+	Gran. kidney	Rhombs crystallized in meshes of mucus.
Fine pink	—	—	—	+	Dyspepsia	Fine tables and cylinders.
B. Urate Ammonia.						
Deep lilac	—	—	—	+	Pregnancy	Amorphous powder.
Brown	—	—	—	+	Phthisis	Ditto.
Bronze tint	—	—	—	s. +	Phthisis	Ditto.
Pale pink	—	—	—	s. +	Gran. kidney	Ditto.
Ditto	—	—	—	s. +	Pregnancy	Ditto.
Fine purple	—	—	—	+	Morbus Cordis and ascites	Ditto.
Pink	—	—	+	+	Rheumatism	Ditto.
C. Cystic Oxide.						
—	—	—	s. +	+	Calculus	Six-sided plates of cystine.
Ditto	—	—	s. +	+	Calculus	Ditto.
Pale lilac	—	—	—	+	?	Ditto, and roundish plates.
D. Oxalate of Lime.						
—	—.	—	—	+	Calculus	Splendid octahedrons, mixed with urate of ammonia.
Bronze tint	+	—	+	+	Dyspepsia	Copious octahedrons.
Pink	—	—	—	+	Ditto emaciation	Ditto, but small.
Ditto	—	—	—	+	Ditto	Dumb-bell shaped crystals, finely striated.
Ditto	—	—	—	+	Ditto	Minute copious octahedrons.
Ditto	—	—	—	+	Ditto	Very large octahedrons.
E. Earthy Phosphates.						
—	—	—	s. +	s. +	Injury to back	Amorphous powder.
Deep lilac	—	—	+	+	Diseased kidney	Fine prisms of triple.
Pale ditto	—	—	+	+	Excessive fatigue	Amorphous by heat.
Ditto	—	—	+	+	Gran. kidney	Fine prisms.
Rose	+	—	+	+	Extreme old age	Prisms with puriform globules.
—	coagulate	+	—	+	Calculus	Amorphous powder, with acicular crystals.

d : *s = slight*, + *a precipitate*, — *no change.*

PLATE I.

Fig. 1. A section of a large oxalate-of-lime calculus, remarkable for its cubical figure : it consists of two portions ; one, a tolerably oval nucleus, formed of radiating needles, deposited in the centre of the concretion. Both nucleus and body possess the same composition (No. 2138).

Fig. 2. An uric acid circular calculus, remarkable for the absence of distinct nucleus, and for its hollow mammillated centre (2113).

Fig. 3. Section of a calculus (2171), of which the centre consists of oxalate of lime, of its usual irregular form, concealed by a subsequent amorphous uric deposit.

Fig. 4. Section of a small calculus (2136^{50}), apparently divided into two portions, and subsequently united and framed in by a deposit of urate of ammonia.

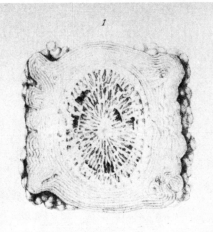

1

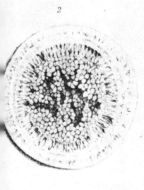

2

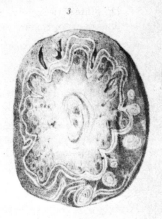

3

PLATE II.

Fig. 5. Section of a compound calculus, consisting of two green zones of cystic oxide, separated by a layer of urate of ammonia, and deposited on an oxalic nucleus (No. 2168).

Fig. 6. The large cystic oxide calculus described and figured by Dr. Marcet twenty-five years ago, shewing its structure, and present blueish-green colour. (2143.)

Fig. 7. Cystic oxide calculus, of a greyish colour, and ear-drop figure (2145^{35}).

Fig. 8. Compound calculus of uric acid and oxalate of lime; the irregular figure of the latter deposit concealing the smooth central portion of the former substance (2166).

Fig. 9. Section of a calculus, having a nucleus of uric acid followed by a layer of oxalate of lime, again succeeded by the former deposit. This is remarkable for the delicate pencillings of the pink deposit (purpurine) with which the different layers are marked (2170^{50}).

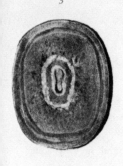

5

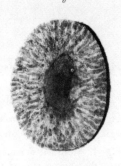

6

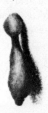

7

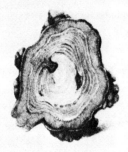

8

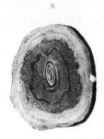

9

st. del et lith.

Printed by M & N Hanhart

Published by S Highley, Fleet Street.

PLATE III.

—

Fig. 1. Natural rhomboïd lozenges of uric acid : the internal structure is shewn at *b*.

Fig. 2. Modified rhomboïds, resembling spindles and fleur-de-lis.

Fig. 3. Uric acid approaching a cubic figure : at *a* the transparent margins : and at *b* the interior markings, are figured.

Fig. 4. Modified serrated tables of uric acid found in very acid urine : the shorter curved variety is shewn at *b*.

Fig. 5. Serrated crystals of uric acid shewing the crescentic structure, obtained by precipitating urine by an acid. The serratures are figured much too widely : in the crystals, they resemble a compact series of dark lines.

Fig. 6. Tables and lozenges of uric acid in rosettes and crosses.

Fig. 7. Diverging fasciculi of linear tables of uric acid.

Fig. 8. Uric acid in cylinders.

Fig. 9. Compound crystalline laminæ of uric acid.

Fig. 10. *a,* Crystals of oxalate of lime, resembling two superposed cubes. *b,* Acute octahedrons of oxalate of lime found in deposits.

[The three dumb-bell-like crystals unnumbered, beneath Fig. 12, represent the newly-observed form of oxalate-of-lime crystals.]

Fig. 11. Various forms of crystals of triple phosphate.

Fig. 12. Foliaceous laminæ of bi-basic phosphate.

Fig. 13. Stellar crystals of bi-basic phosphate.

Fig. 14. Normal crystals of cystic oxide.

Fig. 15. Serrated tables of cystic oxide, more frequent in deposits than Fig. 14.

Fig. 16. Laminæ of common salt slowly evaporated from urine.

Fig. 17. Daggers and croslets of salt obtained from urine by rapid evaporation.

Fig. 19. Crystals of hippuric acid, obtained by precipitating the urine of a patient taking benzoïc acid, by muriatic acid.

The Figures in this Plate were drawn from specimens preserved in balsam between slips of glass, by means of a mirror of Sömmering.

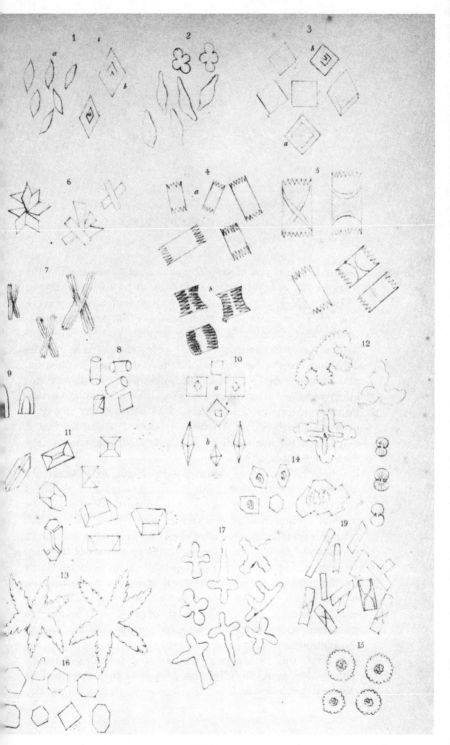

REMARKS

ON

CYSTINE, or CYSTIC OXIDE,

AND

ITS EXISTENCE IN URINARY DEPOSITS.

BY MR. GOLDING BIRD.

———

Cystic Oxide is not of very frequent occurrence in calculous formations; and was quite unknown, until its discovery, in 1810, by Dr. Wollaston; since which period, with the exception of a few instances, chemists have not had an opportunity of examining it for themselves: and we were indebted for our knowledge of the properties of this curious substance to the researches of Drs. Marcet and Wollaston, and, more lately, of Dr. Prout; and hitherto it was not known to exist in urinary deposits. From some late investigations, however, I am inclined to believe, that not only does it occur as a constituent of urinary deposits, but that it enters into the composition of calculi rather more commonly than has been imagined.

Cystic oxide, or, as it has been perhaps more correctly termed by Berzelius, cystine, in its physical and chemical characters differs from all the other constituents of calculous matter. When in mass, it is sectile; and if pure, quite white; insoluble in alcohol, water, or acetic acid; readily soluble in alkalies and their carbonates, with the exception of the carbonate of ammonia; and precipitable from these solutions by the mineral acids, which, when in excess, re-dissolve it: when recently precipitated, it is white and crystalline, presenting, under a lens, the form of six-sided prisms, so truncated as to resemble six-sided plates. When heated on platinum foil, cystine blackens; evolves a very peculiar fetid and rather acid odour; and inflames, burning with a blue, scarcely fuliginous flame, without shewing the slightest tendency to fuse; leaving a very minute quantity of ash, which is probably owing to the presence of a trace of phosphate of lime.

Calculi containing cystine generally possess a waxy lustre, with a tint, varying from the *cold sea-green* of sulphate of iron, to a pale mulberry-brown : their surface is generally more or less tubercular ; and their section presents a crystalline appearance, not unlike cholesteric calculi, from which it differs in the absence of the zeolitic arrangement of the crystals so peculiar to biliary calculi. The cut surfaces of nearly all the cystine calculi, that have been described, appear to have possessed a blueish-green tint of varying intensity ; but I had lately an opportunity of examining a calculus of this kind, whose section was of a yellowish-brown tint, bearing no distant resemblance to the colour of the fawn-coloured urate of ammonia calculi. Nothing is known concerning the cause of this difference of colour : but, for my own part, I should rather attribute it to some diversity in its crystalline structure influencing its optical properties, than to any chemical difference; more particularly as both varieties, when reduced to fine powder, become perfectly white.

One of the calculi described by Dr. Marcet in his work, being the second in which Dr. Wollaston detected the presence of cystine, is in the Museum of Guy's Hospital, (which probably contains the richest collection of cystic oxide calculi in existence,) being No. 2143 in the Museum Catalogue : it is, I believe, the largest calculus, consisting entirely of cystine, that has been yet met with : its form is that of a flattened ellipse, its long diameter being about 1.5 inch, and its transverse diameter about 1. inch : externally, its colour is yellowish-brown, but its section is of a fine sea-green, verging into a brownish tint in its centre ; which change of colour is not, however, sufficiently abrupt to indicate the existence of any thing like a distinct nucleus. In the same Museum are nine other specimens of this kind of calculus, obtained, I believe, from the same patient : they are all nearly round, very tubercular, and blueish-green *externally,* varying from the size of a pea to that of a small marble. Three of these calculi (No. 2144 of the Museum Catalogue) have been described by Dr. Marcet : the other six (No. 2145) have been placed in the Museum since the publication of his work. Another calculus consisting of cystine, in the same collection (No. 2145ᴬ), is remarkable for its singular shape, in which it exactly resembles a lady's ear-drop, having probably assumed this form during its residence in the pelvis of the kidney: it is about an inch long, and, like the others, possesses a pale-green colour: indeed, from the frequent occurrence of this tint in calculi composed of cystine, it has been looked upon as being quite characteristic of its presence; and this circumstance, I am inclined to think, has been the cause of these calculi, when not possessing this colour, being occasionally overlooked in large collections.

A calculus composed entirely of cystine has been lately added to the collection (No. 2145ᴮ) at Guy's Hospital, by Mr. C. Aston Key; who removed it from the urethra of a private patient: and to whose kindness I am indebted for the following account of the case; which is the more interesting, as the paucity of cases of this form of calculous diathesis, on record, prevents our being so well acquainted with the predisposing or exciting causes of this, as of the other varieties of diathesis.

"The subject of the cystic oxide calculus was a young "gentleman, aged about 12 years, of a delicate complexion, "with hair and eyes inclined to auburn, and in his frame "exhibiting general delicacy of texture. His parents, though "healthy, are not strong persons, but have not been dis-"posed either to calculous disorders or to gout. The pre-"vailing disposition in the family is a tendency to strumous "affection; under which, in a somewhat aggravated form, a "younger member of the family is now labouring. The "boy from whom the stone was taken had never, as far as "his mother could recollect, shewed signs or expressed "symptoms of kidney affection; nor had his urine been "noticed as peculiar. The only circumstance that his parents "had remarked, was, that he could not eat the meat at "school, on account of its being less nicely dressed than that "to which he had been accustomed at home; and his diet, "therefore, had been less nutritious than usual. The attack "which brought the stone to light was sudden. On the "afternoon of the 24th of May 1836, he complained of "difficulty and pain in voiding his urine; and in the evening "he was able to void only a few drops at a time, and at

" frequent intervals. About midnight, the urine ceased to
" flow, even after violent efforts to pass it; and I was requested
" to see him. On attempting to introduce a catheter, I was
" checked by a foreign body lodged in the urethra, just
" anterior to the scrotum, which entirely occupied the canal
" of the urethra, and seemed to be firmly impacted. From
" its size, I judged it to be too large to escape by the glans;
" and therefore extracted it by an incision through the cor-
" pus spongiosum. It proved to be a rather large calculus,
" of an oval shape, and studded with minute tubercles: its
" colour struck me as being peculiar: it had not the nut-
" brown or reddish colour of the lithic acid, but the amber
" tint of the cystic oxide formation, and also the translucent
" appearance characteristic of that species of calculus. The
" wound has healed quickly; and his health remains good.
" He is passing the summer at the sea-side."

The calculus removed by Mr. Key from the patient whose
case has just been detailed, presented, on making a longitudinal section of it, the same confused crystalline structure
as the other specimens of this species of calculus, but does
not possess any of the green colour usually present; its
tint being exactly that of the fawn-coloured urate of ammonia calculus: its specific gravity was 1.777. The following is an account of its behaviour towards re-agents; which
it may be interesting to mention; as this calculus, on account of its unusual colour, might be supposed to differ from
the true cystine, or cystic oxide calculus.

1. When heated on platinum foil, it blackened, evolved
the peculiar odour of burning cystine, without fusing, and
burnt with a blue flame, leaving scarcely a trace of ash.

2. It dissolved readily in a solution of potass; being deposited from this solution in six-sided crystals, on the
addition of acetic acid.

3. Boiled with a little nitric acid to dryness, it left a deep
sepia-brown residue, quite distinct from the pink hue
yielded by uric acid when treated in a similar manner.

4. Sulphuric acid dissolved it, *without* becoming coloured ;
leaving, by evaporation, fine needles of sulphate of cystine.

5. Hydrochloric acid readily dissolved it; the solution

yielding, by evaporation, delicate needles of hydrochlorate of cystine.

These circumstances distinguish this form of calculus from all others yet known ; for had it consisted of earthy phosphates or oxalates, a considerable residue would have been left after incineration, and it would not have dissolved in alkaline solutions ; whilst the absence of uric acid and urates is shewn by the peculiar action of nitric acid, as well as by its solubility in hydrochloric acid, in which, as is well known, uric acid is insoluble.

I could not detect the presence of muriate of ammonia in this calculus; although I have discovered this salt in almost every other species, having always looked for it since reading Dr. Yellowly's Paper upon this subject in the Philosophical Transactions. As the boy, from whom this calculus was removed was under treatment when I received it for examination, I was exceedingly anxious to obtain specimens of his urine, to ascertain whether it deposited any thing, and if so, what this deposit consisted of. On mentioning this to Mr. Key, he very kindly procured for me, at different intervals, specimens of the urine ; in which I very readily detected cystine, not only as a deposit (as I had anticipated), but also in solution. This urine was pale, of low specific gravity, generally being about 1.0148, without any action on litmus or turmeric papers ; and contained, in diffusion, clouds of mucus, mixed with a white, crystalline deposit, which readily subsided to the bottom of the vessel, and closely resembled a deposit of the ammoniaco-magnesian phosphate ; from which it was readily distinguished by a microscopic examination, presenting the appearance of flat six-sided tables, which I have already mentioned as quite characteristic of cystic oxide. On applying a boiling temperature to the urine, after the deposit had been diffused by agitation, it did not become clear, until after the addition of a considerable quantity of muriatic acid : acetic acid did not, under similar circumstances, dissolve it ; as it would have done had the deposit consisted of earthy phosphates or oxalates. Ammonia, with the aid of heat, readily dissolved this deposit.

On submitting this urine to quantitative analysis, after

being freed from the deposit by filtration, I found it to consist of,

Water 974.444
Urea, with alkaline chlorides, phosphates, and lactates, 5.7
Aqueous extract, with alkaline sulphates 14.7
Albuminous matter and earthy phosphates 4.8
Uric acid and adherent mucus 0.016
Cystine (cystic oxide) 0.340
                                              1000.

I was surprised to find cystine in *solution* in this urine, knowing its total insolubility in water : for this circumstance I am unable to offer any very satisfactory explanation. Perhaps it might be held in solution by the excess of acid in the biphosphate of ammonia, which is a constant constituent of urine ; or even by means of carbonic acid, which exists in every specimen of urine I have hitherto examined ; and which certainly appears to be the solvent for the earthy phosphates, when they exist in urine in an anormally large proportion ;—a fact that has been, in my estimation, fully proved by the late experiments of my friend Mr. R. H. Brett (*Med. Gaz. March* 1836). I may remark, that the urine, of which the analysis is above mentioned, was passed by the patient on May 28th, being four days after the removal of the calculus. I examined different specimens of the urine passed by the same patient at different intervals ; viz. June 7th, 14th, and 27th ; which differed from the first specimen, in the gradual decrease of albuminous matter and cystic oxide, and increase of urea : indeed, in that passed on June 27th, not a particle of cystic oxide could be detected : but whether this circumstance indicates the removal of the diathesis, or the formation of another concretion, must be left to time to determine. Before concluding this paper, I may perhaps be permitted to correct what I believe to be an erroneous opinion connected with the composition of cystic oxide calculi, which was put forth by the late Dr. Marcet, and adopted by Dr. Prout ; viz. " that the cystine diathesis " generally exists, to the exclusion of other diatheses ; and " that this diathesis does not seem readily to change into any " other" : both of which assertions I have good reason to believe to be incorrect : and in this I am supported by the examination of the section of a calculus which I met with in the Museum of Guy's Hospital.   This specimen (No. 2168), is very curious, and quite unique: it was placed among the mulberry calculi, and had been in the collection some length of time.   Externally, it was of a pale-fawn colour, scarcely tubercular: its section presented a series of concentric layers, of which two exactly resembled crystals of green sulphate of iron.   I carefully examined this curious calculus; and found it to consist of the following substances, arranged in distinct and separate zones:

1. A nucleus of oxalate of lime.
2. A zone of green cystic oxide, about $\frac{1}{30}$ inch thick.
3. A zone of urate of ammonia, *mixed* with fawn-coloured cystic oxide, $\frac{1}{10}$ inch thick.
4. A zone of green cystic oxide, about $\frac{1}{20}$ inch thick, resembling No. 2.
5. A layer of the urates of ammonia and soda, $\frac{3}{10}$ inch thick.
6. Alternating layers of urates of ammonia and soda, with oxalate of lime, about $\frac{1}{10}$ inch thick.

The section of this calculus thus acquaints us with some very interesting and important facts; that not only can the cystic oxide *replace* other diatheses, but it can exist *simultaneously* with them.   Thus, when this calculus was *first* formed, the oxalate of lime diathesis must have prevailed;— that this must have been replaced by the cystic oxides;— that, subsequently, the urate ammonia diathesis must have existed for a time contemporary with that of the oxide, and then disappeared, again leaving the cystic oxide diathesis prevailing: this, in its turn, had again been replaced by the diathesis of the alkaline urates; which finally alternated with the oxalate of lime, until the calculus ceased to increase. The examination of this calculus thus effectually disproves the assertions of the two chemists above mentioned, respecting the *exclusive* nature of the cystic oxide diathesis.

With regard to the treatment of this diathesis, I have nothing new to offer.   If the chemical action of remedies taken internally is adopted, neither the administration of alkalies nor mineral acids is objectionable, as the cystine is equally soluble in both these menstrua: but probably in this, as in all the other forms of calculous diathesis, more is to be expected by combating the derangements of the stomach and chylopoietic viscera generally, than by the *chemical* action of any supposed lithontriptics.

ON THE

PATHOLOGY OF CELLS.

BY THOMAS WILLIAMS, M.B.

———

THE following article is intended to form the commencement of a series of Reports of facts and observations obtained
and accumulated in the Microscopical Department of this
Hospital; more especially by the examination of *Morbid Structures*, which the dead-house almost daily affords. From the
comparative shortness of the time since these observations
were first instituted, it will be seen to have been impossible to
have amassed material enough for attempting any systematic
classification of the numerous and diversified objects com-
prised within the limits of the present subject. Since, however, they are designed to bear only the character of "Reports,"
and to participate little in the higher qualities of "Essays,"
it will signify little in what order the subjects are treated.

1. A most remarkable æra in the history of modern Physiology is the period at which Schleiden and Schwann gave
definite expression to the discovery, that all animal and
vegetable tissues derived their common beginning from *cells.*
The brief interval of time which has elapsed since the publication of Schleiden's *Phytogenesis*, and Schwann's more elaborate work, has been characterized by an extraordinarily
rapid progress in the development and collection of facts in
the department of physiology, which the genius of these two
great observers had so successfully opened to view. But,
notwithstanding the essential and important office which *cells*
perform in the original formation and subsequent metamorphosis and regeneration of animal and vegetable structures,
and the definite and intimate knowledge of their natural
history which science now commands, with few exceptions,
no systematic attempt has hitherto been made towards rendering prominent the great value and importance of the

microscope, as a means for the study and investigation of
disease. Müller led the way in this interesting department, by
the publication of his well-known work on morbid growths[1].
Dr. Grüby, of Vienna, has more recently published the results of his observations on some pathological fluids, in a
little work[2] which can be considered by no means an unimportant acquisition to the literature of pathology. Raspail,
too, in his Lectures, and in some of his later works[3], has pro-
pounded certain abstract theorems in regard to the pathological susceptibilities of the ultimate " vesicles" or " cells"
of tissues, which, if they add nothing to the treasury of *facts*
which the microscope has already unfolded, are calculated to
imbue the minds of less philosophical observers with principles
as important as facts themselves, in the further prosecution
of the subject. The recent laborious work[4] of Rokitansky,
however, while it abounds in much novel and useful imfor-
mation in relation simply to the *external character* of morbid
structures, presents us with few proofs of the author's having
cultivated that more recondite division of the science of
morbid anatomy, which seeks, by the assistance of the microscope, to resolve the solid products of disease to the simplicity of their elementary components. The names of many
excellent observers in this country are identified with isolated contributions of no inferior value to the subject of the
pathology of cells. In the list of casual contributors, the
names of Gulliver[5], Bowman[6], Addison[7], Dalrymple[8], Smee[9],

([1]) On Carcinomatous Growths.

([2]) Observationes Microscopicæ ad Morphologiam Pathologicum, auctore Dr·
David Grüby, 1840. See also Microscopic Journal.

([3]) Le Nouveau Système de Chimie Organique, 1838. Lectures on Physiology of Health and Disease, &c., in Medical Times, by M. Raspail.

([4]) Handbuch der Pathologischen Anatomie. *Wien*, 1842.

([5]) Gerber's Anatomy. See also Papers in Medical Gazette, read before
the Medico-Chirurgical Society, 1841--42.

([6]) Lancet, January 1842, on Fatty Degeneration of the Liver.   Philosophical Transactions, Part I., 1842.   Cyclopædia, Anatomy and Physic: Art.
"Mucous Membrane."

([7]) Papers in Medical Gazette and Lancet, 1840--43, on the Red Particles
of the Blood ; read before the Microscopic Society, 1843.

([8]) On the Mode of Ossification of Encysted Tumors ; read at the Medico-
Chirurgical Society. Reported in Medical Gazette, May 1843.

([9]) On the Structure of Normal and Adventitious Bone.—Medical Gazette,
Nov. 20, 1840.

and Wharton Jones[10], are the most prominent; to each of
whom science is indebted for communications of greater or
less value and interest. At this early stage, in a field illi-
mitably prolific in materials of study and research, the duties
of the historian must abruptly cease. A singular distrust
in the accuracy and fidelity of the microscope, as an instrument of investigation and discovery, has so alienated the
taste of many well-informed pathologists, as to induce them
to regard the facts ascertained directly through its assistance
as something like the spectres of an imaginative eye, or the
refined delusions of a complex optical mechanism, or, at best,
the obscure shadows of infinitely-divided particles of organic
matter, in reference to which it would be impossible to establish, with precision, either the figure or the size. Such
unphilosophical scepticism is a libel upon the character of
those whose lives have been ardently devoted to the furtherance of microscopic science. Under the shelter of a classic
adage—*Nequeunt oculis rerum primordia cerni*—they seek to
circumscribe the domain of observational science to the
straitened limits of those grosser aggregations of matter,
whose properties are cognisable enough to unimproved and
ordinary sense. There is something unworthy of the present
age in the puerile superstition which, with the complacency
and boldness of " little knowledge," attaches, by its imputa-
tions, the character of doubt, uncertainty, and mystery, to a
process of research which is strictly demonstrative in its
pretensions. In this statement it is not desired to claim for
it any supernatural immunity from error. Fallibility will
continue to be the indelible attribute of every ramification of
human science, so long as the qualities of men's minds will
continue to exhibit variations in degrees. Philosophers, of
any acumen and discrimination, have always perceived and
taught, from Wollaston and Ehrenberg to the least-pretending
microscopists of the present day, that the endowments and
capabilities of the senses, like those of the mind, present palpable individual differences. In the examination of a morbid structure by the aid of a modern achromatic microscope,
which enables the observer to resolve the object of study into

([10]) Observations on the Anatomy, Physiology, and Pathology of the Blood.—
Foreign Review, 1842.

its *ultimate* and integral *cells* and *filaments*, and *their parent* molecules and capillary system—conducting thus the eye, and therefore the mind, into nearer approach to those more hidden and deeper elements, in the definite characters of which it may read the incipient and secret changes which, by their silent continuance, lead to an accumulation of diseased product, which soon and sensibly proclaims a departure from the healthy state—contrasted with that coarser and more summary method of examination which obliges the pathologist, however inquisitive he may be, to rest contented with simply looking at, handling, and dissecting, a compound mass of heterogeneous mischief, in the combined and collective characters of which there is little which can be recognised and interpreted with exactitude—it becomes at once evident, that this invaluable instrument should be in future accepted as the inseparable companion of the morbid anatomist.

The difference between a primitive cell and a mass of organized structure is not simply one of proportion or magnitude. Although not strictly an elementary body, an ultimate vesicle, even if it were endowed with a nucleus, and this with a nucleolus, is, in its mechanical construction or organization, infinitely less complex than the mass. And does it not follow, as an obvious inference from the enunciation of this fact, that an organ so simple must, under the conditions of disease, present changes and phænomena *proportionably* more satisfactory and intelligible than a complex organ of more elaborate manufacture. There is, however, another point of view in which the dissimilar relations of the primordial cell and the compound organ assume surpassing interest, when contemplated by the pathologist. By the concurrent labours of Valentin, Purkinge, Henle, Müller, Wagner, Turpin, and, above all, by the more recent and conclusive investigations of Dr. Martin Barry[1], Mr. Goodsir[2], and Mr. Bowman[3], the position has become fundamental in philosophy, " that nearly all the animal tissues, however great the alterations they may have undergone in

[1] Phil. Transactions, 1839.
[2] Edin. New Phil. Journal, July 1842.
[3] Phil. Transactions, 1842.

structure and properties, have their immediate origin in cells; and that in animals, as in plants, *all the changes in which organic life essentially consists* are performed by *cells*[4]." A *Cell* is the ultimate limit of organized structure. When the formative blastema—a structureless substance more or less fluid—assumes the attributes of organization, this is the first visible form under which it presents: it is an atom of organized matter, beyond the limits of which division would be as impracticable as it would be incompatible with the idea of elementary unity. A primogenial cell abruptly assigns the confines of microscopic analysis; but the diversities of size allowed to this primitive organismus range from dimensions of immeasurable minuteness to the magnitude of a cell visible to the naked eye. The component organs of a polygastric animalcule, the whole bulk of whose body does not equal the dimensions of a nucleated cell, must occupy an inconceivably minute extent of space: an object of indisputable corporeity, which can be contained within a point of space measuring less than the $\frac{1}{376,000}$th of an inch[5] is indeed, though a *small fact*, quite ample enough to kindle in every contemplative mind unqualified sentiments of wonder at the unfathomable profundity of organization. These refined depths of analysis, however, since they occur in the remoter regions of animate nature, which the morbid anatomist will be seldom required to visit, need scarcely intimidate the honest inquirer, or deter him from industry and exertion in more accessible departments of useful and available knowledge. As formerly stated, the primitive or ultimate cells of organs are the immediate agents of all the *organic processes :* the elaboration of nutrient matter, in all its stages and its disintegration, for the purposes of secretion and elimination, are essentially *cell*-phænomena. The circulating system, even its capillary segments, accomplishes the subsidiary and secondary purpose only of mechanical conveyance. It must not, however, be forgotten, that the *blood* itself, during its incessant circuits through this complex system, undergoes changes of organic composition preparatory and necessary to the

([1]) Carpenter. ([5]) Ehrenberg.

subsequent steps of *solid* organization[1]. It requires no prophetic vision to perceive that the remarkable advances which these discoveries have effected in physiology are destined to produce correspondingly-important changes in the character of pathological science, and to widen the limits of those narrow bounds within which the routine morbid anatomist has hitherto been accustomed contentedly to circumscribe his inquiries.

The conclusion is obvious, that the *same* organic laws preside over the combinations and resolutions of the minutest, as of the most colossal aggregations of living matter— a monad, as of an elephant—a simple primordial *cell*, as of a voluminous compound organ. It is therefore difficult to enunciate a proposition more rational than that which inculcates, that the most fruitful materials for the successful extension of pathological science lay hidden in the integral elements of structure, and veiled from the eye of the cursory observer by the ponderous mass which progressive changes may have accumulated. If not the *principia*, cells unquestionably are the *seminia morbi*—the machinery of propagation.

It is scarcely necessary to present an hypothetic delineation of the origin and progress of a morbid growth, in order to render them intelligible ; but let it be conceived, that the eye of the microscopist recognises the indications of the disease, on the minutest possible scale, in *one* of the elementary *cells* of an organ[2]: this may be either *functional*, or it may be so far organic as to have deranged and altered the physical character of the little organ : if the morbific causes were to cease at the incipient stage of their operation, it is evident that the little cell might have undergone disease, and eventual decay, without causing any conceivable departure from

---

([1]) For a lucid analysis of the subject, I beg to refer the reader to the " Report of Dr. Carpenter on the Physiology of Cells ;" Forbes's Foreign Review, Jan. 1843 ;—and Mr. Wharton Jones's " Report on the Blood," in previous Number.

([2]) The *cell* of an acephalo-cyst is believed by Professor Owen to be an actual illustration of this idea. See Lectures on the Comparative Anatomy of the Invertebrata, p. 44.

the total sum of the organ's function. It would furnish a pointed example of what is popularly described as "molecular death." Let, however, this imaginary case be further extended ; and suppose that the disorganizing process, having its point of origin in the remoteness of this primordial cell, were to communicate to the affected particle the morbid power of propagating the same diseased tendency to all the contiguous vesicles ;—by this work of silent invasion, a sum of accumulated consequences would soon result, which at length would openly pronounce the presence of disease. Thus, disorder of an organ, or a part, is manifestly proclaimed only after the lapse of a considerable interval of time, during which the number of the affected organs (cells) has undergone palpable multiplication. When the process of disorganization originates in the focal point of a minute and isolated cell only, with what multiple profuseness may not the mischief extend when it spreads the subtle principles of contagion to every vesicle within the reach of its poisoning secretion. It cannot, therefore, be maintained that such a source is a germ too inconsiderable to produce those giant consequences of disease which are required to endanger the stability of the whole body. But suppose the existence of a morbid cause, operating from the beginning on a more extensive scale, and myriads of these ultimate cells to suffer at once from impaired or suspended function, what formidable magnitude may not the mischief rapidly assume ! Does not fever, in all its phases, present us with a striking instance of a disease which prosecutes the work of destruction on the grandest and most formidable scale ? All the organic processes are involved in one common consequence : whatever its nature, or in whatever quarter it may originate, it cannot be questioned that it affects injuriously the nutrient and secerning agency of every *cell* in the body. A morbid growth, confined only to a small part, deriving its commencement from a diseased action, which some accidentally-applied cause may have entailed upon a few of the ultimate cells of the affected structure, furnishes an example of local deviations from the healthy standard which may occur in the character and office of the ultimate organs of nutrition.

Before proceeding to the consideration of the particular

cases of disease which the microscope succeeds in demonstrating in these miniature organs, it is desirable to state briefly the organic laws to which they, in common with larger masses, are subjected.

A definite scale of development is assigned to the primary organic cells proper to the various structures of the body. The cells of the blood, the liver, the mucus, and other structures, therefore pass systematically through prescribed gradations of growth; and, in the natural state, the duration of their life-period is equally pre-limited and ordained. The parenchymal cells of all glandular organs demonstrably attain a given stage of evolution when the natural consequence of dehiscence occurs, by which their contents are contributed towards the general sum of the secretion. The typical elements of an organic primary cell are three only:

Fig. 1.

Primitive Cell.

a Cell-membrane.   *b* Nucleus.   *c* Nucleolus.

first, an external sac, then a smaller vesicle, which contains a third. In general physiological language, when speaking of the ultimate cells of the various structures of animals and vegetables, the first is designated the cell-membrane; the second the nucleus; and the third the nucleolus. When, however, the description is intended to apply to the *ovum*, although the several parts are identical in absolute and relative characters at this primordial stage, the first is distinguished as the *vitelline capsule*, " membrana vitelli," which contains the yelk intervening between it and the next, which is called the *germinal vesicle*, enclosing the *third*, the *germinal spot* of Purkinge. Raspail employs the terms, " chorion," " amnios," and " embryo," in allusion, respectively, to these three organic elements of the ovum. In the phanerogamic department of the vegetable kingdom, the amnial sac of the ovulum is nearly the counterpart of the *ovum*, contained in the capsule of De Graef in the ovary of the higher animals.

By the significant assistance of three small concentric lines, it is thus practicable definitively to express the profound truth, that a slender tripartite cellule is typical of the common germ from which all animal and vegetable existence proceeds. It is the universal focus of parentage to every individual within the confines of organic nature.

Primary cells propagate themselves by the reproduction of cells similar to themselves. In its pathological relations, this is a very important circumstance: for although it were at present visionary to anticipate any discovery with reference to the nature of that subtle formative agency, which, under one set of condition, obliges the primitive cell to undergo metamorphosis into bone, under another into muscle, and under others into nervous and mucus tissues, &c., it is quite philosophical to acknowledge the authority of this law within certain limits. When the malignant tendency, for example, has been once established in a part, by the organization of a *cancerous primary cell*, in virtue of this extraordinary power, which, from the beginning, inheres in the cell of multiplying its kind, the continuance of the destructive process in the part is certain and inevitable.

Every ultimate vesicle is so far a unity, as that it is capable of isolation from the surrounding cells, yet dependent for its nutrition upon the general circulation. The vital currents of the circulation, therefore, are channels of direct communication, by which every part and cell in the fabric are brought into relation with a common centre, and by which the compound unity of the whole body is established.

These are considerations which will be constantly involved into all subsequent pathological inquiries. Although not susceptible of positive demonstration, all analogy conducts to the inference, that *every cell* is the scene of two descriptions of circulation:—one which may not inappropriately be distinguished by the term "diasmotic[1];" the other *intrinsic*, and strictly nutrient and vital. What can be demonstrated in the example of the simple cells of the *chara*, and

---

([1]) Διὰ, "through," ὠσμὸς, "impulsion;" which signifies simply the transit of a fluid through a membranous partition, without specifically denoting whether the current enters into, or escapes from, a cavity.

many others of the confervæ, is also probably true in regard to the ultimate vesicles of all vegetable and animal structures. The following plan may serve to indicate the principle of this microscopic circulation.

Fig. 2.

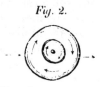

Plan of Cell Circulation.

The nutrient fluid transudes the septum of the *cell* membrane; and either undergoes a concentric movement along its internal surface, or enters into combination with its contents—the vitelline structure—to undergo a preparatory elaboration, before fulfilling the more important office of nourishing the *germinal* vesicle and its contained part. The observations formerly made by Mr. Grainger with respect to the liquefaction of the yelk, preparatory to its absorption by the vasa lutea[1], afford a direct confirmation to this view. It is now obvious, that one of two circumstances may produce disease in those delicate organisms, of which one may affect simply the quality of the nutrient circulating fluid, and the other may be associated with some impediment to its circulation. Under the operation of either of these causes, disease will be entailed on the cell. The labour of primary and secondary assimilation, to employ the language of Prout and Liebig, devolve exclusively upon these ultimate cellules of organic structures. By this cursory physiological analysis of the subject, the desirable service may have been rendered of imbuing the minds of those unfamiliar with microscopic study with the first principles upon which microscopic pathology must found and rest all its future pretensions.

2. It was maintained, for a long period subsequently to the writings of John Hunter and Cullen, that a disordered state of the capillary circulation, called inflammation, was

(¹) Müller's Physiology, by Baly, p.1559: Note by Mr. Grainger and Mr. Dalrymple.

necessary, as a prelude to the occurrence of all morbid organic changes. It is sufficient here to state, that the microscope has introduced, within a comparatively recent period, important revolutions into the doctrines prevalently entertained in regard to the essential character of this process. For present purposes, all the phænomena of which the process consists may be viewed under two divisions; of which the first includes all the changes, *mechanical*, chemical, and vital, which the blood undergoes *before* its escape from the channel of the capillary vessel; the second, those organic, or rather organizing changes which the *plasma* (liquor sanguinis), the material which has transuded the parietes of the capillary vessel as a *consequence* of the antecedent condition of the blood *within* the vessels, more or less rapidly puts on. This appears to be a determinate and natural classification of the familiar phænomena constituting the sum of this singular and useful organic process. Whatever may be the attendant conditions in relation to the chemical and vital composition of the liquor sanguinis, the truth of the circumstance may be admitted, as Magendie expresses it, that " du moment qu'il existe un défaut d'harmonie entre le diamètre des capillaries et le volume des molécules sanguines, des obstructions surviennent, et *alors* apparaissent les caractères de l'inflammation[2]." It is scarcely necessary to contend, that there can be no direct relation between the process of organization which proceeds in the effused plasma, and the conditions affecting only the *contents* of the capillaries which led to that effusion : of course, the *quality* of the pabulum will impose a corresponding stamp upon the character of the organizing process which it is designed to maintain. This circumstance, however, it will at once be seen, does not alter the meaning of the preceding statement. Now the whole tendency of modern innovations in the fundamental doctrines of physiology countenances no other view than that which requires that the process of organization, through the inter-agency of cells, which takes place in all cases in the inflammatory product, should be regarded as essentially one of nutrition, ultimately conforming, in all its necessary conditions, with those which

(2) Lectures on the Blood.

regulate and determine the process of primary "assimilation" (structural renovation), at every moment and in every part of the body. The term "inflammation," therefore, whatever meaning it may etymologically or practically convey, is applicable only to the abnormal phænomena which are referable to the deviations from health, which happen *within* the channels of the capillary system. On this occasion it is proposed only to investigate the changes which the liquor sanguinis undergoes subsequently to its effusion upon the open inflammatory surface.

So far there is some concurrence and agreement in the results of observations, as conducted by Professor Gerber, Mr. Gulliver, and Dr. Martin Barry, that they describe the presence of corpuscles which arise in and from the semi-fluid plasma, primitively under the character of minute amorphous molecules, which enter into determinate groups and combinations, out of which corpuscles of considerable magnitude are evolved, for which the name of *exudation-corpuscle* has been proposed.

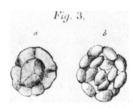

Fig. 3.

a Exudation-corpuscle, in process of division into pus-corpuscles.
b More advanced stage : mag. 1300 diameters.

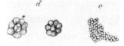

d Exudation-corpuscles in contact with the inflamed living surface.
e Granules found in liq. sanguinis, when removed from the influence of the living surface.

These bodies, according to the views of Gerber and Gulliver, are destined, under favourable conditions, to undergo transformation into *cells*, and other organic elements of more elaborate structure than themselves ; but under the opposite circumstances of disease, they are stated to resolve themselves into *pus-globules*[1]. When the effusion occurs in sufficient quantity upon the free surface of an inflamed part, these peculiar corpuscles are formed in corresponding abundance, and, adhering to each other in a stratiform manner, form successive orders of superimposed layers, presenting the steps of organization in different stages of advancement.

By many observers these exudation-corpuscles are maintained to be identical with the colourless corpuscles of the blood: their identity, however, is by no means obvious. The theory of transformation proposed by Gerber is implicitly adopted by Dr. Carpenter; advocated on a much more extended scale by Dr. M. Barry; and, after submitting it to certain modifications, wrought out to further applications by Mr. Addison. It is not here presumed to impugn the general accuracy of these excellent observers; but since every endeavour to re-observe these alleged metamorphoses uniformly proves fruitless, it certainly by no means can be expected, that a servile admission of their truth should be made. Whatever may be their source, or the mechanism of their production, pus-globules, as defined by the superior instrument in use at this hospital, present the following physical characters:—

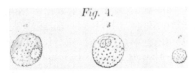

Fig. 4.

a   Corpuscle, with single nucleus: Cell-membrane, crenated, but not mulberry-like, as shewn by Gerber, *Fig.* 3. *b.*

b   The double nucleated corpuscle.

c   Non-nucleated, smaller-sized corpuscle.

They are more or less perfectly orbicular *cells;* the *external* surface of which is studded with granules, which sometimes are so obvious as to impart a *crenated character* to the cell-capsule, for the most part furnished with a nucleus, sometimes with two nuclei: under other conditions it is altogether destitute of nucleus. Generally, the cell

([1]) I have here introduced the figures in Gerber's work, illustrative of the exudation-corpuscle in the act of resolving itself, by fissiparous multiplication, into pus-corpuscles. (Fig. 3.)

contains but few primitive molecules; according to the number
of which, its degree of pellucidity and transparency is determined. The three varieties, here represented as the most
common and prevalent modifications which the true pus-
corpuscle assumes, appear, from the local and constitutional
circumstances under which the peculiarities are respectively
generated, to be determined essentially by differences in the
organic qualities of the matrix or blastema from which they
immediately spring. The uni-nuclear corpuscle, which exhibits all the indications of a definitively-organized structure,
is always found in the secretion which bathes the surface of
a recent healthy suppurating wound : it may indeed, in conformity with the vernacular conventionalities of surgery, be
called a *laudable corpuscle*. The second variety—the binu-
cleated—is most frequently discovered in recent phlegmo-
neous collections of pus in a healthy actively-produced
abscess. The third form, in which the nucleus body is altogether absent, occurs in the ill-conditioned secretion of old
chronic and unhealthy wounds : the cell capsule also, in this
description, is very attenuated, and the contained granules
few in number ; all conspiring as indications of an inferior and
imperfect organization. It is evident from these facts, which
so clearly tell the tale of the patient's condition — or, in
more scientific language, which so explicitly express the measure of organizing power possessed by the product of the
local excitement—that it would obviously harmonize with the
best principles of surgery to maintain that the *double nuclei*
are evidences of a high standard of organization in these
varieties of corpuscles. No pupil in this school requires to
be lessoned into a knowledge of the elementary truth, that
the state of an ulcer is a significant and valuable exponent of
the measure of organizing or healing power enjoyed by the
general system. It is by the detection of such happy coincidences between the demonstrations of this splendid auxiliary
(the microscope) to man's limited and myopic sense, and the
results of rational and inductive experience, that its practical value and useful applications can be rendered convincing.
There is a remarkable analogy between the most inferiorly-
organized pus-corpuscle and the *mucous* globules.

Fig. 5.

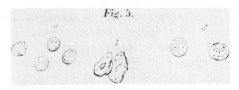

a Globules of healthy mucus from the nose.
b Epithelium scales.   *d* Other varieties.

a Mucous globules.   *a′* Most numerous in inflamed mucus.
b Altered epithelium scale.

These likewise are orbicular bodies, sometimes endowed with a nucleus, and sometimes destitute of this part. In pus, as well as mucous globules, the position of the nucleus, with respect to the mathematical centre of the vitelline capsule, presents several variations: sometimes it is quite central; sometimes more or less excentric; and frequently it is observed to be adherent to the parietes of the vitelline or cell-membrane. There is no doubt that this little circumstance should be interpreted into a proof, whether normal or diseased, of organic distinction between these varieties of corpuscles. It is a remarkable and most interesting fact, that the corpuscles found in inflamed and healthy mucus, as indicated in the preceding sketches, manifest no structural, physical differences: in mucus, however, produced by an inflamed surface, they are considerably more numerous than in the healthy secretion. Without observing the homage which the fascinating plausibilities of many ingeniously-pictured theories almost constrain us to pay, may it not be safely said of the fact just expressed, that it proves that *inflammation*, especially when attacking an extended open surface, like a mucous tract, consists essentially of nothing more than a preternatural stimulus or impulse received by the affected part, under which its natural functions acquire such an unusual augmentation, that the process is typically and truly one of *vigorous nutrition*.

When an effusion of liquor sanguinis, dissolved in a large quantity of *serum*, takes place, as in pleurisy, peritonitis, and

pericarditis, a membranous *layer* of tenacious substance is
deposited upon the inflamed surface, in quite a mechanical
manner.   This is found to consist of extremely delicate filaments, intersecting each other in every possible direction,
and corresponding in every particular with the fibrils existing
in any clot of fibrine.

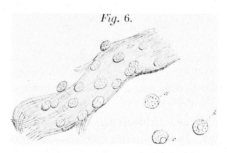

Fig. 6.

*Plastic Product of Peritoneal Inflammation, a fasciculus of delicate
fibrils, including numerous non-nucleated pus-corpuscles.*

a Detached corpuscle.   *b* Pus-globule, with central nucleus.
c Pus-globule, with excentric nucleus.

The meshes of the filaments are occupied by globules of pus,
which bear a very close resemblance to the corpuscles of
mucus, or to the low-organized pus: this circumstance probably depends upon the dilution of the liquor sanguinis with
serum.   But whether so or not, these microscopic analogies
between the solid organized constituents of certain varieties
of pus and mucus may certainly be regarded as proofs additional to, and confirmatory of, the results originally obtained
by the experiments of Dr. Babington[1]; and subsequently, by
the observations of Dr. Golding Bird[2] and Dr. Rees, in reference to the ready convertibility of pus and mucus.   In diameter, the corpuscles of pus exceed by about three times those
of the red particles of the blood.   By most physiologists, this
fact is construed into an evidence of the mechanical difficulty
which must oppose the escape of the corpuscle, as such,
ready formed, from the interior of the capillary vessel: and
since, by the recent improvements in the art of minute injection, anatomists, having acquainted themselves with the

(1) **Guy's Hospital Reports**, October 1837.   (2) Ibid. April 1838.

measurement and characters of nearly all the capillaries of
the body, have now the means in their possession of ascertaining the relation between the volume of the red particles
and pus-corpuscles, and the diameter of the capillary channel; and therefore of determining and settling the question,
that it is impossible for a full-grown pus-corpuscle to *circu-
late* through a capillary vessel; and consequently, that it could
not have thus originated in the liquor sanguinis whilst yet
contained within the vessels. It is well known, that Müller long
since, with his characteristic labour and originality of argu-
ment, which in the present day would be deemed supereroga-
tory, has gravely marshalled every fact, orthodox in physiology
at the period at which he wrote, in maintenance of the position
that pus-corpuscles are *generated* by a process of organization
in the *product* of the disordered secretion of the part; —
a theory which is directly opposed to the views of those, who
regard pus as a morbid *secretion* proceeding immediately,
and ready elaborated, from the blood. The rapid advances,
which the *cell theory* of nutrition and secretion has recently
made, have rendered quite untenable the idea that elaborated
pus can pre-exist in the blood. The ascertained evidence
with respect to the production of pathological fluids is yet
too limited to allow any generalisations; but it may be
confidently stated, that the ultimate pus-corpuscle finds no
corresponding element or analogue in any normal tissue or
fluid in the body. In the developed state, therefore, it is unquestionably heterologous from, and alien to, all the healthy
and ordinary ultimate constituents of structure. Its departure in physical characters from the cells normal and proper to the part, on which the pus-corpuscle is formed, may be
due to the operation of one of two causes: either the corpuscle, ab origine, must be produced, constructed in its earliest germ on faulty principles, and from a matrix of morbid
quality; or its first production must be in strict accordance
with the natural cell-forming process of the part, but that
subsequently, under the agency of some unhealthy influence,
the development of the particle is completed on a perverted,
although determinate, plan [3].

[3] In a *future Report,* a further and more matured microscopic history
will be given of the various pathological fluids, or morbid secretions.

Considerable labour and attention have recently been devoted to the subject of the chemical analysis of purulent fluids by the French chemists M. Darcet and M. Conte. They appear to concur in the conclusion, that these fluids contain but a very small proportion of fibrine, whilst they afford a considerable proportion of albumen. Is it not probable that this circumstance—the paucity, namely, of *organizing material* (fibrine)—may afford some explanation of the *slender* inferiorly-organized character of the pus-corpuscle?

Cells of the Liver [1].—The liver abounds in large, well-defined, spheroïdal cells, having distinctly a biliary tinge, and a considerable quantity of granular amorphous material. These are the elements which the microscope recognises, whenever a portion of the organ is torn up and examined with the higher powers. The accompanying figures are designed to exhibit the characters of these cells; which may be appropriately called the parenchymal cells of the organ, since they constitute a considerable portion of the mass of the liver, and possess distinctive characters. They present the peculiarity

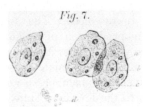

Fig. 7.

Ultimate Glandular Cells of the Liver, having a yellow tinge.

a Nucleus.   *b* Nucleolus.   *c* Adipose particles.
d Primitive molecules surrounding and contained in the cells.

of having in their interior, as one of their normal constituents, adipose particles, which vary remarkably in number and size.

From the unusual magnitude of these cells (varying from $\frac{1}{1500}$th to $\frac{1}{2000}$th linear), which may be completely defined by the $\frac{1}{4}$th objective and low eye-piece, and the tenuity and trans-

<hr />

([1]) The following observations on the morbid anatomy of the cells of the liver were commenced and prosecuted mainly at the request of Dr. Addison; to whom a separate ward in the hospital has been appropriated, for the investigation of hepatic disease.

parency of the cell-capsule, rendering thus practicable a clear examination of their contents, the changes wrought by disease can be most satisfactorily observed. Indeed, the liver should be selected, as the organ which affords the best opportunities for the prosecution of the interesting subject relating to the *pathology* of cells. The existence of fatty particles in the interior of the hepatic cells was determined indepently by Henle and Erasmus Wilson; but the credit of first demonstrating the pathological bearing of this discovery is due to Mr. Bowman[2]: (Medical Gazette, Jan. 1842.) In his short communication on this subject he announced the fact, that in the proportion of one-third of the total number of cases of phthisical disorganization of the lungs, the epithelium cells of the liver become gorged more or less with adipose particles. Mr. Bowman's inquiries appear not to have extended beyond the simple determination of this fact —a fact which, it may here be remarked, has been repeatedly verified at this hospital during the progress of our microscopic observations. There are, however, several interesting points, both as respects the morbid anatomy of the cell itself, and the general considerations associated with this state of fatty degeneration to which it is liable, which yet remains to be stated.

(2) It must, however, be remembered, that Mr. Bowman's claim to discovery relates only to the microscopic fact of having shewn that the accumulation of fat in this state of the organ is due to its preternatural formation *within* the hepatic cells. But as far as my acquaintance with the literature of the subject extends, it is to Dr. Addison that the Profession is indebted for materially adding to our knowledge with respect to this state of *fatty degeneration* to which the liver is liable. In a former number of Guy's Hospital Reports, he pointed out that this species of degeneration was not a constant attendant upon phthisical disorganization of the lungs;—that it could not be regarded as a *necessary* and direct consequence of the pulmonary disorganization, for it may happen when the lungs are quite healthy. He conceives that its production is associated with a scrofulous predisposition, of which the formation of tubercle is but a *local* indication, *like the fatty change in the liver;* but that the occurrence of this latter change is *facilitated, rendered more probable,* when preceded by tuberculous disorganization of the lungs. In that communication, also, Dr. Addison enumerated the diagnostic marks which, according to his experience, were the most valuable evidences on which to predicate the existence of this fatty condition of the organ.

Fig. 8.

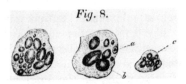

Hepatic Cell gorged with fat.

a Atrophied nucleus.　　　　　*b* Adipose cells.
c Hepatic cell arrested in its development by the undue formation of fat.

The simple condition of fatty engorgement is illustrated
in the accompanying cut. It is a singular circumstance in
the history of the parenchymal cell in this disease, that a
fat globule, however minute, has never yet been discovered
in the interior of the *nuclear cell*. It invariably occupies and
thrives in the interval between the nucleus and the *outer*
capsule or cell-membrane: so that its situation precisely
corresponds with that cavity of the *ovum* which is occupied
by the vitellus. What distant physiological analogy or correlation there may be between the fat in the hepatic cell and
the vitelline, or *oil* globules in the ovum, is an interesting
proposition, which may be referred to the genius of those
skilled in the science of inductive philosophy: but the
coincidence of anatomical position is certainly not unworthy
of remark. In regard to the mechanism of the secerning
process, of which these ultimate cells are unquestionably the
seat, the circumstance relating to the situation of the fat
appears to sanction the following conclusions;—that the
adipose matter is either *secreted*, as a ready-elaborated proximate principle, by the vitelline or cell membrane; or that
the elements of fat, unelaborated, attain in common, and
mingled with other principles, the chamber of the *outer cell*,
when its elements spontaneously individualise themselves,
and enter into new and high combinations: that the *nuclear*
capsule is either proof against the entrance of the adipose
principles, or that the nucleus has not yet attained that degree of development, at which it is endued with the property
of secreting *fat*. Then, if the former corollary be admitted, it
must be further allowed that the outer cell-capsule possesses
the power of *determining the production* of the numerous
primitive molecules and the bile-coloured fluid, which its
chamber contains.

During these observations, the following positions were also arrived at: that the nucleus completely disappears under the *pressure* of the increasing fatty accumulation;—that the primitive molecules, which, in the healthy condition, the hepatic cell contains in obvious quantity, undergo absorption, and disappear in proportion as the adipose particles augment in number and volume;—that with the disappearance of the primitive molecules, the *yellow tinge* or *bile-colour* of the cell also disappears. During the prosecution of these observations, the idea was suggested and sustained, by various kinds of evidence, that in these cells the *nucleus* could not be viewed as *parentally*, but rather as filially related to the vitelline capsules; that it was rather the expanding germ of a future generation of cells, than the withered remnant of one passing away; consequently, that the *nucleus* participated in no way in the secerning operation of the developed cell. Several facts will be adduced in the following account, which tend to support the validity of the preceding positions. During the progress of fatty degeneration of the liver, there is no difficulty in establishing the circumstance, that the parenchymal cells, in which considerable distention by the fat produced has occurred, can no longer retain the power of sustaining their accustomed part in the process of secretion, and that eventually they must *burst*. As these disorganizing changes—for they must be actually regarded as such—proceed, it is quite evident that a universal suspension of the secreting agency will take place; so that the last avenue for the elimination of carbon from the blood suffers fatal obstruction, and the lungs and the liver, being thus involved in the common ruinous incapacity for labour, the whole body is precipitated in the wreck, which the rapid and unrestrained accumulation of carbon in the blood must occasion. At the earlier stage of the history of this complicated succession of changes, the undue development of fat in the liver, under the gradual failure of the respiratory agency of the lungs, was obviously a protective alternative; but during the subsequent steps of their progress the remedy becomes a poison; and the struggling system, now deprived of the agency of two important organs, is soon overwhelmed by the consequences. Fat contains about 80 per cent. of carbon;

and carbonic acid contains 6 of carbon in every 22 parts. It is therefore not difficult to perceive, that when these two great channels for the removal of carbon from the system are blockaded by accumulated disease, the injurious influence of the retained carbon must be as fatal as its production is rapid. No enlightened pathologist can question the value of these considerations, with respect to the *effects* on the general system, and the pathology of tuberculous disorganization of the lungs, to which these consequent changes in the structure of the liver so obviously conduct.

Additional proofs to those hitherto adduced by microscopic physiology, tending to establish the true *glandular* agency of the hepatic nucleated cells, which appear to possess no inconsiderable physiological value, were recently brought to light in this hospital, during the examination of a person[1] who died of a malignant disease of the duodenal extremity of the pancreas; which exerted such forcible pressure upon the common excretory duct, that the passage of the bile into the duodenum had become almost impossible; at all events, it could only have escaped by very slow degrees, and in very small quantity. The consequences which directly resulted from this obstruction were manifest in the extreme distention of the biliary ducts and gall-bladder, which necessarily caused a considerable increase in the volume of the whole organ: the liver had lost its fragile, solid character, and had become soft, flabby, and not capable of being easily broken down by pressure. On the application of the microscope for the purpose of examining the ultimate structure, the extraordinary fact was developed, that scarcely a *single* nucleated glandular cell, in a perfect state, could be found. Different portions of the organs were carefully and repeatedly prepared, in order to remove every possibility of mistake or mis-observation: the conclusions were uniformly the same, that the true parenchymal cells of the organ were certainly *not present*. These preparations were also seen and examined

(1) For the particulars relating to the examination of this person (Anne Seymour, Lydia Ward, May 22, 1843, patient of Dr. Addison) I must direct the reader to the "Post-mortem Register" kept by Mr. King. Preparations of the liver are contained in the microscopic cabinet of the hospital, by means of which the changes described in the text may be demonstrated and authenticated.

by several excellent observers about the hospital. In each portion of the organ mounted for inspection, nothing more than minute *free* fatty particles, and equally free, floating, amorphous, granular matter, could be discovered: it was very seldom that a *whole* nucleated cell could be seen. The following cut may serve to convey a conception of the microscopic characters of these objects.

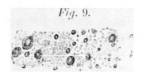

Fig. 9.

Ultimate Structure of the Liver in Jaundice from nearly complete obstruction.

a Fat particles, free.   b Primitive molecules, free.

There seems to be but one inference to be deduced from the indisputable facts which the microscope has elicited in this case; that, namely, in consequence of the excessive distention from retained secretion, to which the whole organ was subjected, the ultimate cells, exposed to the *arrière* force of this universal pressure, whilst the process of adding to their contents by secretion suffered no cessation, had undergone universal dehiscence. It is evident, that if a continually-acting mechanical obstacle to the *gradual* escape of their contents, or if their *progressive* and natural dehiscence be rendered impossible, the consequences of the universal rupturing of the pregnant cells must inevitably follow. But whatever may be said of the adequacy of the proposed explanation, it would be scarcely reasonable, with reference to this case, to dispute the two circumstances, that the mechanical obstruction created by the pancreatic tumor *produced* the effects in the structural elements of the liver, the details of which have now been described. The adipose particles are normal and legitimate *inmates* of the cells; and when they are observed in a liberated state, what other conclusion can be supported than that they have escaped by the mechanical dissolution of the *cell* capsule? The history of these singular facts reminds us strongly of how adroitly nature sometimes, when the science and skill of the physician are no more than ornamental sounds, mitigates the severity of consequences which cannot be averted, by blending their occurrence with others of an opposite tendency. The extensive injury, which the liver must have sustained by this extensive and violent dehiscence of its cells, had the temporary effect of preventing further accumulation of secretion, by suppressing the stream at its origin. The fact of this dehiscence appears conclusively to prove that the secretion of the liver is really and immediately due to the agency of these nucleated cells, and that the contents of these cells consist of *bona-fide* bile.

That the *adipose* contents of these cells is destined to constitute a portion of the hepatic secretion may be regarded as fully determined by the recent analyses of bile carefully conducted by Berzelius himself. He has shewn that this secretion, as obtained from the gall-bladder, contains oleate, margarate, and stearate of soda; or, in other language, saponified fat. To complete the determination of its presence, he has further proved that the glycerine, separated from this saponified fat, is also present. In these examinations, it has been several times observed, that when the obstacle to the outflow of the secretion is only partial[1], the parenchymal cells are seen as more prominent objects, exhibiting evidently the indications of an increased size from retained secretion. In these cases the *yellow colour* is most obvious. The conclusion has been invariably arrived at, that the depth of the yellow colour, which most probably is dependent upon the collection within the cells of actually elaborated bile, is proportionate to the *number* or quantity of granular matter which the *cell* contains; and is equally diffused throughout the cell, *excepting the interior of the nucleus*, which appears yellow only so far as it derives its tinge from the surrounding molecules.

In *fever*, the adipose globules almost completely disappear from the cells of the liver. In its relation to organic chemistry no trifling interest attaches to this fact.

[1] Several cases of jaundice, from biliary calculi, have been examined.

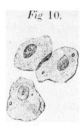

Hepatic Cells in Fever, almost entirely destitute of fat particles.

The absorption of fat from the hepatic cells in fever may be viewed as a circumstance, in reference to its physiological relations, which depends upon conditions exactly the converse of those obtaining in cases of disorganization of the lungs. The latter organs being reduced to a state more or less completely of disuse, the liver becomes burdened by vicarious labour. In *fever*, on the contrary, from the exalted condition of the respiratory agency, the rapid circulation and highly-oxidized state of the blood, the decarbonizing function of the liver is little required. All the stagnant carbon of the body, and consequently that situated in the interior of the hepatic cells in the form of fat, submitted thus to the direct chemical agency of an immense amount of the free or unemployed oxygen with which the blood is impregnated, is pressed into rapid chemical combination, and carbonic acid and water are the products[2]. An equivalent of fat consists of $\begin{Bmatrix} C. & 11 \\ H. & 12 \\ O. & \end{Bmatrix}$: it would therefore require, to produce the transformations of which we speak, 30 equivalents of oxygen; 22 equivalents to convert 11 equivalents of carbon into carbonic acid; and 12 equivalents to produce water with the hydrogen. From this estimate, an approximative conception may be formed of the unnatural excitement which must pervade all the organic processes in fever. Of course, this accelerated state of the respiratory and circulating systems must be sustained by secondary and hidden *organic* changes in the structural composition of the several elements of the body. These are

[2] A similar view, in reference to the hyperoxidized state of the blood in fever, has been ingeniously supported by Mr. Coventry, Surgeon, of Clapham.— *Medical Gazette, Aug.* 26, 1842.

changes, however, which pathological science has not yet
unfolded, even to the most foresighted inquirer. The preceding explanation of the conditions leading to the removal
of the fatty particles from the cells of the liver, in fever, is
rendered probable by the truths derived from comparative
anatomy. In insects and birds the hepatic apparatus is relatively small; but this inferior size, and therefore its limited
decarbonizing agency, has immediate reference to the proportionably increased development of the breathing system.
In mollusca and fishes, in which the standard of respiration
is low and aquatic, the reverse of these physiological depen-
dencies prevails. This view likewise comprehends the
theory, as Liebig has already shewn, on which the greater
morbid liabilities of the liver in intra-tropical countries are
to be explained.

There is one more fact, in connection with the morbid
anatomy of the *hepatic cells*, which it seems desirable to communicate. The liver is liable to a disease which is called
simply a " granular state of the organ." These granules are
small bodies of the same size precisely with the lobuli of the
liver, projecting in relief from the surface of the organ, as
dirty-white, changed *lobuli*, or white scrofulous tubercles.
By selecting, by means of a pointed instrument, nothing but
a portion of these white bodies, their microscopic structure
can be separately inspected. The whole substance of each
portion examined consisted of cells of varying figure and
magnitude, of which *many*, however, exhibited all the characters of the true hepatic *cell*, but differing from the latter
in the *absence* of that most obvious of all its distinguishing
marks, the yellow colour. In all instances in which no
healthy part of the liver had been taken up with the diseased, the cells were wholly destitute of the yellow colour.
The following sketch will shew the characters of these objects.

Fig. 11.

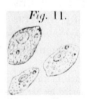

*Hepatic Cells in Granular Liver, transparent: molecules few, and
destitute of the yellow tinge.*

Notwithstanding the absence of that *colour*, which is naturally imparted to the *cell* by the presence of the bile in its interior, there was no difficulty in identifying these as really altered hepatic cells: the other varieties may be still further modifications. It will be seen that the adipose particles are present; and this is a striking identifying circumstance. From the *pale* transparent state of the particle, and the small proportion of primitive molecules contained, the inference appears quite legitimate, that the condition of the ultimate cell observed in this case realizes all the physical appearances which the simple circumstance of the *suppression of bile* could induce. It further leads to the suspicion, that *originally*, in the chamber of the primitive elaborating cell, the *adipose* is produced independently of the other principles of the bile, although subsequently, in the process of elimination, they become mutually admingled. The idea of an actual suppression of an organ's function can only be entertained by reference to the remotest, the very first *link* in the complicated succession of parts, the integrity and harmony of which are presupposed in its proper execution. These cells, according to the testimony of every species of evidence yet obtained, are actually engaged in the process of secreting the bile. Disease, therefore, seated in them, mutilates the tenderest elements in the machinery of the gland, and those, too, most essential to the continuance of the secerning process.

Morbid growths.—There are two significations in which the term "heterology" may be used in pathological science: the first may be illustrated by a formation anatomically different from the structure in and from which it grows. When the coat of an artery, the subpleural tissue, or the dura mater undergoes ossification, the osseous product of the change is *heterologous* from the part in which it is formed. Yet, although alien to this particular spot, it is, notwithstanding, *homologous* to the structure of some *other* system of *organs.* In structural character, therefore, it is not *absolutely*, but only relatively heterologous. If, however, an organ, or part, become the seat of an unnatural growth, the structural characters of which are essentially and wholly *unlike every form of tissue* which is natural to the body, such a morbid production becomes *absolutely* heterologous and heteromorphous. This definition is not sufficiently unexceptionable to justify, upon its basis, the construction of a syllogistic generalization, although the approximative proposition may be expressed, that malignant formations are all absolutely heterologous: all varieties of carcinoma are malignant, therefore they must be absolutely heterologous. In the succeeding observations, it will be presumed that the reader is familiar with the doctrines of Müller in relation to the growth and propagation of malignant disease by the multiplication of *cells.* These views are implicitly founded upon the discoveries of Schwann with reference to the anatomical and physiological history of *cells.*

A malignant growth, although heteromorphous, is not parasitical, for its vessels and nerves are continuous with, and part of, the body: viewed as a *whole,* it is not structurally independent of the general system; but if a single one of its ultimate cells be taken, it may, with undoubted accuracy, be said, with respect to it, that it was an independent and separate organism, as much so as an hydatid. The very same statement, however, may, with equal correctness, be made of *every* ultimate cell in the body; so that the whole body, in actual reality, is a vast compound fabric, like the habitation of alcyonidal polypes, the integral parts of which are made up of separate and individual existences, which are united by the bonds of common centres of sympathy and nutrition. But the *cell* of a malignant growth is distinguished by this singularity: it not only departs in microscopic figure from the normal surrounding cells, it violates also the laws of increase and multiplication, which regulate all the ultimate elements of the economy; it usurps the power of multiplying its species on a new and independent plan, a plan over which the principles of organic nutrition have no controul: so far, then, the morbid growth possesses a *physiological* independence of the body in which it is found. There is no capricious and singular irregularity in its modes of production and growth. This is established by the historical circumstance, that cancer, in all its formidable varieties, occurs under precisely the same characters in the present day as a hundred years ago. *All varieties* of carcinoma are reducible to *three species*—the encephaloïd, the schirroïd, and the colloïd. The microscope proves that the ultimate elements of structure in these several species, in all cases, present a striking uniformity of character. Chemical analysis has repeatedly confirmed the position, that all cancerous tumors abound in albumen (Hecht). Gelatine is contained in greater proportion in schirroïd than the encephaloïd species. Fat has never yet been demonstrated as an element of carcinomatous tumors. Malignant disease is distinguished by the peculiarity, that, after artificial removal, it manifests the constant tendency to re-appear in the same part. In true malignant disease, the system exhibits proofs, in the universal disturbance of its organic processes, that its various functions are involved more deeply than *simple* local irritation and local pain could possibly occasion. There is no indefinite mysticism or vagueness about these facts. In their collective testimony, they may be regarded as a ground, on which confidently to rest the anticipation, that the time will come, when all the phænomena of malignant disease will be assembled under, and referred to, fixed and determinate laws; and it is by the assistance of the microscope that this great object is mainly to be accomplished. The opportunities hitherto afforded at this hospital of examining malignant disease by means of the microscope have been limited: as formerly stated, therefore, the present article is designed only as the introduction to future and more matured and repeated observations. In his valuable monograph on morbid growths, Müller's merit appears in the capacity of a simple descriptive microscopist. He has not opened to view one really new position in regard to their essential organic relations—*why* and *how* a malignant growth is originally formed. Hypotheses are the beacons of discovery. They should be regarded as theorems resting on doubtful conditions: they thus become objects of direct consideration to the mind, and all the force of its concentrated attention is devoted to their establishment or refutation. This exertion must redound to the advantage, if not to the extension, of science. There are two plain and intelligible propositions to be enunciated, in introducing ourselves to the study of this difficult subject.

When a malignant disease commences in a part, the *cell* which is its germ may originally be physically the same as those of the cells of the healthy structures around ; but, that, in consequence of a perversion of growth, its development may become arrested at a particular stage, or it may assume, *in the progress of growth*, a permanently new and hetero-morphous figure.   This form of cell, immediately assuming the character of permanency, may rapidly multiply, and transmit its type to all succeeding generations of cells pro-duced by the diseased part, the accumulated sum of which constitutes the morbid growth.   The second position requires that the changes tending to the production of the morbid growth should commence at a state of more refined remote-ness : it supposes that the *material*—the blastema, or perhaps, in plainer terms, the *liquor sanguinis*—being vitiated in *quality*, in virtue of the *cachexia cancerosa*, the *cell* is faulty, *ab ori-gine*, formed upon an abnormal plan from the earliest be-ginning ; and not, therefore, a monstrosity of the natural *cell*, but an absolutely new and superadded organism.

It is not difficult to perceive that this question, as thus presented, abounds in *nugæ difficiles* numerous enough to gratify the most ardent admirer of hypothetic and erudite enigmas.   When, however, they are soberly viewed, as so many *heads* under which to range all the facts and phæno-mena relating to this profound and important subject, they at once acquire the character of usefulness.

Professor Owen has recently advocated the theory, that an acephalocyst or hydatid " should be truly designated as a gigantic organic cell, and not as a species of animal, even of the simplest kind :" this view he founds upon the circum-stance, that " the knowledge we now possess of the primitive embryonic forms of all animals, and of all animal tissues, places us in the position to take a true view of the nature of the acephalocyst [1]."

An acephalocyst consists of a sub-globular oval vesicle, filled with fluid, exhibiting a few pellucid points on its external

[1] Hunterian Lectures on the Comparative Anatomy and Physiology of Invertebrate Animals, 1843.

Fig. 12.

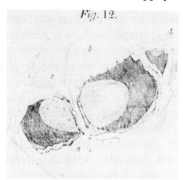

Acephalocyst (after OWEN).
a   The containing cavity of condensed tissue.
b b   Acephalocysts.   c Germs of future cysts.

surface, which Professor Owen, from their analogy to the "hyaline" of Dr. M. Barry, believes to be the germs of *new cells*; but which Dr. Hodgkin [2] considers as points of morbid products. An acephalocyst is filled with fluid; and has no *nucleus*, or the remains of one, like the cell of the protococcus, to which Professor Owen compares it : it however bears this resemblance to these low orders of cryptogamia, that the adult cells among these vegetables produce sometimes embryo cysts from their external surface.   Young hydatids do not always escape externally : they are frequently detached into the interior of the primary vesicle in the capsule of which their germs originated; constituting thus the variety which John Hunter called the pill-box hydatid, and Kuhn and Cruvelhier the acephalocystis endogena.   These hydatids have the power of rapidly reproducing their kind, and, in fact, realise all the particulars given in the definition of malignancy; yet surgeons maintain the doctrine, that hydatid testicle is not malignant, but only incurable.   It must be admitted, with Professor Owen, that there is a remarkable similarity between the larger cells of cryptogamic plants and the vesicle of an acephalocyst; but the question is, where is the *proof* that an hydatid is a gigantic organic cell ?   The cell-capsule of an hydatid may consist and be formed of many nucleated cells.   Professor Owen does not state that the

(2) Lectures on Morbid Anatomy, 1836, vol. I. p. 189.

hyaline points, which he describes as the embryo of future
hydatids, really are simple cells — a circumstance which
should be proved, in order to give strength to the resemblance which he points out; or we might as plausibly assert
that the urinary bladder was only a gigantic organic cell,
because it happens to be a hollow viscus containing fluid.
Before proceeding further into the consideration of this subject, it becomes desirable to ascertain what are the real characters of a malignant cell, and the varieties which it is capable
of assuming. A little familiarity with the microscopic history
of the several varieties of carcinoma would be enough to
satisfy any observer that the cells of all the soft or encephaloïd varieties approach more or less obviously to the spindle-
shaped and oval, of which the caudate and orbicular are the

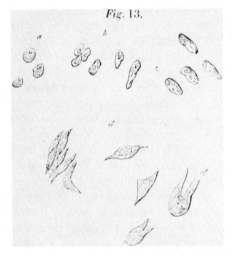

Fig. 13.

Cells characteristic of the Encephaloïd Species of Carcinoma.

a b c d Varieties depending partly upon the age of the cell, and partly upon
differences of anatomical structure in the varieties of the same encephaloïd
species. All partake more or less of the spindle-shaped and caudate figure :
a b c may be viewed as the embryonic stage of *d*, the development of which
may be arrested at the stage *a*, or may be extended until the cell attains the
stage *d* (some of these are copied from Müller).

two extremes of modifications. All the encephaloïd varieties
of cancer, or medullary growths, when examined with the
microscope, are found to present three principal varieties of

cells, differences in the relative proportions of which occasion the varieties of form and general character which the species of carcinoma assumes.

The first variety, as established principally by the observations of Müller, has *cells* of a round and slightly elongated figure, which contain very minute nuclei and granules (fig. 13 *a*): in addition to which, tender transparent fibrils intersect these tumors. This variety is always distinguished by the rapidity of its formation, and its soft, brain-like consistence : examples of it are afforded in struma fungosa testis, medullary sarcoma, and fungus hæmatodes.

The next variety of encephaloïd disease is marked by pale elliptical cells, with a slight tendency to a tail-like or caudate prolongation (fig. 13 *b*). According to Müller, this is a very rare variety : the corpuscles are destitute of nuclei. The third variety is characterized by the spindle-shaped or caudate corpuscles (fig. 13 *d*) : these tumors are always more dense and fibrous than the former. The linear aggregation of these elongated cells would, if compactly disposed, evidently produce fibrous bands. In some instances, therefore, the *filaments*, as well as the cells, must be regarded as truly malignant. In the same specimen it is not unfrequently found that all the varieties of ultimate cells shewn in fig. 13 are present. From this circumstance, it appears quite legitimate to conclude that this series essentially belongs to one and the same order of cells, and that the apparent dissimilarities manifested by the several individuals depend upon differences simply of age. In process of development, *a* probably becomes *b*, and this subsequently assumes the more matured characters of *c*, until, ultimately, the adult characters represented at *d* would result. Now, let the supposition be hypothetically entertained, that *a*, the first and youngest of these varieties, after having vigorously attained the stage of childhood, were suddenly to sustain an arrest or check of growth, but, notwithstanding its dwarfish and diminutive proportions, it were still to enjoy the power of reproduction — of reproducing, *too, its kind*, although it may be the *dwarf* only of a larger species ;—is it not evident, that a tumor made up of such cells would be distinguished by mechanical and anatomical characters extremely unlike another whose component cells were long,

spindle-shaped, or caudate and bicaudate, admitting thus of
more compact aggregation than the weakly-organized circular variety?—and can it be affirmed that the history of development affords no grounds, no principles, on which to advo-
cate the tenability of such views?   Although, on a more
palpable scale, the principle of development is in no particular
different from that which checks the prescribed evolution of
the palate or the lip—from that which operates on the insig-
nificancy of an ultimate cell, and forbids the progress of its
destined growth.   Let the examination, however, be extended to other species of malignant formation.

Fig. 14.

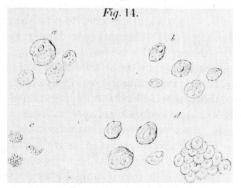

Cells characteristic of the Schirroïd Species of Carcinoma.
Shewing the circular—round—to be the prevailing figure, generally provided
with a well-marked nucleus. Sometimes this is double, sometimes absent, the
cells assuming a transparent pellucid character.

In the schirroïd varieties of carcinoma, the prevailing or
predominant figures in the ultimate cell are the orbicular
and circular.   In all the sub-varieties, the cells are more or
less completely reducible to this conformation: the stone-
like density of schirrus is due to the fibrous stroma, in the
meshes of which the true cancerous cells are contained.
These intersecting stromatous fibres, according to the opinion
of the best authors, cannot be considered a part of the malignant growth: they contend that they consist of the proper
structures of the part, thickened, tightened, and otherwise
altered by the local agency of disease.
    The cells of schirrous carcinoma are furnished, for the
most part, with nuclei and nucleoli.   It should never be

forgotten, that the presence or absence of a nucleus, or even difference in its *size* and *position*, constitute real and organic dissimilarities between individual cells. It may be observed, from the varieties of cells here shewn, that in one, *a*, the nucleus is small, pellucid, and indistinct; the cell altogether being large, and enclosing *few* primitive molecules: in another, *b*, the *cell* is smaller, and the nucleus larger. Sometimes, too, an orbicular group of primitive molecules, *destitute* of an enclosing *capsule*, are observed: on other occasions the *cells* are endowed with a double nucleus, and present all the indications of a high standard of organization. It is a singular circumstance in the history of *schirrus*, that it occurs solitarily—confined, that is, to one locality: it is slow in its growth, and rarely attains a very large size. The pancreatic sarcoma of Abernethy, the carcinoma reticulare of Müller, the chondroïd cancer of Recamier, are examples of varieties which belong to the species *schirrus*. *Colloïd carcinoma* constitutes a distinct species, and presents an organization more characteristic and distinctive than any of the preceding[1]. It consists of a gelatiniform mass, the structure of which is composed of several orders of definitely-disposed cells, thus:

Fig. 15.

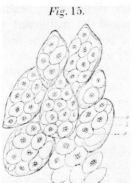

Plan of Cells in Colloïd Carcinoma.

a Primary order of cells.   *b* Secondary.   *o* Tertiary (after Müller).

[1] No examination of this species has recently taken place in this hospital. The account in the text is given on the authority of Müller.

Fig. 16.

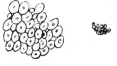

Carcinoma Tuberosa of the Liver, magnified
170 *diameters,*
shewing simple orbicular, nucleated, and
rapidly-multiplying cells.

Mucedinous fungus.

The primary order of cells, fig. 15 *a*, appear under the character of capacious areolæ, enclosing a secondary series, *b*: and, finally, a third system appears as granular nuclei to the second, *c*.

This species manifests a remarkable preference for the muscular structure of the stomach: the characteristic cells are generated at a very early stage, and are less visible at the more advanced.

Fig. 16. is a sketch of the remarkably uniform *orbicular*, nucleated cells, which almost exclusively compose the substance of malignant tubercles of the liver—carcinoma tuberosa of Dr. Farre. It is an important fact in the history of these tubercles, that they implicate very little the proper glandular structure of the liver: healthy hepatic tissue may immediately surround the malignant growth: the tubercles arise in different portions of the organ, from independent centres of growth; and the cells proceed rapidly on the work of multiplication. These observations were made upon a case which some time since occurred in this hospital. The cells are as uniform and regular as those of the colloïd species of cancer. In encephaloïd disease of the *ovarium*, as it was lately shewn in our observations, a species of compound cell may be found which bears no distinct analogy in plan to those of colloïd cancer. It consists of a large oval capsule, measuring $\frac{1}{785}$ of an inch in its long diameter; and distended with small orbicular nucleated cellules, measuring about $\frac{1}{3000}$ linear. In addition to which, however, this ovarian tumor abounded in the characteristic encephaloïd caudate cells. The very counterpart of this compound cell was also discovered here, lately, in the yellowish deposit or transformation which is found in the cortical segment of the *kidney* at the more-

Fig. 16ᴬ.

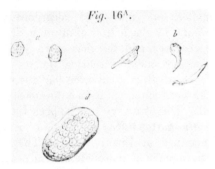

Cells found in very large and old malignant disease of the Ovary (Encephaloïd).

  a Pus-globules.
  b Caudate cells, frequent in encephaloïd varieties of carcinoma.

advanced stage of albuminous disorganization of the organ. There is a true malignant stamp in the aspect of these compound cells, although little is yet known of their natural history.

A specimen of *epulis*, and another of semi-ossified tumor attached to the inferior maxilla, were recently examined by the microscope, at the request of Mr. Key. The examinations led to extremely instructive distinctions between the microscopic structure of those growths which are truly malignant —that is, those local growths, which, during their progress, radically and organically involve all the component systems of the body; and those tumors, which are simply heterologous, which acquire, however, the undue power of implicating the surrounding structures. The ossified tumor was composed of cells which throw important light upon the process of ossification. Numerous cells of this description were found,

Fig. 17.

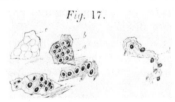

  a Ossified cell.   *b* Secondary sacculi.
  c Same cell acted upon by dilute hydrochloric acid.
  d Fibres of the fibrous portion of tumor interspersed : free calcareous points.

in which smaller solid masses of calcareous matter were
clearly made out: by the action of dilute hydrochloric acid,
effervescence occurred, and the masses in great part disappeared.   On subsequently treating the preparation with
acetic acid, it was distinctly observed that the masses of calcareous matter were contained in membranous *sacculi* within
the larger cell.   This is a very near approach to the plan on
which the *gritty* matter in the *pineal gland* is organized, as
recently determined at this hospital.   The effervescence
which, under the agency of hydrochloric acid, occurs, indicates
that the masses are principally composed of carbonate, and not
phosphate of lime.   To Mr. Dalrymple the merit belongs of
first proving that ossification may take place by the collection
of sclerous material within the sac of a *nucleated cell;* but
Mr. Dalrymple has made no allusion to the membranous sub-
celluli in which the osseous deposit is contained[1].   Properly
speaking, however, it is not ossification; for the deposit che-
mically differs from the hard portions of true bone.   It
should therefore be designated simply as an abnormal secretion of carbonate of lime; just as urate of soda, in rheumatic
diatheses, is secreted in the neighbourhood of joints[2].   These
cases of morbid growth, whose heterologous character is
simply local, are those which, if once completely removed by
surgical operation, never exhibit a disposition to re-appear.

As the limits allotted to this article are already trans-
gressed, the points desired to be inculcated, with reference
to the question of malignancy, may be briefly expressed in
conclusion.

That as science advances, the probability becomes corre-
spondingly stronger, that general laws will be developed on
which to account for the production and unmanageable progress of malignant disease.

That the facts and principles, which modern physiology has
already unfolded, warrant the inference that *malignancy* is
originally synonymous with a local perversion of nutrition;

[1] Mr. Dalrymple, however, does not appear to be aware of the fact, that
true *organic*, as well as calcareous molecules, are removed by dilute hydrochloric
acid from the interior of nucleated cells.

[2] All the further details and sketches relating to these observations may
be found in the " Record of Microscopic Observations" kept at the hospital.

but that, under a continuance of the process, a *re-action* of its influence upon the general system occurs; after which all hopes of recovery, from surgical removal of the part, are blighted.

That the *mechanism* of growth in cancer differs in no particular from that of *normal* nutrition; but that the organic *elements* at work in the two cases are dissimilar.

That the *cells* of malignant growths are only monstrosities of the normal cells, produced by a *perversion* of the *moulding* agency during the process of growth.

That the *degree* of malignancy is proportionate to the simplicity and uniformity manifested by the ultimate elements of the tumor: that on this, the encephaloïd species of carcinoma exhibit proofs of lower standard of organization than the scirrhoïd—of being *less* under the controlling agency of the general system.

CASE

OF

FEMORAL ANEURISM,

FOR WHICH THE

EXTERNAL ILIAC ARTERY WAS TIED BY SIR A. COOPER, Bᵀ.

WITH

AN ACCOUNT OF THE PREPARATION OF THE LIMB, DISSECTED AT THE EXPIRATION OF EIGHTEEN YEARS.

TAKEN FROM

SIR ASTLEY COOPER'S NOTES.

———

WILLIAM COWLES, aged 39, in the spring of the year 1808, walked the distance of five miles with a heavy burden, which fatigued and strained him, and caused an uneasiness in the right groin. On examining the part of the thigh where he felt pain, he discovered, a fortnight afterwards, a hard tumor about the size of a hazel-nut, which throbbed violently under the finger. As the pain was inconsiderable, he disregarded it for six weeks, during which time the swelling had increased to the size of a large marble. He observed, that, whenever he drunk more than usual, the throbbing was much stronger, and the pain from tension much greater. He continued to work at his business as a gardener, but suffered great inconvenience in the act of stooping. In about three months the swelling had become as large as a walnut, beating with increased force; and in six weeks more it had acquired the size of a pullet's egg. He now left off work, in consequence of the great pain which he suffered. The swelling continued to increase in size; and the suffering became so intense, that he came to town, for the purpose of obtaining advice. In the course of his journey on the outside of the coach, he fell asleep while lying on his abdomen, and the pressure on the swelling in his thigh produced some discoloration on its surface.

At this time he came to Guy's Hospital, walking occasionally from Brompton, where he resided on his arrival in town. On examination, the tumor was found to be situated close below Poupart's ligament, and, by its pressure, to raise it considerably; the artery was dilated to the size of a small pint-bowl, and the skin covering it had become extremely thin, tense, and irregular on the surface. The more prominent parts of the swelling had become changed in colour, presenting several hues of purple. From the advanced state of the tumor, it was evident that no time was to be lost in performing the operation of securing the vessel, and the patient was admitted into the hospital. The thigh and leg were of their natural temperature, and exhibited no deviation from their healthy state.

The operation was performed on the day of his admission, 22d of June 1808. The first incision commenced an inch and a half from the superior spinous process of the ilium, and extended obliquely inwards, towards Poupart's ligament. The tendon of the external oblique muscle, being laid bare, was divided so as to expose the free edges of the internal oblique and transversalis muscles. These were turned up by the finger, with the peritoneum; so that the external iliac artery could be felt distinctly pulsating at the bottom of the wound. The handle of the scalpel was then employed, to separate the artery from the surrounding parts. This became the most difficult part of the operation, on account of the depth of the vessel, and the difficulty of bringing it into view. The division of the lower fibres of the transversalis and internal oblique muscles facilitated this part of the operation; and the artery was then exposed to view, detached from the surrounding structures. An aneurismal needle, armed with a double ligature, was passed under the vessel; and the two ligatures applied so as to include about three-quarters of an inch of the artery between them. The upper ligature was first tightened; and one end carried, by means of a needle, through the artery, and secured to the other end by a knot. The lower ligature having been tightened, the artery was divided midway between the two. The coats of the vessel appeared quite healthy. The external wound was closed with straps of plaster, supported by a fold of linen and a T bandage.

Towards the conclusion of the operation, the temperature of the limb sensibly diminished, but soon regained nearly its former height. The patient was laid in bed, on his left side, with a pillow between his knees to support the right limb; and his leg was covered with a thick stocking and a double fold of flannel. On being questioned, he did not complain of any numbness in the lower part of the limb, nor sense of coldness. In the evening, his pulse was 85: he was free from complaint, and expressed himself as being comfortable. The dark colour of the tumor had somewhat diminished, since the operation.

June 23. He had passed a restless night; and complained of soreness at the lower part of the abdomen, just above the wound: his pulse was excited: the temperature of the limb natural. In the evening, a dose of sulphate of soda and senna was prescribed, to act on his bowels; and a clyster was ordered, in case the bowels should not be moved before twelve o'clock.

On the following day—He had been relieved by a free evacuation of his bowels on the preceding evening, and he had passed a comfortable night. His pulse, however, rose considerably towards the evening.

On the succeeding day, his pulse rose to 108; and he complained much of having passed a restless night, and of great commotion of his bowels, without any evacuation: he was ordered a purgative dose of senna. In the evening, a small discharge of pus began to ooze from the wound, and there appeared to be great constitutional disturbance.

June 26. He had been delirious during the early part of the night; and required an attendant constantly, to prevent his getting out of bed: his bowels were relieved towards the morning, and he fell into a quiet sleep. He awoke relieved—expressed himself altogether free from pain. The wound had discharged a large quantity of pus, which was probably the cause of the relief he had experienced: the granulations looked healthy. The straps of plaster were loosened, and in part removed, to allow the escape of matter. The tumor was reduced in size; but remained very soft, as if its contents consisted of nearly fluid blood. The suppurative stage being established, and his pulse being inclined to fall, supporting diet was allowed.

On the 30th, the aneurismal sac, which had gradually become softer, opened, and began in the night to discharge a quantity of dark-coloured blood; which, on pressure, oozed out freely, leaving the sac flaccid, and nearly empty. He complained of pain and rheumatic

sensations about his limbs and other parts of his body. His respiration was quick, and his pulse jerking, but not exceeding 108 in a
minute. Discharge from the wound, thin and less copious. A
sponge, with vinegar and water, was ordered to be applied over
the sac.

On the following day, more grumous blood came away from the
sac, mixed with some coagulated fibrin. He seemed anxious and
restless, and his skin indicated fever. Some opium at bed-time
was ordered.

From this time to the 8th of July his symptoms remained much
the same. His appetite increasing, he was allowed meat and bread,
of which he partook freely: the sac continued to discharge an icho-
rous and offensive fluid. On this day, when the sore was dressed,
the inner surface of the sac came away in a mass, as if it had
sloughed; and exposed a rather healthy granulating surface at the
bottom of the wound. Common poultice was applied, to encourage
healthy suppuration and granulations. The wound of the operation
continued to discharge, but appeared healthy; and the sac, or rather
its remains, gradually diminished in volume, and improved in appearance.

On the 8th of July, the upper ligature came away; and was followed by the other ligature on the following day, without any
hæmorrhage. From this time a pint of porter was added to his diet,
and his health and strength began to improve: the sac continued to
granulate, and to contract in size; and the incision looked healthy, and
inclined to close.

In the second week of July he left the hospital, under the impression that a better air would restore his strength.

In a week after he left the hospital, the sac had entirely closed, as
had also the wound, and he was able to take exercise: but he began
to complain of feverish sensations, especially at night, attended with
pain in the limb, which shot across the abdomen from the wound.
In a week after the wound had closed, the scab was accidentally struck
off, and a small quantity of matter oozed from the opening. The sore
again closed; and his fever, which had slightly remitted, returned
with more violence than before, accompanied by the pain in the
limb, and across the belly.

This state continued till the 25th. On this day he walked a
quarter of a mile. A profuse discharge of pus took place from the
incision, and also from the opening of the sac, and continued throughout the night.

The discharge from both openings by degrees diminished; and by
the 1st of September had entirely ceased, the wounds being both

healed. On the afternoon of the same day, they re-opened, and about four ounces of matter again were evacuated through both openings. This discharge was attended with a severe diarrhœa, which lasted seven days; and was checked by grain doses of ferri sulphas with pulvis opii, given him at bed-time. The diarrhœa left him with some degree of fever and a white tongue, which were relieved by mild rhubarb purgatives.

He continued in the same state, with an occasional return of the purging, and a continuance of discharge from both openings, till the 23d of the same month; when a fresh abscess formed at the seat of the operation, and emptied itself at the outer extremity of the incision. About half a pint of matter made its escape.

From this period he suffered no relapse, with the exception of occasional pains in his limb, on which he continued to walk during the discharge of the abscess. The wounds gradually healed, under a a free allowance of wine and water, with two pints of porter a day.

This patient went to reside in a distant part of the country, and continued to enjoy a good state of health for some years.* In the autumn of the year 1826, eighteen years and a half after the operation, he died: and an opportunity of examining the limb offering itself, it was injected from the common iliac artery, and the anastomosing vessels carefully exposed by-dissection. The drawing shews the vessels principally concerned in carrying on the circulation. The preparation from which it is made is in the museum of the School. The following account, drawn up by Mr. Cock, will render the route of the circulation intelligible.

Description of the Preparation.

In order that the course of circulation through the limb might be examined and preserved, an injecting pipe was introduced into the aorta, just above its bifurcation. The left common iliac artery was tied, and the arteries of the right side were filled with wax. The vessels were then traced from the bifurcation of the aorta, as far as the knee-joint: the limb, including the os innominatum, the sacrum, and the lower portion of the spine, was removed from the body, and the leg was separated just above the condyles of the femur. The preparation, which we shall now endeavour to describe and explain, consequently comprises the right

* A brief account of this case was published in the Fourth Volume of the Medico-Chirurgical Transactions, in the year 1813; the patient being at that time alive, and perfectly well.

common iliac artery, the internal iliac and its branches, the external iliac on which the operation was performed, and the whole course of the femoral.

In describing the result of this dissection, we shall speak, 1st, Of the condition of the iliac trunk above the point where the ligature was applied. 2dly, Of the appearances presented by the vessel immediately below the ligature; together with the situation and remains of the aneurismal tumor, and the femoral artery as restored by the influx of blood from anastomosing branches both above and below the sac. 3dly, The manner in which the restoration of the femoral trunk had been effected by collateral circulation.

Condition of the External Iliac Artery.

The external iliac artery was pervious, to the extent of rather more than an inch from the bifurcation of the common iliac; but had become somewhat diminished in size, and altered in shape. No branches were given off from this portion of the vessel, which, when filled with injection, presented a conical form, tapering downwards to a mere point, and terminating in a rounded cord, which constituted the remaining part, or the obliterated portion of the artery, and was continued down to the spot where the operation had been performed. The ligature had probably been applied just above the origin of the circumflex and epigastric branches, although no evidence remained to indicate the precise spot. Just above Poupart's ligament, the iliac trunk became suddenly restored (apparently by the influx of blood from the branches mentioned above), and assumed about half its natural size. The obliterated vessel presented the appearance of a continuous unbroken cord, from the cessation of the iliac above, to its restoration below.

Condition of the Iliac and Femoral Artery, below the Ligature.

It has already been stated, that the iliac trunk became restored just above Poupart's ligament, by the retrograde circulation established through the circumflex and epigastric branches, which received their blood from the branches of the internal iliac above. The vessel having thus regained about half its natural size, passed into the thigh, and was continued without receiving any accession from collateral vessels, until it reached the origin of the profunda. From this branch (*i. e.* the profunda) the trunk appeared to derive a large supply of blood, sufficient to restore it to the ordinary extent of calibre which the femoral possesses in a stout muscular limb; the remaining portion of the femoral artery, below the profunda, presented nothing unusual in its appearance, and bore no indication of having received any further influx of blood through collateral branches. Just above the origin of the profunda, the femoral artery had become distorted, and irregular in shape; and was rendered somewhat obscure by its connexion with what appeared to be the remains of the aneurismal sac, adhering to the anterior surface of the vessel, and gluing it to the adjacent muscles and fascia. There can be but little doubt, that the original opening of communication between the sac and the femoral trunk had existed at this spot, viz. just above the profunda branch; but it would seem equally apparent, that, as the aneurismal tumor became obliterated in the progress of the cure after the operation, the opening into the vessel also became closed, while the integrity of the arterial trunk, above and below the sac, was maintained continuous and entire.

The manner in which the restoration of the femoral trunk had been effected by the collateral circulation.

The collateral circulation had, in this instance, been established by the junction of the ileo-lumbar, obturator, gluteal and ischiatic branches, from the internal iliac, with the circumflex and epigastric of the external iliac, and the profunda of the femoral. They consisted of three sets of communicating vessels, which descended, respectively, over the fore part, the internal side, and the posterior surface of the hip-joint; and may be described as forming a vascular plexus around the articulation, ramifying amongst the muscles of that region.

The anterior set consisted—1. Of a very large branch from the ileo-lumbar artery, which descended along the crista of the ilium, to terminate in the circumflexa ilii and circumflexa ilii externa. 2. Of another branch from the ileo-lumbar, which became joined by a small artery from the obturator, and divided into a number of small and exceedingly tortuous vessels. These connected themselves to the anterior crural nerve; and, descending under Poupart's ligament, terminated in the external circumflex branch of the profunda. 3. Of two other branches from the obturator, which turned over the brim of the pelvis, and formed a plexus similar to the last, which, after communicating with the epigastric, descended on the inner side of the femoral trunk, and terminated in the internal circumflex branch of the profunda.

The internal set consisted of the branches, given off by the obturator after it had left the pelvis, which ramified amongst the adductor muscles on the inner side of the hip-joint, and joined most freely with the divisions of the internal circumflex from the profunda.

The posterior set of anastomosing vessels was constituted— 1. By three large branches from the gluteal; two of which crossed the dorsum of the ilium, in close contact with the bone, and anastomosed near the anterior and superior spinous process, with the ascending branches of the external circumflex; whilst the third descended in a direction more nearly vertical, between the gluteus maximus and medius muscles, to join with the middle branches of the same artery, just below and behind the trochanter major. 2. By several slender and very tortuous vessels from the ischiatic, which surrounded the great nerve of that name, and thus, descending behind the thigh, communicated with the internal and external circumflex, and finally terminated by joining the perforating branches of the profunda.

In this preparation, the ileo-lumbar, obturator, gluteal and ischiatic arteries will be seen enormously dilated. The internal pudic is also of large size; but it does not appear to furnish any direct communication with the femoral. Doubtless, however, in the dissection of the limb, many small branches were removed, which, during the life of the individual, lent their tributary streams to swell the femoral trunk, and assisted in restoring to the limb that supply of blood which enabled it to maintain its muscular developement, and carry on its functions with undiminished vigour.

51

PLATE I.

a   The Common Iliac Artery.

b   The External Iliac.

c   The Internal Iliac.

d d The Femoral Artery.

e   The Arteria Profunda.

f   The External Circumflex.

g   The Internal Circumflex.

h   The Iliac Artery, which had been tied, and had become a Cord.

i   The remains of the Aneurismal Sac.

k k Anastomosing Branches of the Circumflexa Ilii.

l   Anastomosing Branches of the Circumflexa Externa.

m   Obturator Artery, anastomosing with

n   The Circumflexa Interna.

o   Numerous Branches of the Obturator Artery, anastomosing with the Circumflexa Interna, under Poupart's Ligament.

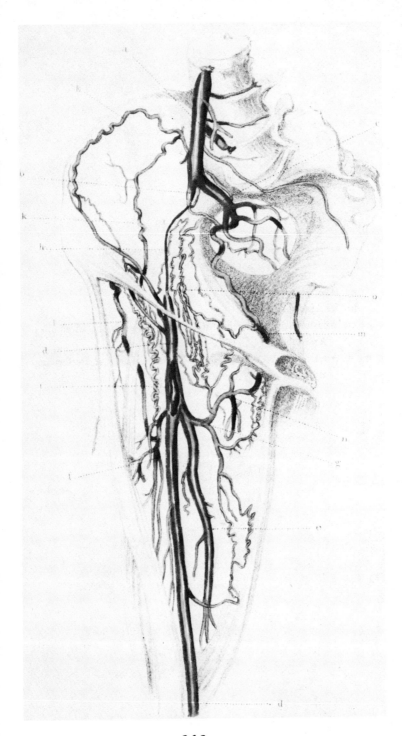

52

PLATE II.

POSTERIOR VIEW OF THE SAME PREPARATION, SHEWING THE PELVIS
AND BACK PART OF THE THIGH.

a   The Gluteal Artery.

b   The Ischiatic Artery.

c c c c   Anastomosing Branches of the Gluteal, with the Circumflex
Artery.

d d d   Anastomosing Vessels of the Ischiatic, with the Perforating
Branches of the Arteria Profunda.

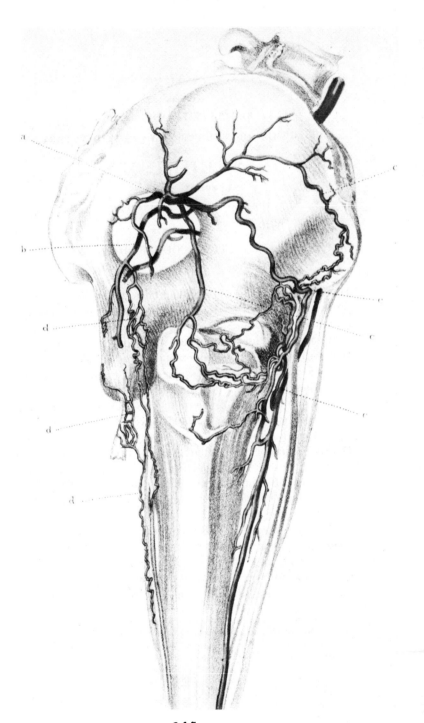

53

ACCOUNT

OF THE

FIRST SUCCESSFUL OPERATION,

PERFORMED ON THE COMMON CAROTID ARTERY,

FOR

ANEURISM,

IN THE YEAR 1808 : *

WITH THE POST-MORTEM EXAMINATION, IN 1821.

FROM THE NOTES OF

SIR ASTLEY COOPER, BART.

H. HUMPHREYS, aged 50, who had been used to carry heavy burdens in the streets of London, perceived, about six months ago, a tumor, about the size of a walnut, possessing a pulsatory motion, on the left side of the neck, just below the angle of the jaw, and extending down as low as the thyroid cartilage. It was productive of great pain on the same side of the head, and the left eye-lid appeared to contract over the globe of the eye. The pain in his head was first felt about a month after he discovered the swelling, and was attended with a sense of pulsatory motion in the brain. His speech had become, of late, somewhat affected, being less distinct than it formerly had been, and hoarse ; and he also complained of some difficulty in breathing, apparently from the pressure of the swelling on the larynx. His appetite had of late become impaired. He had a sense of coldness, succeeded by heat, in his left ear ; and he often became sick when eating, but did not vomit. Upon attempting to stoop at any time from that period, he had an insupportable feeling as if his head would burst, a giddiness, loss of sight, and almost total insensibility. The only remedy he had tried

---

* The first operation for Carotid Aneurism was performed by Sir Astley Cooper two years and a half before, but proved unsuccessful : this was therefore the second operation for Carotid Aneurism. The two cases are reported in the First Volume of the Medico-Chirurgical Transactions.

for the relief of the pain, was a blister on the head, which gave him ease for a few days. He did not discontinue his usual occupation. The internal carotid appeared to be dilated just where it comes off from the common carotid : the tumor was about the size of a pullet's egg, and very prominent about its centre.

The operation of tying the common carotid was performed on the 22d of June, in the theatre of the hospital. The pulsation of the tumor was remarkably strong on that day : when pressure was made on the artery below the tumor, the latter was emptied ; and when the pressure was removed, it filled at one impulse of the heart.

The external incision was begun opposite to the middle of the thyroid cartilage, and continued down to within an inch of the sternum, along the inner side of the sterno-mastoid muscle. On raising the edge of the muscle, the omo-hyoideus could be distinctly seen crossing the carotid sheath, and the descendens noni lying upon it. On separating the sterno-mastoid and omo-hyoideus, the internal jugular vein became immediately apparent, and, dilating at each exspiration, spread itself over the carotid artery : the vein being drawn aside, the par vagum came into view, as the artery was cleared from its sheath. A double ligature was then carried under the artery, by means of a blunt iron probe constructed for the purpose, and the lower ligature was tightened. The artery was then detached from the surrounding parts, to the extent of an inch upwards, and the upper ligature secured, so as to include, between the two, the detached portion of the vessel. The artery was divided midway, between the ligatures ; and the blood contained in the vessel was found to be already coagulated. Each ligature was carried, by means of a needle, through the coats of the artery, and secured by a knot, in order to prevent the force of circulation from disturbing it.* The incision was dressed, by placing a pad of lint over it, and securing it by straps of plaster ; the ligatures hanging out of the wound.

Dr. Vose, dresser in the hospital, took charge of the patient ;

---

* This practice was adopted, in consequence of a fatal hæmorrhage that had occurred in a case under the late Mr. Cline, occasioned by the ligature having been forced from the artery.

and reported, that, immediately after the operation, he had been entirely relieved of the pain which for two months he had incessantly experienced, together with the throbbing of all the arteries in the left side of the head. This pain never returned. The pulsation did not wholly cease in the tumor, after the artery was tied, but was distinctly felt, though very slight, by Mr. Forster, Mr. George Young, and Mr. Dubois, jun., who were present at the operation. It was thought to be caused by the recurrent circulation through the internal carotid from the brain, in consequence of the free anastomosis which exists between the blood-vessels within the scull.

The patient's head was supported by a pillow; and slightly bent forwards, to relax the sterno-cleido-mastoid muscles.

3 p.m. Pulse moderate: skin cool: little pain in the wound: pulsation in the aneurism distinct ; but inconsiderable, when compared with what it was before the operation.

8 p.m. Pulse natural, and skin cool.

June 23. He has passed a comfortable night; and is otherwise free from complaint, with the exception of a slight cough. The tumor to-day is more tender, and still slightly throbbing: its contents feel more solid, as if the blood were coagulating.

25. The patient says he is quite easy, with the exception of a slight rattling, from an accumulation of mucus in the larynx: pulse tranquil. The tumor is diminishing in size, and gives him little or no uneasiness. No constitutional irritation.

26. Report good ; the same as yesterday.

27. Has passed a very restless night: has coughed much, and had pain generally over the head: his spirits are depressed, but otherwise free from disturbance.

28. His symptoms of yesterday have been relieved, by his bowels having been opened: pulse 84 : free from pain : slight pulsation still to be felt in the aneurismal tumor, which is diminished in size.

29. Pulse natural: no pain: pulsation still perceptible: tumor is so much shrunk, that the skin over it is wrinkled : wound dressed for the first time, and looking healthy.

On the following day, he was very hoarse, and hardly able to speak in a tone above a whisper. This symptom was again relieved by a purgative, which freely unloaded his bowels.

On the following day the hoarseness was diminished. He continued in the same favourable condition up to the 12th.

On that day, the ligatures were observed to have projected farther from the wound, which had begun to discharge more profusely.

On the two following days, the ligatures came away, as Dr. Vose was dressing the wound. The upper ligature separated first.

On the 17th of July, the patient walked out of his ward. The tumor had hardly any pulsation, and was gradually getting smaller. The wound was cicatrizing favourably: the sac was reduced more than one half in size.

The wound was a long time in healing, owing to a small sinus remaining in the track of the ligature; and a small projecting fungus required to be touched often with caustic. He was discharged from the hospital in September.

He called on Sir Astley Cooper on the 16th of October following: the tumor could no longer be distinguished by the eye: he felt quite well, and in no respect different from what he was before the occurrence of the disease. The eye, which had been very much closed, had regained nearly its former appearance. The facial and temporal arteries on the same side could hardly be felt, particularly the former: the latter beating slightly. Those on the opposite side pulsated with more than usual vigour.

This man continued to work, in the employment of a large ironmaster, Mr. Crawshay, in Upper Thames Street, and enjoyed good health, till towards the year 1821; when he had pains in the head, which led eventually to a fatal attack of apoplexy, in the following year. In his last illness, he was attended by the late Mr. Ankers, surgeon, in the city; who immediately requested, and obtained permission, for Sir Astley Cooper to inspect the body.

For this purpose, Sir Astley Cooper, accompanied by Mr. Key, went, after surgical lecture, late in the evening, to make the inspection.

POST-MORTEM EXAMINATION.

The aorta was opened, and an injecting-pipe introduced into the arch, for the purpose of filling the anastomosing vessels with coarse common injection; the subclavian arteries being tied externally to the scaleni. The head was then opened and examined, for the purpose of discovering the seat and cause of the fatal effusion. On cutting away the hemisphere of the left side of the brain, a large semi-fluid clot was discovered, filling an apoplectic cell in the substance of the brain, just above the corpus striatum, and close to the corpus callosum: the size was that of a hen's egg. A little further examination discovered the source of hæmorrhage to be a large branch of the middle cerebral artery, the trunk of which vessel appeared more dense and white than usual, as if undergoing the change prior to ossification. The disease of which he died sufficiently attested the freedom of the circulation, as well as its force in the cerebral vessels, on the side on which the carotid had been tied. The arteries on the left side of the brain were rather larger than those on the opposite side. The anterior cerebral artery was of the same size as its fellow : the middle cerebral larger than that on the right side, which was filled with a coagulum, and did not admit the injection, as the drawing shews.* The large size of the latter vessel is accounted for by the increased size of the communicating branch ; which, receiving its blood from the basilary, had become as large as an ordinary radial artery. The basilary appeared to be of its usual capacity, although it was evidently the channel which supplied the middle cerebral artery. The blood probably found an easier course from the basilary, through the left communicating branch, than into the right corresponding vessels, which appeared rather diminished in size. From an inspection of the base of the brain, after the vessels had been injected, it immediately struck the observer, that the left side of the arterial circle of Willis was much more developed than the right, and that the left side of the brain received its full share of arterial blood. The anterior cerebral artery received its supply from its fellow by means of the transverse branch : these vessels seemed to be of their usual size. The internal carotid artery was pervious for about half an inch, and of its ordinary capacity.

The external vessels were not so well displayed. Those of the face did not receive the injection. The common carotid trunk was impervious throughout its whole extent, being reduced to a mere cord. The external carotid was injected at its commencement; and the superior thyroïdeal was also filled from the arteries of the opposite side : but beyond this the branches were empty, and therefore could not be satisfactorily traced. The free communication, however, of the branches of the external carotids, in their natural state, affords an ample channel of supply, when the circulation in one is cut off. The aneurism must, as Sir Astley Cooper suspected, have been situated in the internal carotid artery.

* See Plate III. page 58.

PLATE III.

A VIEW OF THE UNDER PARTS OF THE BRAIN, IN THE CASE OF CAROTID ANEURISM.

The Four Lobes of the Cerebrum.

The Two Lobes of the Cerebellum, and the Medulla Spinalis.

a a   Internal Carotid Artery injected.

b b   Vertebral Artery.

c   Basilary Artery.

d   A Vessel of the Circulus Arteriosus upon the right side.

e   A Branch of the Circulus Arteriosus upon the left side, much enlarged, it being the principal anastomosing vessel to the Internal Carotid Artery, after operation.

Plate 3.

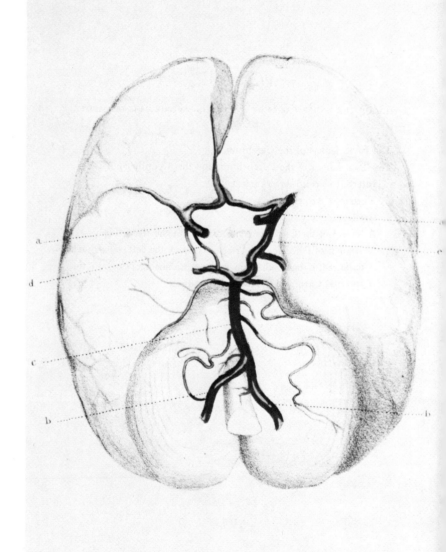

a

d

c

b

e

e

b